Gastrointestinal Pathology

Editor

RAUL S. GONZALEZ

SURGICAL PATHOLOGY CLINICS

www.surgpath.theclinics.com

Consulting Editor
JASON L. HORNICK

September 2020 • Volume 13 • Number 3

ELSEVIER

1600 John F. Kennedy Boulevard • Suite 1800 • Philadelphia, Pennsylvania, 19103-2899

http://www.theclinics.com

SURGICAL PATHOLOGY CLINICS Volume 13, Number 3
September 2020 ISSN 1875-9181, ISBN-13: 978-0-323-75880-2

Editor: Katerina Heidhausen
Developmental Editor: Donald Mumford

Surgical Pathology Clinics (ISSN 1875-9181) is published quarterly by Elsevier Inc., 360 Park Avenue South, New York, NY 10010. Months of issue are March, June, September, and December. Business and Editorial Office: Elsevier Inc., 1600 John F. Kennedy Blvd., Ste. 1800, Philadelphia, PA 19103-2899. Accounting and Circulation Offices: Elsevier Inc., 3251 Riverport Lane, Maryland Heights, MO 63043. Periodicals postage paid at New York, NY and at additional mailing offices. Subscription prices are $219.00 per year (US individuals), $294.00 per year (US institutions), $100.00 per year (US students/residents), $272.00 per year (Canadian individuals), $335.00 per year (Canadian Institutions), $263.00 per year (foreign individuals), $335.00 per year (foreign institutions), and $120.00 per year (international students/residents), $100.00 per year (Canadian students/residents). Foreign air speed delivery is included in all *Clinics'* subscription prices. All prices are subject to change without notice. **POSTMASTER:** Send address changes to *Surgical Pathology Clinics*, Elsevier, 3251 Riverport Lane, Maryland Heights, MO 63043. **Customer Service: 1-800-654-2452 (US). From outside the United States, call 1-314-447-8871. Fax: 1-314-447-8029. E-mail:** JournalsCustomerServiceusa@elsevier.com **(for print support)** and JournalsOnlineSupport-usa@elsevier.com **(for online support)**.

Reprints. For copies of 100 or more, of articles in this publication, please contact the Commercial Reprints Department, Elsevier Inc., 360 Park Avenue South, New York, NY 10010-1710. Tel. 212-633-3874; Fax: 212-633-3820; E-mail: reprints@elsevier.com.

Surgical Pathology Clinics of North America is covered in *MEDLINE/PubMed (Index Medicus)*.

Contributors

CONSULTING EDITOR

JASON L. HORNICK, MD, PhD
Director of Surgical Pathology and
Immunohistochemistry, Brigham and Women's
Hospital, Professor of Pathology, Harvard
Medical School, Boston, Massachusetts, USA

EDITOR

RAUL S. GONZALEZ, MD
Director of Gastrointestinal Pathology, Beth
Israel Deaconess Medical Center, Associate
Professor of Pathology, Harvard Medical
School, Boston, Massachusetts, USA

AUTHORS

LODEWIJK A.A. BROSENS, MD, PhD
Pathologist, Department of Pathology,
University Medical Center, Utrecht, Utrecht
University, Utrecht, The Netherlands;
Department of Pathology, Radboud
University Medical Center, Nijmegen, The
Netherlands

NORMAN J. CARR, FRCPath
Consultant Pathologist and Director of
Research, Peritoneal Malignancy Institute,
Basingstoke and North Hampshire Hospital,
Basingstoke, United Kingdom

NOOSHIN K. DASHTI, MD, MPH
Department of Pathology, Microbiology and
Immunology, Vanderbilt University Medical
Center, Nashville, Tennessee, USA

EMMA ELIZABETH FURTH, MD
Professor of Pathology and Laboratory
Medicine, Hospital of the University of
Pennsylvania, Philadelphia, Pennsylvania, USA

JEFFREY D. GOLDSMITH, MD
Department of Pathology, Boston Children's
Hospital, Harvard Medical School, Boston,
Massachusetts, USA

RAUL S. GONZALEZ, MD
Director of Gastrointestinal Pathology, Beth
Israel Deaconess Medical Center, Associate
Professor of Pathology, Harvard Medical
School, Boston, Massachusetts, USA

NOAM HARPAZ, MD, PhD
Professor, Departments of Pathology,
Molecular and Cell-Based Medicine, and
Medicine, Icahn School of Medicine at Mount
Sinai, New York, New York, USA

MELANIE JOHNCILLA, MD
Adjunct Assistant Professor, Department of
Pathology and Laboratory Medicine, Weill
Cornell Medicine, New York, New York,
USA

JONATHAN A. NOWAK, MD, PhD
Associate Pathologist, Brigham and Women's
Hospital, Assistant Professor of Pathology,
Harvard Medical School, Boston,
Massachusetts, USA

ALEXANDROS D. POLYDORIDES, MD, PhD
Professor, Departments of Pathology,
Molecular and Cell-Based Medicine, and

Medicine, Icahn School of Medicine at Mount Sinai, New York, New York, USA

JUAN PUTRA, MD
Department of Laboratory Medicine and Pathobiology, University of Toronto, Division of Pathology, Department of Paediatric Laboratory Medicine, The Hospital for Sick Children, Toronto, Ontario, Canada

MICHELLE D. REID, MD, MS
Professor, Department of Pathology and Laboratory Medicine, Emory University Hospital, Atlanta, Georgia, USA

CHANJUAN SHI, MD, PhD
Department of Pathology, Duke University School of Medicine, Durham, North Carolina, USA

ANGELA R. SHIH, MD
Assistant Professor of Pathology, Harvard Medical School, Department of Pathology and Laboratory Medicine, Massachusetts General Hospital, Boston, Massachusetts, USA

RACHEL S. VAN DER POST, MD, PhD
Pathologist, Department of Pathology, Radboud University Medical Center, Nijmegen, The Netherlands

SHOKO VOS, MD, PhD
Pathologist, Department of Pathology, Radboud University Medical Center, Nijmegen, The Netherlands

CHRISTA L. WHITNEY-MILLER, MD
Vice Chair, Anatomic Pathology, Director, Surgical Pathology, Associate Professor, University of Rochester School of Medicine and Dentistry, Rochester, New York, USA

YUE XUE, MD, PhD
Associate Professor, Department of Pathology and Laboratory Medicine, Northwestern University, Chicago, Illinois, USA

RHONDA K. YANTISS, MD
Professor, Department of Pathology and Laboratory Medicine, Weill Cornell Medicine, New York, New York, USA

LAWRENCE ZUKERBERG, MD
Associate Professor of Pathology, Harvard Medical School, Department of Pathology and Laboratory Medicine, Massachusetts General Hospital, Boston, Massachusetts, USA

Contents

Although the features of lower gastrointestinal tract inflammation associated with ulcerative colitis and Crohn disease are generally familiar to pathologists, there is less awareness of and familiarity with the manifestations of inflammatory bowel disease in the esophagus, stomach, and duodenum. Nonetheless, their diagnosis has therapeutic and possibly prognostic implications, potentially foretelling severe complications. The recognition that ulcerative colitis can affect gastrointestinal organs proximal to the large intestine and terminal ileum represents a revision of concepts ingrained among generations of physicians. This article reviews the pathologic features and clinical significance of esophagitis, gastritis, and duodenitis associated with inflammatory bowel disease.

This review provides an overview of different types of gastric epithelial polyps. The polyps are classified based on their cell or epithelial compartment of origin. Some of these polyps can be considered reactive or nonneoplastic, whereas others are neoplastic in origin, are sometimes associated with a hereditary polyposis/cancer syndrome, and may have malignant potential. The aim of this review is to provide a pragmatic overview for the practicing pathologist about how to correctly diagnose and deal with gastric epithelial polyps and when (not) to ponder, and when (not) to panic.

The ampulla of Vater gives rise to a versatile group of cancers of mixed/hybrid histologic phenotype. Ampullary carcinomas (ACs) are most frequently intestinal or pancreatobiliary adenocarcinomas but other subtypes, such as medullary, mucinous, or signet ring/poorly cohesive cell carcinoma, may be encountered. Ampullary cancer can also be subclassified based on immunohistochemical features; however these classification systems fail to show robust prognostic reliability. More recently, the molecular landscape of AC has been uncovered, and has been shown to have prognostic and predictive significance. In this article, the site-specific, histologic, and genetic characteristics of ampullary carcinoma and its precursor lesions are discussed.

Mucinous appendiceal tumors include low-grade appendiceal mucinous neoplasm, high-grade appendiceal mucinous neoplasm, and mucinous adenocarcinoma. Nonmucinous adenocarcinomas are less frequent. Recent consensus guidelines and the latest edition of the World Health Organization classification will allow consistent use of agreed nomenclature. Accurate diagnosis is important not only for patient management but also to allow comparison of results between centers and tumor registries. Serrated polyps are the most common benign polyp in the appendix. They need to be distinguished from low-grade appendiceal mucinous neoplasm, which can also mimic other benign conditions. Goblet cell adenocarcinomas are a distinctive type of appendiceal neoplasm.

SURGICAL PATHOLOGY CLINICS

SERIES OF RELATED INTEREST

Clinics in Laboratory Medicine
https://www.labmed.theclinics.com/
Medical Clinics
https://www.medical.theclinics.com/

THE CLINICS ARE AVAILABLE ONLINE!
Access your subscription at:
www.theclinics.com

Preface

Updates and Challenges in Gastrointestinal Pathology

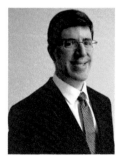

Raul S. Gonzalez, MD
Editor

Gastrointestinal pathology accounts for a large portion of the specimens encountered in most surgical pathology departments. There are several reasons for this, including the wide availability of colonoscopy and esophagogastroduodenoscopy and the high incidence of gastrointestinal carcinomas. Many of these cases can be fairly straightforward and present little challenge to most practicing pathologists. However, the larger a case volume, the more likely a pathologist is to encounter a challenging case, meaning that one day's stack of gastrointestinal pathology specimens can throw several curveballs.

The past few years have seen new editions of both the *American Joint Committee on Cancer Staging Manual* and the World Health Organization Digestive System Tumors classification. Their impact on daily practice has been incremental, mostly creating subtle nuances and distinctions rather than seismic shifts. As a result, such updates may be easily overlooked or not entirely understood, underscoring the need for familiarity with these and other important updates.

This issue of *Surgical Pathology Clinics* focuses primarily on the challenges faced daily by pathologists signing out gastrointestinal pathology specimens, whether it is the sole scope of their practice or one slice of their daily caseload. This includes focuses on ever-updating terminology (such as for neuroendocrine and appendiceal neoplasms), cases with subtle but key distinctions (such as ampullary lesions and gastric polyps), often-overlooked considerations (such as difficulties encountered when grossing complicated specimens and inflammatory bowel disease affecting the upper gastrointestinal tract), and specimens that may lie beyond the typical comfort zone of gastrointestinal pathologists (including pediatric specimens, anus biopsies, and mesenteric lesions). Known interobserver variability in gastrointestinal pathology is also covered, as well as important prognostic considerations in colorectal carcinoma histology. Finally, there is an article discussing the relevance of HER2 assessment in colorectal carcinoma; pathologists who have not yet been asked to perform such a workup may not wish to hold their breath.

All the articles in this issue have been written by experienced gastrointestinal pathologists with deep knowledge of the topics presented. I am grateful for their contributions, and I hope the reader finds these articles informative and valuable to daily practice.

Raul S. Gonzalez, MD
Department of Pathology
Beth Israel Deaconess Medical Center
330 Brookline Avenue
Boston, MA 02215, USA

E-mail address:
Rgonzal5@bidmc.harvard.edu

Surgical Pathology 13 (2020) ix
https://doi.org/10.1016/j.path.2020.06.003
1875-9181/20/© 2020 Published by Elsevier Inc.

surgpath.theclinics.com

Grossing of Gastrointestinal Specimens
Best Practices and Current Controversies

Emma Elizabeth Furth, MD

KEYWORDS

• Grossing • Anatomy • Staging • Margins • Tissue sections

Key points

- With every case, think about the patient and form the questions to be answered to create a logical approach to handling the case.

- Know the anatomy to help orient the specimen.

- Specimen margins are those aspects that had to be cut/transected to remove them from the body. The presence or absence of circumferential radial margins varies along the luminal gastrointestinal tract.

- Not all that appears grossly normal is normal.

ABSTRACT

The proper handling of the gross specimen is imperative, as it is the most important first step in providing excellent patient care. Our diagnoses depend on the correct description and submission of tissue sections for histologic analysis. A logical and problem-solving approach to handling the gross specimen is presented.

The proper handling of the gross specimen is imperative, as it is the most important first step to enable us as pathologists to care for our patients. As physicians, we strive to render accurate, precise, and meaningful diagnoses. Although the microscopic analysis of our tissue sections encompasses a predominant proportion of our time diagnostically and in teaching our residents, fellows, and colleagues, the time and effort devoted to the handling and care of the gross specimen has unfortunately diminished. Our correct diagnoses depend on the correct description and submission of tissue sections for histologic analysis. If the handling of the specimen at the outset is wrong, everything downstream, including our diagnoses, will be wrong, with subsequent impact

on patient care. Our reports and diagnoses drive patient care as we provide prognostic and therapeutic data. In short, for each case, we want to be able to answer the following questions: (1) What is going on? (2) What caused this problem? (3) What should be done to treat the issue? (4) What is the prognosis?

Understanding how to handle the gross specimen is often a daunting endeavor, especially to trainees; however, by knowing a few fundamental principles, one may build a framework to approach our cases. Although scripted menus of descriptions and tissue submission are at times helpful, they cannot cover every situation and in themselves do not necessitate critical thinking. We will take a careful, problem-solving, and when available, data-driven approach to the care of the gross specimen.

From the outset, attending to paperwork to ensure concordance with identifiers is critical, as even the best dissection and diagnosis, if given to the wrong patient, is horrendous. Next, by asking yourself "What are the questions to be answered?" you will be driven to create a logical plan derived from first principles and reasoning. Answering this question may be layered by

---

Department of Pathology, Hospital of the University of Pennsylvania, 6 Founders building, 3400 Spruce Street, Philadelphia, PA 19104, USA
E-mail address: EEF@PENNMEDICINE.UPENN.EDU
Twitter: @EMMA_FURTH (E.E.F.)

Surgical Pathology 13 (2020) 359–370
https://doi.org/10.1016/j.path.2020.04.001
1875-9181/20/© 2020 Elsevier Inc. All rights reserved.

additional questions as one works with the case. That being said, more often than not, there are many situations for which the "answers" of what to submit for examination are not really known, although guidelines may exist. For example, everyone would agree that a polypectomy specimen should be entirely submitted for histology. On the other hand, given a colectomy with hundreds of polyps from a patient with a germline mutation in *APC,* will you submit every polyp for evaluation? Although one may argue that complete submission may logically extend from the prior polypectomy case, we certainly do not submit every polyp in the second scenario. Thus, we in actuality do and should use our handling and care of the gross specimen to inform and guide our clinical decision making of which tissue sections are needed.

For both neoplastic and non-neoplastic cases, we can and should apply some fundamental principles: (1) identify proper specimen, (2) obtain history, (3) identify organ(s) and margins, (4) frame the questions needed to be answered, (5) complete documentation including measurements by descriptions and photography (ruler) during dissection, and (6) submit tissue. Regardless of the disease, for resection specimens, we should identify margins, open the lumens to study the mucosal aspect, identify lesions, and serially section to be able to examine all aspects of the case. For "lesions," be they depressed or raised, submitting sections of the center of the lesion and sections with respect to the normal (ie, transition areas) will yield informative data. For example, the viral inclusions of cytomegalovirus are often found in the center of an ulcer, whereas herpetic inclusions are often found at the juxtaposition of ulcer bed and normal. Keep in mind that a normal gross appearance of a mucosal surface does not always equate to histologic normality. For example, in sleeve gastric resections done for obesity, the vast majority are normal in gross appearance. The grossly identified abnormalities when present are usually fundic gland polyps; however, clinically important diagnoses such as *Helicobacter pylori* and autoimmune gastritis are indeed present in these seemingly normal specimens.[1]

It is important to place a ruler in the frame with the specimen during photo documentation. For example, the designation of a malignancy as being in the anal canal or distal rectum is dependent on its geographic relationship with the dentate line; those >2 cm proximal are not in the anal canal whereas those malignancies proximal to the perianal skin, as defined by the presence of adnexal elements, and not above 2 cm from the dentate line are staged as anal canal malignancies

regardless of lineage differentiation. Thus, anal canal malignancies deriving from the 2 epithelial components (squamous and colonic type), are most often squamous cell carcinoma and adenocarcinoma, respectively. The importance of this anatomic distinction is twofold: first, the anal canal lymphatics drain to the inguinal lymph nodes, whereas the rectal drain to the peri-aortic ones; second, the 2 tumor locations require different tumor-staging protocols. As another example, the determination as to a malignancy being esophageal or gastric is dependent on its relationship to the gastroesophageal (GE) junction. In the past, tumors with an epicenter ≤5 cm distal to the GE junction were classified as esophageal; currently, this number has been changed to 2 cm. By having this explicit numerical documentation in our reports, we have the data needed to review cases and their diagnoses rendered according to the "rules" followed and set at that particular time period. A "gastric carcinoma" in the past may now be designated as an esophageal carcinoma purely on the basis of shifting definitions and not diagnostic error. Such an understanding of changing diagnostic geographic criteria and the impact on disease prevalence and incidence is important in all academic data set constructions and studies.

For any tumor resection, our sections are aimed at its diagnoses and TNM staging according to the American Joint Committee on Cancer Staging Manual.[2] The staging schemes vary depending on tumor type (eg, adenocarcinoma vs neuroendocrine tumor) and site (eg, rectum vs anal canal). Regardless, the gross examination is critical to guide tissue submission. For previously treated carcinomas, however, it is expected that complete submission of the entire tumor bed and at least 1 cm adjacent to the tumor bed is done to allow assessment of an accurate yT stage and tumor regression score.

Anatomy is important. Knowing the anatomy of organs is imperative to properly handling resection cases. Specifically, identifying every margin is important for both neoplastic and non-neoplastic cases. We define a margin as those areas for which a cut was needed to remove the specimen from the body. Thus, serosa-lined areas are not margins, as no knife was needed to excise that specific aspect from the body. Even when an adenocarcinoma has invaded into and through the wall of the colon and is present on the serosal surface, this involvement does not equate to a positive margin; we designate the importance of this feature by the T stage of T4a. However, for the luminal gastrointestinal tract we always, with the exception of blind pouches, have proximal and distal margins. In addition to the proximal and distal margins, identification of the radial margins may not be as obvious. Additional margins include a mesenteric margin for gastric, small bowel, and colon resections. Because the descending and ascending colon are secondary retroperitoneal, they have an additional radial margin located along their posterior aspects; to remove these parts of the colon, the surgeon must cut, that is, dissect, their posterior aspects off the retroperitoneum. In contrast, the transverse colon is entirely intraperitoneal and is identified by its omentum (**Fig. 1**). Similarly, the sigmoid colon and appendix are entirely intraperitoneal. We benefit from the secondary retroperitoneal location, as it helps to anchor the colon, mitigating free intra-abdominal movement and subsequent torsion. Although most of the small bowel is entirely intraperitoneal in location, the proximal part of the duodenum adjacent to the pancreas is partly retroperitoneal in location. The esophagus has a completely circumferential radial margin, as it is entirely embedded in adventitia. The rectum proximally along the anterior aspect has a serosal surface that is lost asymmetrically proceeding distally. Posteriorly, the rectum sits against the sacrum and is devoid of serosa. Thus, the rectum proximally has an anterior aspect that is not a

margin but its posterior aspect always has a radial margin. The junction of the sigmoid colon and rectum is therefore that point at which the circumferential serosa becomes posteriorly lost (**Fig. 2**). In summary, margins need to be identified and may vary depending on location. Consideration for margins should include the following: (1) proximal, (2) distal, (3) mesenteric, and (4) radial.

Photo documentation is an extremely helpful adjunct and tool. Photographing the external surfaces of specimens before and after any application of ink is important documentation before subsequent dissection and opening of the lumen. Ruler placement in the field is critical, as geometric data are important. Once opened, the luminal aspects may be photographed with closer images in areas of interest. Apart from documentation, these images may help if mapping of tissue sections is done and aid if additional tissue sectioning in specific areas is needed. To mitigate glare, especially in the fresh state, one may apply for about 30 seconds to the surface a paper towel soaked in alcohol, which serves to dehydrate the tissue. Particularly compelling is photographing abnormalities juxtaposed to their normal counterpart, particularly in the same specimen. After fixation, the texture and color of the specimen may

Fig. 1. Anatomy of abdominal colectomy specimen: the proximal margin is identified by the presence of a small segment of terminal ileum and therefore the distal margin is identified as the opposite end of the specimen. By identifying the omentum, the transverse colon is located with the ascending and descending portion of the colon subsequently identified flanking this area. The transverse and sigmoid portions of the colon are entirely intraperitoneal in location and therefore lack radial margins. The secondary retroperitoneal location of the posterior aspects of the ascending and descending colon are radial margins, as surgical sectioning was needed to excise these regions from the body.

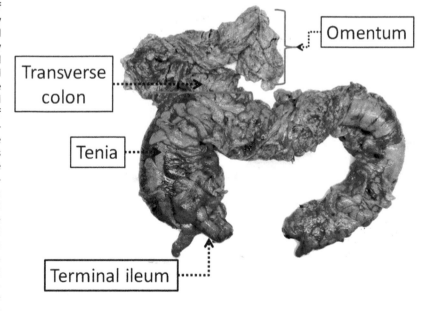

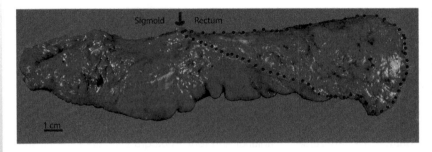

Fig. 2. Rectum and sigmoid colon: the dotted line outlines the mesorectal envelope, which is a radial margin. Posteriorly, the rectum sits against the sacrum and lacks a serosal surface; anteriorly and proximally, the rectum is lined by serosa. Thus, proximally, the rectum has a partial circumferential margin that becomes completely circumferential distally. The sigmoid colon is entirely covered by serosa, making the junction of the sigmoid and rectum easily identified (*arrow*).

change and in many cases add to the photographic documentation. For example, after fixation, subtle mucosal abnormalities may become accentuated (**Fig. 3**). After serial sectioning of the specimen, the relationship of lesions and abnormalities to the wall will become evident and thus photographing this geometry is helpful by laying the sections flat, capturing the entire aspects of the lumen, wall, and surrounding tissues (**Fig. 4**).

Examination and documentation of the external surface, coupled with proper preparation before opening the specimen, is critical. For example, this must be done with an appendix resection for a mucinous neoplasm to avoid inadvertent intraluminal mucin from spilling and adhering to the serosa surface, resulting in falsely increasing the T stage (**Fig. 5**). The following method is helpful to avoid this contamination. Before opening the

specimen, gently blot dry its outer surfaces and then apply ink. To fix the ink, spray the surface with acetic acid and gently blot again. Another application of ink is done and then the specimen placed in formalin unopened for at least 1 hour to further fix the ink. At that point, the specimen is removed from the formalin, blotted dry, and the margin taken off allowing the mucin to drain down into a container as the appendix is held above. Carefully lay the specimen down and fully open the appendix along the longitudinal axis. Return the specimen to the formalin container for further and complete fixation. Complete submission is then done.

Submission of "normal" tissue is important. First, establishing a diagnosis of normal in areas, particularly margins, has value. Second, as previously stated, there may be a disconnect between

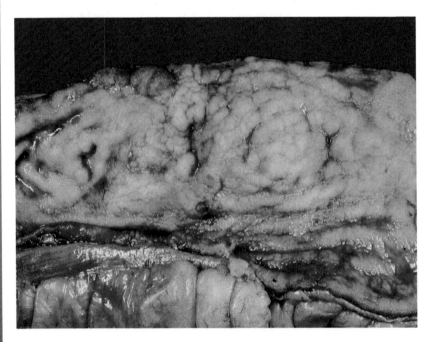

Fig. 3. Dysplastic lesion in ulcerative colitis: mucosal abnormalities are accentuated after formalin fixation. Fixation also reduces glare present in the fresh state.

Fig. 4. Neuroendocrine tumor in small bowel: serial sectioning of the specimen to examine the wall of the specimen often yields important findings. This small tumor was barely visible when inspecting the mucosal surface. However, in the fresh state, the location of the lesion was found by gently palpating the specimen. After fixation, serial sectioning enables documentation of the size and extent of invasion; the tissue sections submitted should follow from the findings from the gross examination.

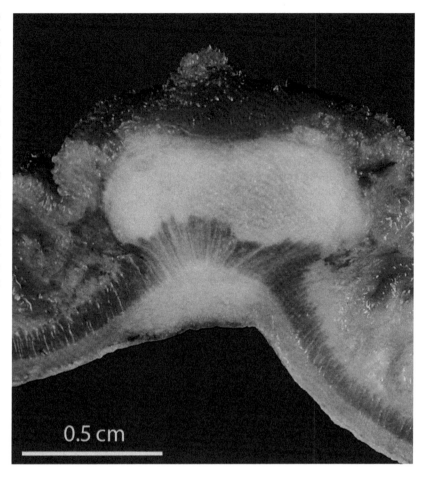

the gross appearance and the histology. For instance, the endoscopic appearance of the stomach may appear normal whereas the biopsy specimen reveals severe *H. pylori* gastritis.[3] On the flip side, there are mucosal "abnormalities" that are simply accentuations of normal structures. For example, with a good bowel preparation, the normally present lymphoid aggregates in the colon

Fig. 5. Low-grade mucinous neoplasm of the appendix: as the T stage is dictated by the presence or absence of mucin on the serosal surface, which completely envelopes the appendix, care must be taken to avoid accidental contamination of the outer surface with luminal mucin.

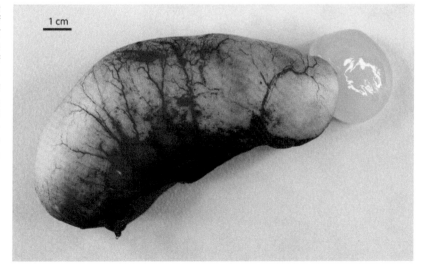

may be easily visualized and mistaken for an aphthous-type ulceration (**Fig. 6**), raising clinical concern for Crohn disease and/or infection.[4] Similarly, the accentuation of normal structures may cause confusion in the terminal ileum, which is replete with Peyer patches and may respond to systemic issues with lymphoid hyperplasia; this expansion may cause these benign lymphoid aggregates to protrude into the lumen, mimicking a polyposis syndrome (**Fig. 7**). Their size, location, and uniformity of shape and spacing are features of benignancy. In contrast, lymphomas usually show marked variation in size and shape of their polypoid projections on gross examination (**Fig. 8**). In treated ulcerative colitis, the mucosal crypt architecture may be restored to a normal appearance, and as well, the inflammatory infiltrate may be abated to the point at which histologic assessment of the mucosal compartment may appear "normal." However, the gross obliteration of the colonic folds leading to "pipe-stem" or flattened mucosa remains (**Fig. 9**). With prompt receipt of resection specimens to the pathology bench, one may actually see the continued propulsive motility of the musculature. In the esophagus, this continued muscle contraction state may create circular folds grossly mimicking the so-called feline esophagus associated with eosinophilic esophagitis (**Fig. 10**). Thus, not all that appears grossly normal is, and not all that appears grossly abnormal is in fact abnormal.

What and how much of the specimen should we submit for histologic examination? We would all agree that for biopsy, polypectomy, and endomucosal resection specimens, the entire specimen is embedded and processed. However, for resection specimens, complete submission and histologic examination for every single case regardless of history and reasons for the resection and gross findings is not only prohibitive from a resource standpoint but, more importantly, illogical. Our challenge, therefore, is to build a logical and data-driven process by which tissue sections from resections are taken. One may think that a general rule may be as follows: "All margins should be submitted for histologic examination." At first approximation, this statement makes sense; submitting the proximal and distal margins from a colectomy is relatively easy, as they usually are submitted in 2 cassettes and their microscopic evaluation is not time-consuming. However, if we consider a partial gastric resection with a distal gastric margin measuring 25 cm in length, will we submit the entire margin? If so, do we submit shaved margin sections or perpendicular sections, each of which may require approximately 20 cassettes and therefore 20 or more slides? Considering the radial margin of an esophagectomy specimen, do we submit the entire radial, circumferential margin, which may require more than 70 cassettes and therefore more than 70 slides? One can therefore understand that even simple and seemingly good "rules" taken to their logical extreme may fail. Regardless of what is submitted for tissue sections, examining and documenting the status of margins grossly is valuable in both

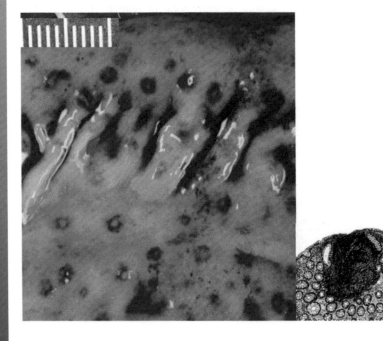

Fig. 6. Pseudo-aphthous ulcerations: with a good bowel preparation, the normally present lymphoid aggregates in the rectum and colon may become easily visible mimicking small ulcers, which may raise concern for Crohn disease and/or infection. The left panel shows the colonic surface with these visible aggregates and the right panel shows the corresponding histology of normal colonic mucosa (Original magnification X100 [right]).

Fig. 7. Terminal ileum and prominent Peyer patches: with varying systemic conditions, the lymphoid aggregates in the terminal ileum may become prominent and create multiple polyps. Note that the distribution of size, spacing and shape is very narrow helping to distinguish this benign process from a lymphoma (see **Fig. 8**).

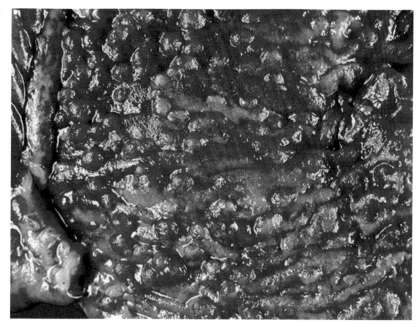

neoplastic and non-neoplastic cases. For example, in resections for Crohn disease, the microscopic status of the margin is not a good predictor of subsequent anastomosis problems,[5] whereas the macroscopic appearance of the margins may serve as a better prognostic feature.

The best way to approach answering the question of what tissue sections to submit is of course based in part on "standards of care," when and if they exist. With most cases, however, we must also think critically about each individual case and tissue sectioning. In addition to framing the key questions to be answered, we must also use the gross appearance of the resection specimen to guide our tissue submission in a thoughtful manner. In the preceding case of the gastrectomy and the question of margin submission, the "correct" answer is dependent in part on the reason for its excision. If we have an intestinal type moderately differentiated adenocarcinoma that

Fig. 8. Follicular lymphoma in terminal ileum: the wide distribution of size, spacing, and shape of these lesions should raise concern for a neoplastic process. Compare with **Fig. 7**.

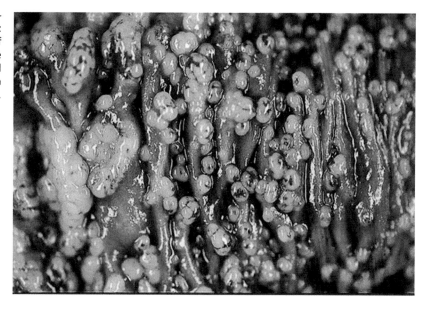

A

B

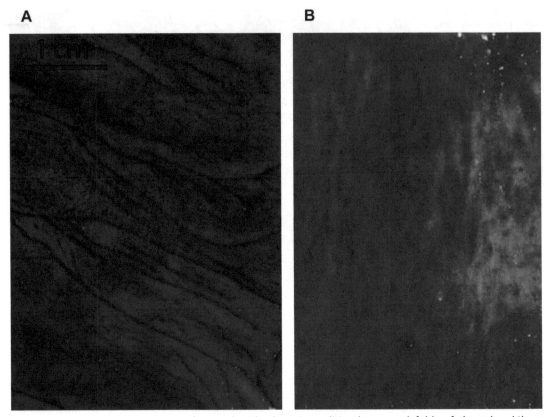

Fig. 9. Colonic mucosa comparison of normal with ulcerative colitis: the normal folds of the colon (*A*) are compared with the flattened mucosa seen in long-standing ulcerative colitis (*B*). Biopsies from patients with treated ulcerative colitis may show relatively "normal" colonic crypts and no inflammation.

forms a well-defined mass that is several centimeters away from the margin, with the margin and adjacent mucosa grossly and texturally normal, then an initial submission of a few shave tissue sections from that long margin may suffice for that margin; one may submit additional sections if a concerning feature is present on histology. If the tumor is a poorly differentiated adenocarcinoma with an insidious growth pattern, complete submission of this long margin at the outset may be appropriate. In the case of the esophagectomy specimen, full-thickness serial sectioning and careful inspection of the relationship of lesion(s) to the wall and beyond to the radial margin is the first step in deciding which sections to submit to assess the radial margin microscopically; one would take sections of this margin at minimum with relationship to the deepest involvement of the lesion. Serial sectioning yielding a few millimeter-thick sections may be accomplished while maintaining the specimen integrity by creating an architecture that resembles pages in a book. Serial sectioning of specimens is equally important in non-neoplastic cases. For example,

in a case of a specimen consisting of loops of adherent bowel, it is impossible to unravel the bowel to then open the lumen longitudinally. By first identifying the margins and taking their sections, one can then serial section the conglomeration of the adherent loops, enabling examination of all aspects of the specimen (**Fig. 11**); the tissue sections submitted will be dependent on the findings but should at least document adhesions and relationships with loops of bowel. Areas of adhesions that appear grossly different from the rest may necessitate additional tissue sections. For example, areas of yellowish/brownish color may reveal on microscopic examination an unexpected neuroendocrine tumor, which are notorious for inciting stromal reactions.

A more nuanced question arises in the following scenario. A 30-year-old woman undergoes total gastrectomy for germline mutation in *CDH1*. On gross inspection, the resection appears and feels entirely normal. What tissue sections "should" be submitted? We know that patients with this germline mutation have an increased risk of signet ring gastric cancer (hereditary diffuse gastric cancer)

Fig. 10. Fake feline esophagus: with continued smooth muscle contractions post resection, the mucosa of the esophagus may be thrown into folds. One should not mistake this finding as evidence of eosinophilic esophagitis.

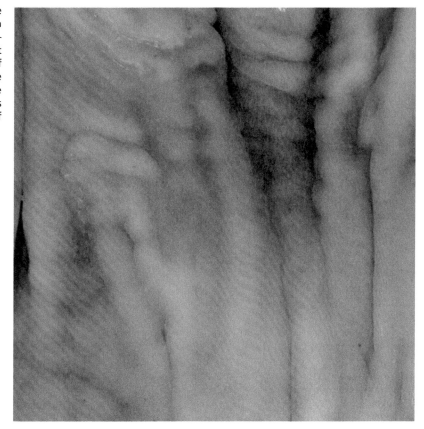

and that women have an additional risk of lobular breast carcinoma.[6] Because of this 70% risk of signet ring gastric cancer by age 60, prophylactic gastrectomy is offered. Given the morbidity of this procedure, the timing of total gastrectomy is important, as optimally one would want to delay resection as much as possible, but before the tumor reaches an advanced stage. It is known that patients with advanced stage signet ring cancer have a 30% 5-year survival.[7] The optimal timing of total gastrectomy to prevent diffuse gastric cancer in individuals with pathogenic variants in *CDH1*

Fig. 11. Adherent and tangled loops of bowel cross section: unraveling entangled loops of bowel is impossible and not necessary. Serial sectioning of the specimen allows complete examination of all geometric aspects of the case.

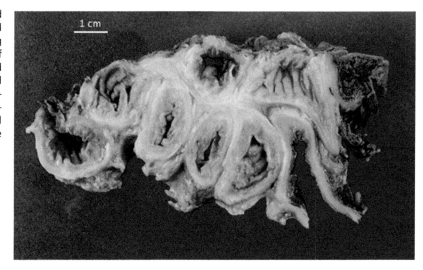

in one study is 39 and 30 years for men and women, respectively.[8] To frame the questions again, we want to know if there is cancer and if so what are the stage and margin status. Academically, we may also be interested in understanding where in the stomach the adenocarcinoma(s) is(are) and the size. Given that these prophylactic resection cases appear totally normal, we cannot depend on gross examination to guide tissue submission. On one hand, one may argue that complete submission of the entire resection specimen is needed; on the other hand, one may argue that submission of at least 16 lymph nodes found at the gross bench coupled with a "generous" sampling on the stomach is sufficient. Total submission is certainly advocated by some.[9,10] In this manner, a nonbiased approached for submission is used and all tissue is examined including lymph nodes for accurate staging. Bear in mind that this total submission may generate more than 300 slides requiring microscopic evaluation. Understanding that many institutions may not be resourced to handle such submission, a tiered approach with partial submission proposal has been put forth.[11] Even if we argue that complete submission is needed, we should realize that we are still reviewing only a fraction of the entire specimen. Considering that each tissue section is 5 μm thick coming from a 2.5-mm-thick submitted tissue section, we review only 0.2% of each section. Thus, even with 100% submission of tissue, we review in fact only 0.2% of the entire specimen. Therefore, complete specimen submission does not equal complete tissue review.

There is a phenotypic spectrum of patients with well-established and studied germline *CDH1* mutations. With increasing advancements and use of sequencing, additional pathogenic variants of *CDH1* are being found with a phenotype that is not well established.[12] Thus, one may argue that complete submission of these prophylactic gastric resections is needed to at least further our understanding of these varying genetic mutations. In addition, if no cancer is found in an incomplete submission, one wonders about the impact of these results on the feelings and well-being of the patient. Even if every single lymph node is submitted with no cancer identified and the stomach partially submitted, from a probability perspective, the chances of cancer recurrence are extremely small. How the patient will feel about this statistical statement is still in question.

What is the "best" approach to submitting lymph nodes in cancer resection specimens and how many is "good enough"? It is very enticing to pick out and submit "just enough" lymph nodes to meet the minimum number from guidelines issued from organizations such as the College of American Pathologists (CAP). Although this approach will meet expectations, we consider several factors. First, choosing only grossly visible lymph nodes is a biased sampling of lymph nodes. This approach would be valid if, for every tumor type in every case, the probability of lymph node metastasis increased with lymph node size. Do large lymph nodes have a higher probability of metastasis compared with small lymph nodes? Perhaps not. The distribution of lymph node size with and without metastasis was identical based on careful histologic measurements in a series of gastric cancer[13]; significantly, metastases were found in lymph nodes measuring 1 mm and thus not grossly identifiable. The use of fat-clearing agents has been proposed to help selective retrieval of lymph nodes. With this approach, smaller lymph nodes were found, a percentage of which had the only site of metastatic disease.[14] In summary, the assumption that large and grossly identifiable lymph nodes are an accurate representation of metastatic disease is in question. The absolute number and/or fraction of metastatic lymph nodes is part of the staging systems and touted to be of prognostic value in several studies; however, these studies are based on a mixture of lymph node retrieval methods. Moving forward, it will be important in developing informative studies to document and take into account how we are retrieving lymph nodes. In contrast, lymph node size determined by preoperative radiology may be a predictor of lymph node metastatic disease.[15] Similarly, imaging (computed tomography) measurements of the short and long axes of lymph nodes were associated with metastatic disease.[16,17] How these radiology metrics correlate one to one with the tissue is not known.

How many lymph nodes are required for evaluation for resections performed for cancer? If we take the approach of submitting at least the entire adipose/soft tissue adjacent to the organ, then the number of lymph nodes is at its maximum number for that case. If we are selective in submission, then we do need to be sure the minimum number of lymph nodes examined as defined by organizations such as CAP are found. Continued submission of adipose/soft tissue in areas enriched with lymph nodes, sites that are organ dependent,[18] regardless of grossly identifiable structures, often yields more lymph nodes and, as discussed previously, in an unbiased manner. What number is truly "sufficient" is organ and study dependent. For gastric cancer, 15 may not be sufficient,[19] and one study suggests that more than 25 lymph nodes improves survival stratification.[20] For colon cancer, the number 12 has been suggested as a minimum.[21] Identifying perirectal lymph nodes in the neoadjuvant setting is often problematic; however, retrieving a sufficient number is important[22] in all cases. In summary, lymph node submission is important especially in neoplastic cases; understanding and being aware of the caveats of the method used for their submission and the origins of given expectations of minimum numbers is critical.

In conclusion, by taking a problem-solving approach to handling gross specimens, we are best equipped to thoughtfully and logically care for our patients. By asking "What are the questions to be answered" coupled with a working knowledge of anatomy, one may then begin to handle appropriately the specimen and understand the reasons for tissue submission. Although cases may follow a certain "script," most cases offer something different, new, and challenging to the unbiased and critical-thinking pathologist. Proper handling of the gross specimen is critical.

Work Flow

a. Cross check paperwork with given specimen.

b. Understand the anatomy and orientation.

c. What are the questions to be answered?

d. Document/photograph external surfaces.

e. Identify all margins including proximal, distal, and radial.

f. Open specimen noting luminal contents.

g. Document luminal surfaces.

h. Serially section to examine full thickness.

i. Sections taken based on "c" and additional gross findings.

KEY ANATOMY TIPS FOR MARGINS

Complete circumferential radial margins are present in the esophagus, distal rectum, and anal canal, and partial circumferential radial margins are present in the proximal duodenum, ascending colon, descending colon, and proximal rectum.

DISCLOSURE

The author has nothing to disclose.

REFERENCES

1. Raess PW, Baird-Howell M, Aggarwal R, et al. Vertical sleeve gastrectomy specimens have a high prevalence of unexpected histopathologic findings requiring additional clinical management. Surg Obes Relat Dis 2015;11:1020–3.

2. Amin MB, Greene FL, Edge SB, et al. The eighth edition AJCC cancer staging manual: continuing to build a bridge from a population-based to a more "personalized" approach to cancer staging. CA Cancer J Clin 2017;67:93–9.

3. Belair PA, Metz DC, Faigel DO, et al. Receiver operator characteristic analysis of endoscopy as a test for gastritis. Dig Dis Sci 1997;42:2227–33.

4. Faigel DO, Furth EE, Bachwich DR. Aphthoid lesions of the rectum. Gastrointest Endosc 1996;43: 528–9.

5. Setoodeh S, Liu L, Boukhar SA, et al. The clinical significance of Crohn disease activity at resection margins. Arch Pathol Lab Med 2019;143:505–9.

6. Kaurah P, Talhouk A, MacMillan A, et al. Hereditary diffuse gastric cancer: cancer risk and the personal cost of preventive surgery. Fam Cancer 2019;18: 429–38.

7. Stiekema J, Cats A, Kuijpers A, et al. Surgical treatment results of intestinal and diffuse type gastric cancer. Implications for a differentiated therapeutic approach? Eur J Surg Oncol 2013;39:686–93.

8. Laszkowska M, Silver E, Schrope B, et al. Optimal timing of total gastrectomy to prevent diffuse gastric cancer in individuals with pathogenic variants in CDH1. Clin Gastroenterol Hepatol 2020;18(4): 822–9.e4.

9. Fitzgerald RC, Hardwick R, Huntsman D, et al. Hereditary diffuse gastric cancer: updated consensus guidelines for clinical management and directions for future research. J Med Genet 2010;47:436–44.

10. van der Post RS, Vogelaar IP, Carneiro F, et al. Hereditary diffuse gastric cancer: updated clinical guidelines with an emphasis on germline CDH1 mutation carriers. J Med Genet 2015;52:361–74.

11. Drake J, Schreiber KC, Lopez R, et al. Establishing a center of excellence for hereditary diffuse gastric cancer syndrome. J Surg Oncol 2019; 119:673–4.

12. Figueiredo J, Melo S, Carneiro P, et al. Clinical spectrum and pleiotropic nature of CDH1 germline mutations. J Med Genet 2019;56:199–208.

13. Noda N, Sasako M, Yamaguchi N, et al. Ignoring small lymph nodes can be a major cause of staging error in gastric cancer. Br J Surg 1998;85:831–4.

14. Hanna GB, Amygdalos I, Ni M, et al. Improving the standard of lymph node retrieval after gastric cancer surgery. Histopathology 2013;63:316–24.

15. Kim DJ, Kim W. Is lymph node size a reliable factor for estimating lymph node metastasis in early gastric cancer? J Gastric Cancer 2018;18:20–9.

16. Hanada Y, Choi AY, Hwang JH, et al. Low frequency of lymph node metastases in patients in the United

States with early-stage gastric cancers that fulfill Japanese endoscopic resection criteria. Clin Gastroenterol Hepatol 2019;17:1763–9.

17. Zhou Z, Liu Y, Meng K, et al. Application of spectral CT imaging in evaluating lymph node metastasis in patients with gastric cancers: initial findings. Acta Radiol 2019;60:415–24.

18. da Costa DW, Vrouenraets BC, Witte BI, et al. Which lymph nodes contain metastases in colon cancer patients? A retrospective histopathological evaluation of 156 patients. Int J Surg Pathol 2015;23:623–8.

19. Kim YI. Is retrieval of at least 15 lymph nodes sufficient recommendation in early gastric cancer? Ann Surg Treat Res 2014;87:180–4.

20. Liu YY, Fang WL, Wang F, et al. Does a higher cutoff value of lymph node retrieval substantially improve survival in patients with advanced gastric cancer? Time to embrace a new digit. Oncologist 2017;22: 97–106.

21. Budde CN, Tsikitis VL, Deveney KE, et al. Increasing the number of lymph nodes examined after colectomy does not improve colon cancer staging. J Am Coll Surg 2014;218:1004–11.

22. Gill A, Brunson A, Lara P Jr, et al. Implications of lymph node retrieval in locoregional rectal cancer treated with chemoradiotherapy: a California Cancer Registry Study. Eur J Surg Oncol 2015;41: 647–52.

Impact of Subspecialty Sign-Out on Interobserver Variability and Accuracy in Gastrointestinal Pathology

Christa L. Whitney-Miller, MD

KEYWORDS

• Gastrointestinal pathology • Interobserver variability • Subspecialty surgical pathology

Key points

- Literature regarding the impact of subspecialization in surgical pathology is limited and shows disparate results.
- Subspecialization within surgical pathology provides modest improvements in report completeness and accuracy.
- Subspecialization within surgical pathology reduces interobserver variability and the need for consultation.

SYNOPSIS

Subspecialty signout is increasingly common in academic medical centers as well as some community practices. Reducing interobserver variability in anatomic pathology is desirable so that clinicians can select the appropriate therapy. Many departments that elect subspecialty signout do so with the assumption that it will improve diagnostic accuracy and interobserver variability – but does it? The literature is mixed.

Subspecialty sign-out is increasingly common in academic medical centers as well as some community practices. A survey of academic pathology departments from the Association of Directors of Anatomic and Surgical Pathology in 2006 showed that 1 department was fully subspecialized, with 70% having subspecialization beyond those with certifying exams (eg, dermatopathology and hematopathology).

Reducing interobserver variability in anatomic pathology is desirable so that clinicians can select the appropriate therapy. In patients with tumors, surgical pathologists determine not only benign versus malignant but also type of tumor and information to prognosticate, predict response to therapy, and identify patients who potentially have a genetic disease. In other settings, they identify infectious disease or identify patients at risk for cancer who need additional screening; they also monitor response to therapy. Given the important role surgical pathologists play in crafting therapeutic decisions, it is critical that interpretations be as precise and reproducible as possible.

With the explosion of medical information, some pathologists have found it difficult to maintain the knowledge required to provide comprehensive reports. This is one reason some departments have elected to transition to subspecialty sign-out, with the assumption that it improves diagnostic accuracy and interobserver variability—but does it? The literature is mixed.

As early as 2000, Farmer and colleagues[1] compared the classification of inflammatory bowel disease (Crohn disease, ulcerative colitis [UC] or indeterminate colitis) by university pathologists versus specialist gastrointestinal (GI) pathologists and showed very poor agreement. The study involved 24 pathologists from 8

University of Rochester School of Medicine and Dentistry, 601 Elmwood Avenue, Rochester, NY 14642, USA
E-mail address: christa_whitney-miller@urmc.rochester.edu

Surgical Pathology 13 (2020) 371–376
https://doi.org/10.1016/j.path.2020.05.001
1875-9181/20/© 2020 Elsevier Inc. All rights reserved.

Table 1
Initial diagnosis compared with review by a specialist gastrointestinal pathologist

General Pathologist's Initial Diagnosis (No. Patients)	Gastrointestinal Pathologist's Diagnosis (No. Patients)
Crohn disease (23)	Crohn disease (19)
	UC (3)
	Indeterminate colitis (1)
UC (70)	UC (40)
	Crohn disease (10)
	Indeterminate colitis (20)
Diverticulitis (1)	Diverticulitis (1)
Normal (6)	No inflammatory bowel disease (4)
	Crohn disease (2)
Inflammatory bowel disease (2)	Crohn disease (1)
	UC (1)
Nonspecific inflammation (17)	Crohn disease (7)
	Indeterminate colitis (2)
	UC (8)

From Farmer M, Petras RE, Hunt LE, *et al.* The importance of diagnostic accuracy in colonic inflammatory bowel disease. *Am J Gastroenterol* 2000; 95:3184-3188; with permission.

institutions evaluating 84 colectomy specimens and 35 biopsy sets from 119 patients with subsequent blinded review by a single GI pathologist. The GI pathologist agreed with the original diagnosis in 45% of surgical cases and 54% of biopsy cases. The κ coefficient for overall agreement was -0.01. The results are summarized in **Table 1**.

A more recent study (Römkens and colleagues)[2] compared the histologic scoring of UC patients with mucosal healing by general pathologists as opposed to expert GI pathologists. They selected this feature because mucosal healing often is a treatment target in clinical trials; 43 biopsy sets from 39 patients were reviewed. After assessment by the generalist pathologist, the

biopsies were rereviewed by 3 GI pathologists, each of whom applied 3 established scoring systems: Harpaz (Gupta) index, Geboes score, and Riley score. The percents of cases classified as histologic remission originally versus the expert GI pathologists is shown in **Table 2**. There was no correlation between the primary assessment and the reassessment by the expert GI pathologists.

In 2002, Baak and colleagues[3] compared general surgical pathologists' grading of Barrett esophagus surveillance biopsies to expert GI pathologists; 143 biopsies were graded as no dysplasia, indefinite for dysplasia, low-grade dysplasia, or high-grade dysplasia by general surgical pathologists. Two expert GI pathologists then blindly reviewed all the biopsies. There was complete agreement in 35% of cases. Results are displayed in **Table 3**; see also **Fig. 1**.

In 2007, Kerkhof and colleagues[4] similarly examined the impact of expert GI pathologists on interobserver variability in Barrett esophagus. They reviewed a large number of biopsies (793) with Barrett esophagus, initially by the local pathologist at 1 of 15 hospitals and then by 1 of 6 expert GI pathologists. When there was disagreement, another expert GI pathologist rendered an opinion and when 2 pathologists were in agreement, that was considered the final diagnosis. Ninety-five of the biopsies were initially reviewed by expert pathologists at the local hospital. The comparison of the initial diagnoses with those of the expert pathologists is shown in **Table 4**. The agreement between nonexpert and expert pathologists was fair if using 3 categories (negative, indefinite + low grade, and high grade + adenocarcinoma) or 4 categories (negative, indefinite + low grade, high grade, and adenocarcinoma) ($\kappa = 0.24$) but did improve if 2 categories (high grade + adenocarcinoma vs negative + indefinite + low grade) were used ($\kappa = 0.62$). Similarly, when comparing the 95 biopsies that initially were read by 1 of the experts with the results of the second review, interobserver variability remained fair if 3 or 4 categories ($\kappa = 0.27$) were used and improved to moderate

Table 2
Percent of ulcerative colitis cases classified as histologic remission

Generalist	Harpaz (Gupta) Index <1	Geboes Score <0.1	Geboes Score <3.1	Riley Score 0
84.7%	88.7%	28.5%	89.1%	25%

From Römkens TEH, Kranenburg P, Tilburg, AV, *et al.* Assessment of histological remission in ulcerative colitis: Discrepancies between daily practice and expert opinion. *J Crohns Colitis* 2018; 12:425-431; with permission.

Table 3
Original and Expert Diagnoses in Barrett Esophagus

		Expert Diagnosis		
		Negative	Indefinite/Low Grade	High Grade
Initial diagnosis	Negative	27	0	0
	Indefinite/low grade	69	22	1
	High grade	6	5	12

From Baak JP, ten Kate FJ, Offerhaus GJ, *et al*. Routine morphometrical analysis can improve reproducibility of dysplasia grade in Barret's oesophagus surveillance biopsies. *J Clin Pathol* 2002; 55: 910-916; with permission.

when negative + indefinite + low grade versus high grade + adenocarcinoma was used ($\kappa = 0.58$).

In another study in 2004 by Komuta and colleagues,[5] 88 cases of endoscopically resected malignant colon polyps were rereviewed blindly by 3 experienced GI pathologists. There was substantial agreement among the expert pathologists regarding T stage, margin status, and Haggitt classification, whereas agreement between initial and expert pathologists was moderate in these areas. Agreement among experienced pathologists with regard to grade of differentiation and lymphovascular invasion was poor. Results are summarized in **Table 5**.

In a 2011 study of report completeness in resections for colorectal adenocarcinoma, Messenger and colleagues[6] showed that reports from GI pathologists were more complete than those from general surgical pathologists. Introduction of a

synoptic template helped the generalists provide more complete reports; the synoptic template had no impact on the completeness of reports from the GI pathologists.

In 2015, Graham and colleagues[7] looked at interobserver variability as part of a study on tumor budding in colorectal adenocarcinoma; 121 cases were reviewed by 2 pathologists with interest in GI pathology; agreement regarding tumor bud score was good ($\kappa = 0.70$). Twenty of those cases also were reviewed by 4 general surgical pathologists and the combined agreement among all 6 was also good ($\kappa = 0.72$). See **Fig. 2**.

In a study comparing diagnoses of anal biopsies, some initially read at a community hospital by a general surgical pathologist and others initially read at the university hospital by a subspecialist pathologist and then all reviewed blindly by a subspecialty pathologist, Roma and colleagues[8] found that the discrepancy rate was higher among

Fig. 1. Low-grade dysplasia (*left side of image*) arising in intestinal metaplasia (Barrett esophagus) (hematoxylin-eosin, original mag-nification ×100).

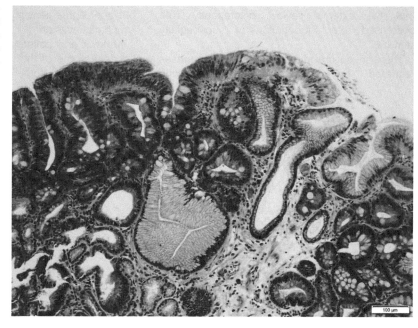

Table 4
Initial versus final diagnoses in 793 Barrett esophagus biopsies

		Final Diagnosis		
		Negative	Indefinite/Low Grade	High Grade/ Adenocarcinoma
Initial diagnosis	Negative	546	19	2
	Indefinite/low grade	111	94	5
	High grade/ adenocarcinoma	0	1	15

the biopsies initially read at the community hospital (20%) compared with the university hospital (16%), although results did not reach statistical significance.

In 2017, as part of a study on the utility of detecting venous invasion in colorectal cancer, Kirsch and colleagues[9] compared interobserver variability between non-GI pathologists and GI pathologists. They found GI pathologists identified vascular invasion more frequently than non-GI pathologists: 30% versus 9.2% on hematoxylineosin alone and 58.3% versus 34.6% with elastic stain (**Fig. 3**).

In their report detailing their experience transitioning to subspecialty sign-out, Conant and colleagues[10] reported on several quality measures overall (not limited to GI pathology). They found the rate of consultation (shown at conference, private internal consultation, and extramural consultation) all decreased after introduction of subspecialty sign-out (**Table 6**). They also showed that the external review discrepancy rate decreased after introduction of subspecialty sign-out.

There are several studies comparing diagnoses rendered by general pathologists with subsequent rereview by an expert GI pathologist that show significant differences, which would be clinically significant. These include Farmer and colleagues' study[1] regarding classification of inflammatory bowel disease (Crohn Disease vs UC vs indeterminate); Römkens and colleagues' study[2] of mucosal healing in UC patients; Baak and colleagues' study[3] of Barrett esophagus biopsies; Messenger and colleagues' study[6] of colorectal cancer report completeness; and Kirsch and colleagues' study[9] of vascular invasion in colorectal carcinoma. Conant and colleagues' report[10] took a slightly different approach and compared quality measures before and after subspecialty implementation and demonstrated improvement in several of them.

Komuta and colleagues' study[5] went farther in their comparison of general versus subspecialty pathologists and showed substantial agreement among the subspecialty pathologists regarding T stage, margin status, and Haggitt classification but poor agreement regarding grade and angiolymphatic invasion.

Kerkhof and colleagues' study[4] is interesting because some of the initial reviews at the local hospitals were done by someone considered

Table 5
Interobserver variability in pathologic assessment of malignant colorectal polyps (k)

Pathologic Feature	Experienced Pathologists	Initial Report vs Experienced Pathologists	P Value
T stage	0.725	0.516	.010
Histologic grade	0.163	0.141	.112
Margin status	0.668	0.555	.051
Haggitt classification	0.682	0.578	.400
Angiolymphatic invasion	−0.017	−0.098	.512

From Komuta K, Batts K, Jessurun J, et al. Interobserver variability in the pathological assessment of malignant colorectal polyps. *Br J Surg* 2004;91:1479–1484; with permission.

Fig. 2. Colonic adenocarcinoma with tumor budding (hematoxylin-eosin, original magnification ×200).

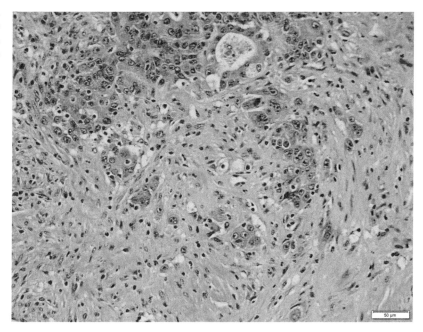

an expert GI pathologist. Depending on the number of categories used, agreement between initial and expert diagnoses was fair to substantial; perhaps surprisingly, this held true regardless of who made the initial diagnosis: a nonexpert, an expert, or the combined group. Along with the findings in Komuta and colleagues' study,[5] this raises the possibility that studies showing discrepancies between generalist and subspecialist surgical pathologists are not due to better diagnoses by subspecialists but rather reflect inherent limitations in classifying disease processes, particularly when trying to categorize a linear process into an ordinal classification.

Graham and colleagues' study[7] is an outlier in that interobserver agreement was good for both subspecialty pathologists and the

Fig. 3. Colonic adenocarcinoma with large vessel involvement (hematoxylin-eosin, original magnification ×100).

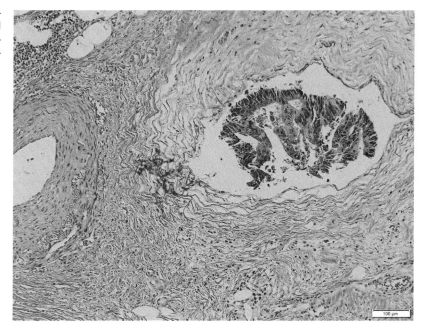

Table 6
Consultation rates before and after subspecialty implementation

Quality Measure	Before	After	P Value
Total cases	49,260	57,294	
Shown at intradepartmental consensus conference	4900 (9.95%)	4678 (8.17%)	<.0001
Internal consult	2931 (5.95%)	2294 (4.0%)	<.0001
External consult	1043 (2.12%)	1106 (1.93%)	.322
Discrepancy after external consult	20 (1.91%)	7 (0.63%)	.008

From Conant JL, Gibson PC, Bunn J, *et al*. Transition to subspecialty sign-out at an academic institution and its advantages. *Acad Patho* 2017; with permission.

combined group of subspecialty and general pathologists.

In summary, the literature regarding the impact of subspecialty sign-out is inconsistent, and study design has a significant impact on the conclusions that can be drawn. There is some evidence that subspecialty sign-out can reduce interobserver variability in selected pathologic features.

REFERENCES

1. Farmer M, Petras RE, Hunt LE, et al. The importance of diagnostic accuracy in colonic inflammatory bowel disease. Am J Gastroenterol 2000;95:3184–8.
2. Römkens TEH, Kranenburg P, Tilburg AV, et al. Assessment of histological remission in ulcerative colitis: Discrepancies between daily practice and expert opinion. J Crohns Colitis 2018;12:425–31.
3. Baak JP, ten Kate FJ, Offerhaus GJ, et al. Routine morphometrical analysis can improve reproducibility of dysplasia grade in Barret's oesophagus surveillance biopsies. J Clin Pathol 2002;55:910–6.
4. Kerkhof M, van Dekken H, Steyerberg EW, et al. Grading of dysplasia in Barret's oesophagus: substantial interobserver variation between general and gastrointestinal pathologists. Histopathology 2007;50:920–7.
5. Komuta K, Batts K, Jessurun J, et al. Interobserver variability in the pathological assessment of malignant colorectal polyps. Br J Surg 2004;91: 1479–84.
6. Messenger DE, McLeod RS, Kirsch R. What impact has the introduction of a synoptic report for rectal cancer had on reporting outcomes for specialist gastrointestinal and nongastrointestinal pathologists? Arch Pathol Lab Med 2011;135:1471–5.
7. Graham RP, Vierkant RA, Tillmans LS, et al. Tumor budding in colorectal carcinoma. Confirmation of prognostic significance and histologic cutoff in a population-based cohort. Am J Surg Pathol 2015; 39:1340–6.
8. Roma AA, Liu X, Patil DT, et al. Proposed Terminology for anal squamous lesions. Its application and interobserver agreement among pathologists in academic and community hospitals. Am J Clin Pathol 2017;148:81–90.
9. Kirsch R, Messenger DE, Riddell RH, et al. Venous invasion in colorectal cancer. Impact of an elastic stain on detection and interobserver agreement among gastrointestinal and nongastrointestinal pathologists. Am J Surg Pathol 2013;37:200–10.
10. Conant JL, Gibson PC, Bunn J, et al. Transition to subspecialty sign-out at an academic institution and its advantages. Acad Pathol 2017;4, 2374289517714767.

Diagnosis and Management of Gastrointestinal Neuroendocrine Neoplasms

Raul S. Gonzalez, MD[a,b,*]

KEYWORDS

- Neuroendocrine tumor • Neuroendocrine carcinoma • Neuroendocrine neoplasms
- Gastrointestinal • WHO classification • Grading • Staging

Key points

- In the new WHO classification, gastrointestinal neuroendocrine tumors and carcinomas are distinguished by histology. Tumors can be any grade; carcinomas are not numerically graded.
- Gastrointestinal neuroendocrine carcinomas are high-grade malignancies with aggressive behavior and poor outcome everywhere along the digestive tract.
- Gastric neuroendocrine tumors may arise in the setting of autoimmune gastritis, where they are small and multifocal. Sporadic tumors have higher rates of patient mortality.
- Small bowel neuroendocrine tumors may be multifocal and may metastasize locally as well as distantly, impacting staging.
- The appendix and rectum are common locations for gastrointestinal neuroendocrine tumors. They are often indolent at these sites, although rectal cases can be aggressive.

ABSTRACT

The latest WHO classification cleanly divides gastrointestinal neuroendocrine neoplasms into neuroendocrine tumor (NET; well-differentiated, any grade) and neuroendocrine carcinoma (NEC; poorly differentiated, high-grade by definition), along with mixed neuroendocrine–non-neuroendocrine neoplasms. NECs are always aggressive, with multiple mutations; they are treated with chemotherapy. NETs have widely different presentations, behavior, and management depending on site of origin. Esophageal examples are vanishingly rare. Most gastric and appendiceal tumors are indolent, as are many colonic and rectal tumors. The duodenum is home to some unusual variants of NET, and jejunal/ileal NETs frequently metastasize, which impacts their staging and clinical management.

INTRODUCTION

Gastrointestinal neuroendocrine neoplasms (NENs) represent a constantly evolving area of gastrointestinal pathology. The nomenclature of such lesions has shifted numerous times, with the traditional term "carcinoid" falling out of favor and grading schemes undergoing numerous revisions. In addition, although well-differentiated neuroendocrine tumors (NETs) look largely similar no matter their organ of origin, their behavior is markedly different from site to site. Accordingly, the new American Joint Committee (AJCC) Cancer Staging Manual offers a separate chapter on staging of NETs for each digestive organ.[1] This review offers a broad overview of gastrointestinal NENs, including updates on naming, grading, staging, and clinical management.

[a] Department of Pathology, Beth Israel Deaconess Medical Center, 330 Brookline Avenue, Boston, MA 02215, USA; [b] Harvard Medical School, Boston, MA, USA
* Department of Pathology, Beth Israel Deaconess Medical Center, 330 Brookline Avenue, Boston, MA 02215.
E-mail address: Rgonzal5@bidmc.harvard.edu
Twitter: @RaulSGonzalezMD (R.S.G.)

Surgical Pathology 13 (2020) 377–397
https://doi.org/10.1016/j.path.2020.04.002
1875-9181/20/© 2020 Elsevier Inc. All rights reserved.

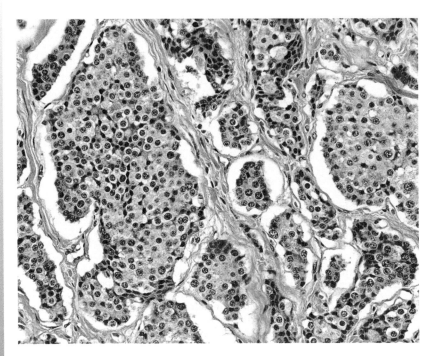

Fig. 1. A classic well-differentiated neuroendocrine tumor of the gastrointestinal tract. The cells are arranged in nests and demonstrate "salt-and-pepper" chromatin and amphophilic cytoplasm. Mitotic figures are sparse, and necrosis is absent (hematoxylin and eosin, original magnification ×400).

NOMENCLATURE AND CLASSIFICATION

The newest edition of the World Health Organization (WHO) Digestive Tumors Classification (5th edition, published in 2019)[2] retains the dichotomy of most gastrointestinal NENs being considered either well-differentiated NETs (**Fig. 1**) or poorly differentiated neuroendocrine carcinomas (NECs), with the latter being subtyped into small cell (**Fig. 2**) and large cell NECs (**Fig. 3**); however, many finer points of the classification scheme have been updated.[3]

NENs are graded using mitotic rate per 2 mm^2 (rather than per 10 high-power fields, which can vary depending on the microscope) and Ki67 immunohistochemical index (**Table 1**). Grade 1 neoplasms have a mitotic rate of less than 2 per 2 mm^2 (WHO recommends counting 10 mm^2 and

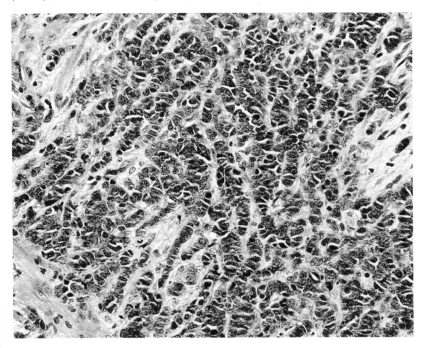

Fig. 2. A poorly differentiated small cell neuroendocrine carcinoma of the gastrointestinal tract. The malignant cells have enlarged, intensely hyperchromatic, molded nuclei and scant cytoplasm (hematoxylin-eosin, original magnification ×400).

Fig. 3. A poorly differentiated large cell NEC of the gastrointestinal tract. The malignant cells have prominent nucleoli and ample amphophilic cytoplasm. Necrosis and mitotic figures are readily visible (hematoxylin-eosin, original magnification ×400).

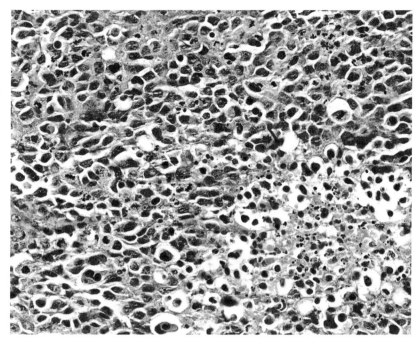

taking the average) or a Ki67 rate of less than 3% (rather than 0%–2% in the previous edition) (**Fig. 4**). Grade 2 neoplasms have a mitotic rate of 2 to 20 per 2 mm^2 or a Ki67 rate of 3% to 20%. A higher rate than these by mitotic count or Ki67 indicates a grade 3 NET. An additional Ki67 cutoff of 55% has been suggested by several investigators, but this has yet to be adopted into any official grading scheme.[4] However, now only NETs are officially graded using this scheme. This fact encapsulates 3 important changes: (1) NETs can now be grade 3, which was not true earlier; (2) NECs are not given a numerical grade, as they are essentially high-grade by definition; and (3) the distinction between NET and NEC is primarily made on histologic appearance (see later in this article). The term "carcinoma" should not be applied just because a NEN is metastatic or is high-grade. In addition, although grade 3 NETs generally have a lower Ki67 index than NECs, some overlap exists,[5] meaning Ki67 should not be used in isolation to justify a diagnosis of NEC. Rare cases of NET with both low-grade and high-grade morphologic regions have been described, although some may represent NETs with variably proliferative foci, as opposed to transformation into NEC.[6]

Table 1
World Health Organization (WHO) grading classification for gastrointestinal neuroendocrine neoplasms

Histology	Mitotic Rate, per 2 mm^2	Ki67 Index (at Least 500 Cells), %	WHO Grade
Well-differentiated neuroendocrine tumor	0–1	<3	1 (low)
	2–20	3–20	2 (intermediate)
	>20	>20	3 (high)
Poorly differentiated neuroendocrine carcinoma	n/a (>20)	n/a (>20)	n/a (not assigned a numerical grade; essentially always high-grade)

Abbreviation: n/a, not applicable.
Adapted from Klimstra DS, Klöppel G, La Rosa S, Rindi G. Classification of neuroendocrine neoplasms of the digestive system. In: WHO Classification of Tumours Editorial Board [Eds]. WHO Classification of Tumours: Digestive System Tumours, 5th Edition. Lyon: IARC, 2019; p. 16-19; with permission.

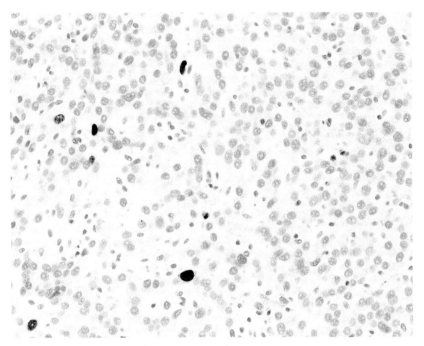

Fig. 4. Immunohistochemistry for Ki67 is required for accurate grading of NETs. Most of these neoplasms are low-grade (grade 1), corresponding to a Ki67 index of less than 3% (Ki67 immunohistochemical stain, original magnification ×400).

Accurate reporting of the Ki67 index of an NET remains a potentially frustrating topic for pathologists.[7] WHO recommends that "at least 500 cells" be counted, and this should be performed in the area of highest staining, also termed the "hot spot" (**Figs. 5** and **6**). There exist several techniques for performing this counting,[8] including (1) the quick but unreliable method of "eyeballing"; (2) printing out a photomicrograph and counting by hand, which is tedious but appears to be the most reliable and reproducible; and (3) using counting software to manually mark and count cells in a digital photomicrograph. Proprietary software programs for counting Ki67 in digital images have been developed, but to date, none are freely or broadly available. If the mitotic rate and Ki67 index indicate different grades, the higher grade should be used; in most cases, the Ki67 index is higher.[9]

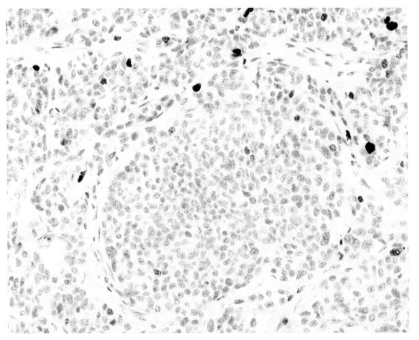

Fig. 5. Compared with **Fig. 4**, more lesional cell nuclei are positive for Ki67 by immunohistochemistry. Tumors with a Ki67 index between 3% and 20% qualify as grade 2 (Ki67 immunohistochemical stain, original magnification ×400).

Fig. 6. This image is from the same lesion as **Fig. 5**, demonstrating the importance of locating "hot spots" with the highest rate of Ki67 staining. This focus clearly shows greater than 20% of cells positive for Ki67, making this tumor high-grade (grade 3) (Ki67 immunohistochemical stain, original magnification ×400).

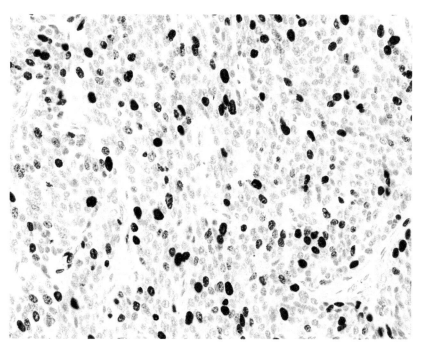

Grade 3 NETs have primarily been studied in the pancreas,[10] which will not be covered here. Data on grade 3 gastrointestinal NETs remain lacking. Our preliminary findings have unsurprisingly indicated that these are rare but aggressive lesions that often metastasize and lead to patient death (Vyas et al, 2020, unpublished data). Most qualify for grade 3 status based on Ki67 index (see **Fig. 6**), although some may show a sufficiently high mitotic rate instead (**Fig. 7**). In the past, most grade 3 NETs were likely diagnosed as, and therefore clinically treated as, NECs, meaning optimal therapy remains to be elucidated.

The old term mixed adenoneuroendocrine carcinoma (**Fig. 8**) has been replaced with mixed neuroendocrine–non-neuroendocrine neoplasm, or MiNEN.[11,12] This term encompasses rare lesions in which the neuroendocrine component is a NET rather than a NEC (**Fig. 9**), as well as lesions in which the nonendocrine component is a squamous cell carcinoma or some other nonadenocarcinoma. WHO still generally advocates that each component represent at least 30% of the lesion, although exceptions can be made for a focal component of small cell carcinoma.[2]

NEUROENDOCRINE TUMORS: GENERAL CONSIDERATIONS

NETs have been increasing in incidence over the past few decades,[13] likely because of a combination of improved detection/diagnosis and an actual increase in baseline frequency. For most gastrointestinal organs, NETs are far more common than NECs.

NETs are composed of rounded, uniform cells with "salt-and-pepper" chromatin and amphophilic cytoplasm, arranged in nests, cords, and/or trabeculae. (In short, they look like "carcinoids.") Mitotic figures are generally sparse, and necrosis should be minimal or absent. Focal "endocrine atypia" may be present, where occasional cells have enlarged or hyperchromatic nuclei. NETs should be convincingly positive for synaptophysin and/or chromogranin. Ki67 immunohistochemical staining must be performed on all NETs, for purposes of accurate grading.

Most gastrointestinal NETs do not cause hormone-based syndromes, with the exception of duodenal NETs (gastrinoma, somatostatinoma) and jejunal/ileal NETs that metastasize to the liver, resulting in carcinoid syndrome due to serotonin secretion into the systemic circulation. (Note: Tumor functionality should be based on clinical symptoms, not on immunohistochemical expression of the hormone.)

Molecular knowledge of gastrointestinal NETs remains somewhat underdeveloped, as opposed to pancreatic NETs,[14] although some advances have been made in recent years. Key molecular findings are mentioned in the text.

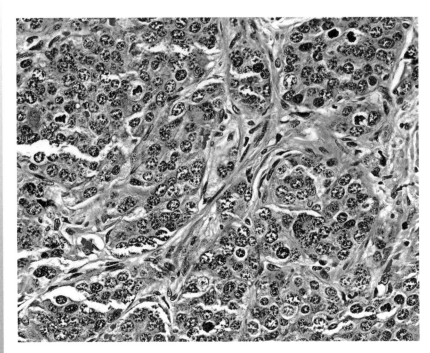

Fig. 7. If neuroendocrine tumor grading by mitotic rate and Ki67 index are discrepant, the Ki67 grading is usually higher. In rare instances, the mitotic rate is higher, such as with this grade 3 NET (hematoxylin-eosin, original magnification ×400). (*Courtesy of* Dr. Andrew Bellizzi.)

NEUROENDOCRINE CARCINOMAS: GENERAL CONSIDERATIONS

NECs in the gastrointestinal tract behave similarly regardless of site of origin; that is, they are aggressive lesions that metastasize rapidly and have a poor prognosis. Small cell NECs are more likely to arise in squamous-lined organs (the esophagus and anus), whereas large cell NECs are more frequent in the rest of the gastrointestinal tract. NECs sometimes can be observed in conjunction with an overlying mucosal adenoma (**Fig. 10**), indicating that the adenoma served as a precursor

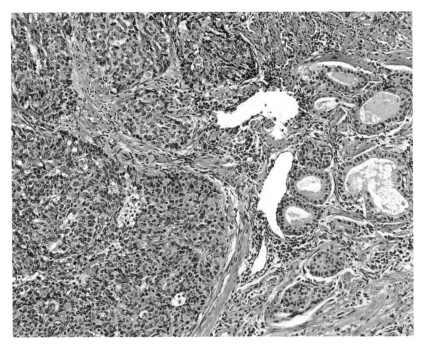

Fig. 8. Most MiNENs are mixed adenocarcinomas and NECs, as in this case (hematoxylin-eosin, original magnification ×200).

Fig. 9. Some MiNENs may consist of an adeno-carcinoma combined with a well-differentiated NET, which was confirmed in this case by a low Ki67 index (hematoxylin-eosin, original magnification ×100).

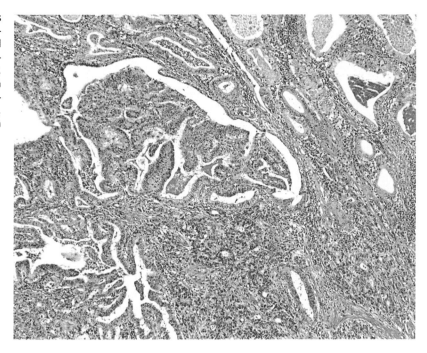

lesion. This distinguishes them from NETs, which do not have a defined precursor lesion, aside from gastric NETs arising in the setting of hypergastrinemia-induced neuroendocrine hyperplasia.

Small cell NECs (see **Fig. 2**) resemble the pulmonary lesions of the same name, consisting of intensely hyperchromatic, small, angulated, molding cells with minimal cytoplasm, arranged in sheets. Necrosis is often seen, either as dying single cells or as large sheets. Large cell NECs (see **Fig. 3**), in contrast, have more open nuclei with prominent nucleoli, as well as amphophilic cytoplasm. Regions of necrosis are also typically

Fig. 10. Gastrointestinal NECs are sometimes seen underneath mucosal adenomas, suggesting progression from a precursor lesion. In contrast, NETs generally do not have a well-defined precursor lesion (hematoxylin-eosin, original magnification ×100).

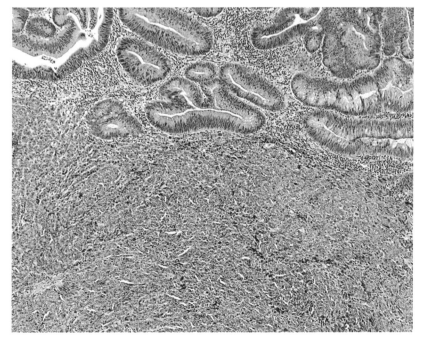

evident. Mitotic figures are plentiful in both types. Small cell and large cell NECs are sometimes difficult to tell apart in the gastrointestinal tract,[15] but the clinical approach and prognosis are generally similar for the two. Prominent immunohistochemical positivity for synaptophysin and chromogranin helps confirm the neuroendocrine nature of these lesions; focal and/or weak staining for these markers should be approached with caution. Ki67 immunohistochemistry usually shows a rate of greater than 80%, although this stain does not need to be performed for these intrinsically high-grade lesions.

From a molecular standpoint, NECs often show mutations in *TP53*, *RB1*, and *SMAD4*. *BRAF* mutations have also been described in colonic NECs,[16,17] and some *BRAF*-mutated NECs may also show microsatellite instability.[18] NECs are not generally considered hormone-secreting lesions and therefore do not cause particular hormone-based syndromes.

Platinum-based chemotherapy is the adjuvant therapy of choice for NECs, particularly small cell NECs.[19] Some patients also may benefit from tyrosine kinase inhibitors.[20] There exists preliminary evidence that PD1 inhibition might confer benefit in patients with gastrointestinal NEC,[21,22] but more study is needed.

Key Features
IN DIAGNOSING GASTROINTESTINAL NEUROENDOCRINE NEOPLASMS

- Well-differentiated neuroendocrine tumors show neoplastic cells arranged in nests and cords. The cells have "salt-and-pepper" chromatin and abundant amphophilic cytoplasm. Patchy endocrine atypia may be present. Mitotic figures are usually uncommon, and necrosis should be rare.

- Well-differentiated neuroendocrine tumors can be any grade, based on WHO criteria using mitotic rate and Ki67 index. They behave differently at different sites of origin.

- Poorly differentiated neuroendocrine carcinomas show malignant cells arranged in sheets, with a high mitotic rate and conspicuous necrosis. Small cell neuroendocrine carcinoma shows intensely hyperchromatic cells that mold to one another, with minimal cytoplasm. Large cell neuroendocrine carcinoma shows cells with prominent nucleoli and some amount of amphophilic cytoplasm. These carcinomas are high-grade by definition and therefore do not require formal grading. They are aggressive no matter the site of origin.

ESOPHAGEAL NEUROENDOCRINE TUMORS

Esophageal NETs are so rare[23] that NECs are quite likely the more common NEN at this location. Still, esophageal NETs share common histologic and immunohistochemical characteristics with NETs elsewhere in the gastrointestinal tract.

GASTRIC NEUROENDOCRINE TUMORS

Unlike for most other gastrointestinal organs, NETs of the stomach often occur in the setting of particular disease states. Because of this, a classification scheme exists for gastric NETs (**Table 2**).[24–26] These tumors do not typically cause symptoms secondary to hormone secretion.

Type 1 gastric NETs, by far the most common type, arise in the setting of atrophic (typically autoimmune) gastritis (**Figs. 11** and **12**). The loss of parietal cells in the fundic mucosa leads to decreased secretion of hydrochloric acid. The antral G cells sense this decreased acid production and increase production of gastrin, in a futile effort to stimulate the absent parietal cells to secrete more acid. This gastrin does, however, stimulate enterochromaffinlike (ECL) cells of the gastric body, goading them into hyperplasia. This hyperplasia can be visualized on a chromogranin stain (**Fig. 13**). Linear hyperplasia is defined as 2 groups of at least 5 ECL cells lined up within a gland, whereas micronodular hyperplasia is defined as at least 5 ECL cells forming a minute aggregate.[27] With continued proliferation, ECL cells form a grossly visible nodule, effectively constituting a NET. Because atrophic gastritis affects the entire gastric body, multiple NETs may arise. Fortunately, these are typically low-grade and indolent, meaning they can be managed with endoscopic surveillance and removal.

Type 2 gastric NETs also arise in the setting of hypergastrinemia, though secondary to a gastrin-secreting tumor (gastrinoma) causing Zollinger–Ellison syndrome. The gastrinoma itself may be sporadic or occurring as part of multiple endocrine neoplasia 1 syndrome. These behave somewhat similarly to type 1 tumors, in that they can be multifocal and are often indolent, although up to 30% can metastasize.

Type 3 gastric NETs occur in the absence of a known precursor and are more aggressive than types 1 or 2. They may be incidentally discovered (as in a sleeve gastrectomy specimen) or cause nonspecific gastrointestinal symptoms. Compared with type 1 and type 2 gastric NETs, these are more likely to be intermediate-grade or

Table 2
Classification system and clinicopathologic features for gastric neuroendocrine neoplasms

	Type 1	Type 2	Type 3
Relative frequency	Common	Rare	Uncommon
Patient age	Usually 50s or 60s	Average in 50s	Average in 50s
Patient sex	Usually female	No sex difference	More often male
Tumor location	Body/fundus only	Body/fundus only	Any site in stomach
Tumor focality	Often multifocal	Often multifocal	Unifocal
Tumor behavior	Typically benign	Up to 30% metastasize	Potentially aggressive
Underlying disease state	Atrophic gastritis	Zollinger–Ellison syndrome or multiple endocrine neoplasia type 1 syndrome	None

Adapted from Delle Fave G, O'Toole D, Sundin A, et al. ENETS Consensus Guidelines Update for Gastroduodenal Neuroendocrine Neoplasms. Neuroendocrinology. 2016;103(2):119-24; and Shi C, Adsay V, Bergsland EK, et al. Protocol for the Examination of Specimens From Patients With Neuroendocrine Tumors (Carcinoid Tumors) of the Stomach. https://documents.cap.org/protocols/cp-stomach-net-17protocol-4001.pdf. with permission.

high-grade, and more likely to metastasize and cause patient death.[24]

In older literature, some investigators categorized gastric NECs as type 4 tumors.[27] Although this terminology has not persisted, there also have been descriptions of a rare form of multifocal gastric NET arising in the setting of achlorhydria and parietal cell hyperplasia.[28,29] If additional studies confirm the unique nature of this lesion, it may become the new type 4 gastric NET.

DUODENAL AND AMPULLARY NEUROENDOCRINE TUMORS

NETs are uncommon in the proximal small bowel. They are generally incidental and indolent, although a sizable proportion of them are functionally gastrinomas and can cause reflux and duodenal ulceration secondary to increased gastric acid. They show classic NET histology, unlike 2 particular histologic subtypes that deserve further mention.

Fig. 11. This type 1 NET of the stomach arose in the setting of atrophic gastritis. Such tumors are small and can be multifocal, but they are generally indolent (hematoxylin-eosin, original magnification ×100).

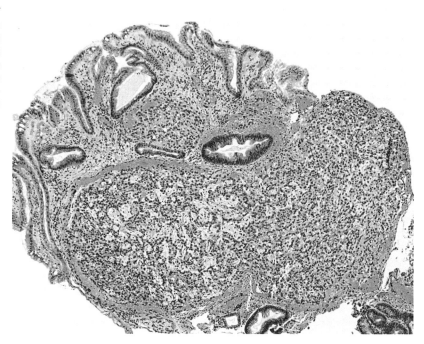

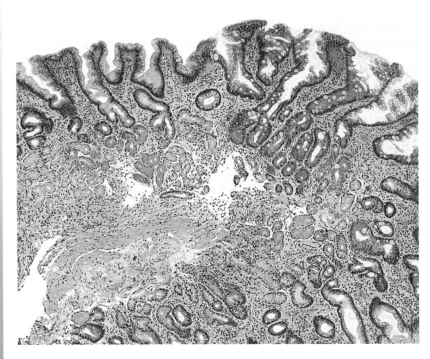

Fig. 12. Atrophic gastritis shows plasmacytic inflammation in the lamina propria, loss of oxyntic glands in the fundus/body, and epithelial metaplasia (usually intestinal, sometimes pancreatic). Patients are at increased risk of developing type 1 gastric NETs (hematoxylin-eosin, original magnification ×100).

Ampullary somatostatinoma is a unique type of NET that has an increased incidence among patients with neurofibromatosis type 1.[30,31] Its production of somatostatin can cause diarrhea, glucose intolerance, and cholelithiasis. This lesion is unique microscopically, as the neuroendocrine cells are arranged in small, angular gland forms rather than nests or cords. In addition, psammoma bodies are readily observed (**Fig. 14**). The cells still resemble classic NET cells, so close observation should prevent misdiagnosis as an adenocarcinoma. It should be noted that although

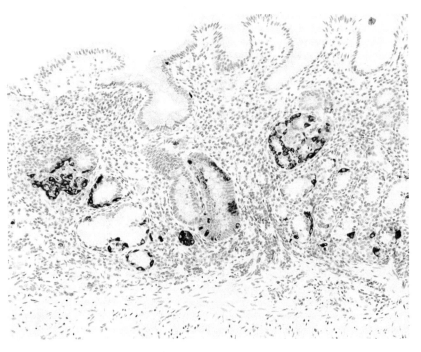

Fig. 13. An immunohistochemical stain for chromogranin can help demonstrate enterochromaffinlike cell hyperplasia in atrophic gastritis. Both linear and micronodular hyperplasia are present in this example (chromogranin immunohistochemical stain, original magnification ×200).

Fig. 14. This ampullary NET consists of cells arranged in a glandlike formation, with psammoma bodies present in the background. This appearance is typical of somatostatinoma at this location. Some patients with these tumors may have neurofibromatosis type 1 (hematoxylin-eosin, original magnification ×200).

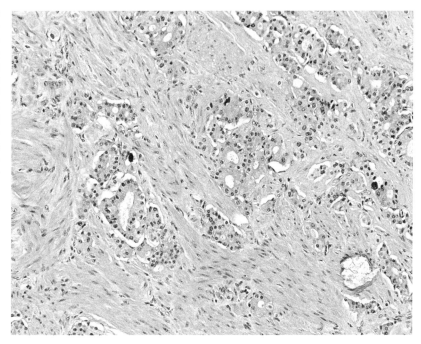

psammoma bodies are a helpful feature, they are not specific to somatostatinoma, even at this location (**Fig. 15**).[31]

Gangliocytic paraganglioma is an enigmatic NEN almost always arising in the ampulla.[31] They are triphasic neoplasms (**Fig. 16**), consisting of nested epithelioid cells (positive for neuroendocrine markers by immunohistochemistry), spindled Schwannlike cells (positive for S100 and neuroendocrine markers by immunohistochemistry), and scattered ganglion cells (positive for synaptophysin and neuron-specific enolase by immunohistochemistry).[32] The proportion and appearance of these 3 components can

Fig. 15. Gastrinomas are the most common functional NET of the duodenum. They have no particular histologic features distinguishing them from other NETs. This particular case happens to demonstrate psammoma bodies, showing that such a finding is not restricted to ampullary somatostatinomas (hematoxylin-eosin, original magnification ×200).

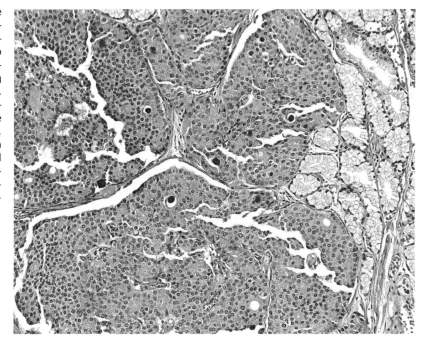

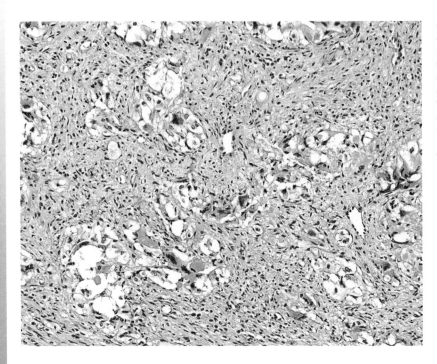

Fig. 16. This triphasic ampullary mass harbors nested endocrine cells, spindled Schwannlike cells, and scattered ganglion cells. This combination is diagnostic for gangliocytic paraganglioma (hematoxylineosin, original magnification ×200).

vary from lesion to lesion, so pathologists should consider gangliocytic paraganglioma whenever encountering an unusual, vaguely neural/neuroendocrine mass in the ampulla. These tumors sometimes metastasize to lymph nodes and have recently been shown to harbor *HIF2A* gain-of-function mutations.[33]

Gastrinomas may sometimes be discovered in lymph nodes (**Fig. 17**) located within the "gastrinoma triangle" formed by the confluence of the

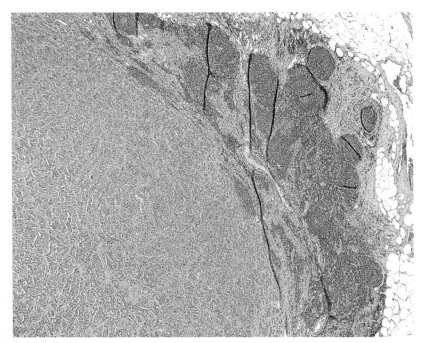

Fig. 17. This NET (clinically a gastrinoma) was identified in a periduodenal lymph node. No primary lesion was identified after thorough examination of the resected duodenum, suggesting the possibility of a primary nodal gastrinoma (hematoxylineosin, original magnification ×40).

cystic duct and common bile duct, the junction of the second and third portions of the duodenum, and the junction of the neck and body of the pancreas. Thorough histologic evaluation of the adjacent duodenum may or may not reveal a putative primary lesion in the form of a submillimeter NET.[34]

JEJUNAL AND ILEAL NEUROENDOCRINE TUMORS

The distal small bowel is the second most common site for gastrointestinal NETs, which are the most common malignancy there, with adenocarcinomas coming in second.[35] NETs at this site have a relatively high propensity for causing patient morbidity and mortality due to metastatic burden and/or induction of mesenteric fibrosis compromising blood flow (which may lead to ischemic bowel[36]). Despite their relatively straightforward histology, distal small bowel NETs have several unique properties.

NETs at this location are often multifocal (roughly one-third, based on various series) (**Fig. 18**), although there is no known "field effect" as with multiple gastric NETs in the setting of atrophic gastritis. Earlier literature indicated that multifocality conferred a worse prognosis,[37] but other reports have found no outcome-related distinction between them and unifocal NETs.[38] Performing Ki67 immunohistochemical staining on only the largest primary lesion seems sufficient for proper tumor grading in most cases.[38] Although grading criteria remain the same as for other NETs, researchers have proposed alternative cutoffs of 5 mitotic figures per 10 high-power fields[39] and a Ki67 index of 5%[40] as superiorly prognostic.

Distal small bowel NETs can often metastasize to lymph nodes (**Fig. 19**) and liver, even when small. In fact, if a NET is detected first in the liver, the small bowel remains a likely site of origin, even if the primary is never found. (Note: Primary hepatic NENs were formally recognized by the newest WHO book,[41] although this diagnosis remains difficult to establish.) These NETs also often metastasize to local soft tissue in the mesentery, forming tumor deposits, analogous to those in colorectal carcinoma. These deposits vary in size and may have an irregular or rounded contour, making them sometimes difficult to distinguish from exuberant lymph node metastases. Abundant perineural invasion is a helpful feature, as large nerves are uncommonly visualized in lymph nodes (**Fig. 20**).

We have shown that tumor deposits confer a worse prognosis than lymph node metastases,[42,43] and other investigators have linked them to increased risk of recurrent/progressive disease.[40] Given this evidence, the eighth edition of the AJCC Cancer Staging Manual created a new pN2 category for small bowel NETs, fulfilled by "[l]arge mesenteric masses (>2 cm) and/or extensive nodal deposits (12 or greater), especially

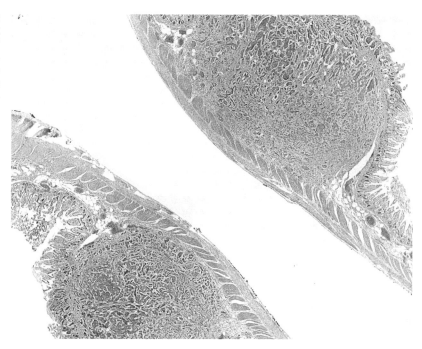

Fig. 18. These sections came from a patient with 8 discrete NETs of the jejunum and ileum. Multifocality is not uncommon in that location (hematoxylin-eosin, original magnification ×20).

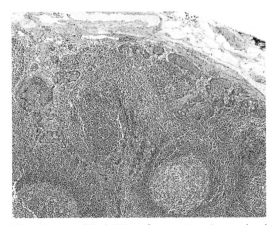

Fig. 19. Jejunal/ileal NETs often metastasize to local lymph nodes, even when the primary lesion is minuscule (hematoxylin-eosin, original magnification ×100).

those that encase the superior mesenteric vessels."[44] These criteria may change in the future, as we have recently demonstrated that tumor deposit size has no impact on patient outcome, whereas multiple tumor deposits portend a worse prognosis than single deposits,[45] and a clinical group has reported worse patient outcome at a cutoff of 4 positive lymph nodes.[46] The new AJCC M-category staging also distinguishes between hepatic and extrahepatic distant metastases.[44] This has been borne out by studies showing a worse outcome for patients with nonhepatic disease, such as peritoneal metastases.[47]

Molecular analysis has delineated 3 subtypes of distal small bowel NET. The analysis found significant differences in patient outcome among the 3 subtypes, although overall this categorization has yet to find widespread clinical use.[48]

Surgery is the primary treatment modality for primary NETs of the distal small bowel. Some centers perform resection of liver metastases, even when multiple, and some patients with unresectable liver disease may benefit from surgical debulking.[49] Resected metastatic deposits should be regraded, as they may show a higher proliferative rate than the primary lesion(s); as with those primaries, staining the largest metastatic focus should be sufficient.[50] Somatostatin analogues are a mainstay of adjuvant therapy,[51] and more recently, peptide receptor radionuclide therapy (such as ^{177}Lu-Dotatate) has emerged as a promising modality for control of metastatic disease.[52,53]

APPENDICEAL NEUROENDOCRINE TUMORS

The appendix is one of the most common sites of NETs in the gastrointestinal tract. They are quite often incidental lesions, discovered by dutifully submitting the tip of the appendix for microscopic examination. They most often show a nested configuration, although trabeculae may be encountered (**Fig. 21**). A minority of appendiceal NETs can metastasize to local colonic lymph nodes, meaning that completion right

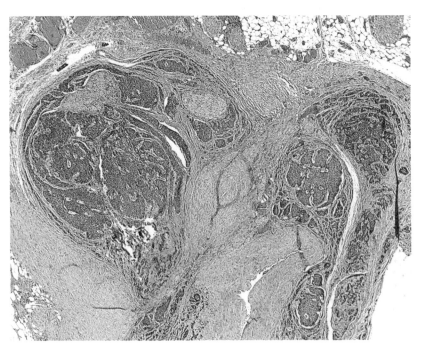

Fig. 20. Jejunal/ileal neuroendocrine tumors may also spawn metastases to mesenteric soft tissue. Such tumor deposits may mimic nodal disease but often display prominent perineural invasion. A large blood vessel is also visible in this example, possibly representing the route of spread (hematoxylin-eosin, original magnification ×40).

Fig. 21. NETs of the appendix are often, but not always, small and incidental. This subcentimeter example was discovered in an appendix removed for right lower quadrant pain (hematoxylin-eosin, original magnification ×10).

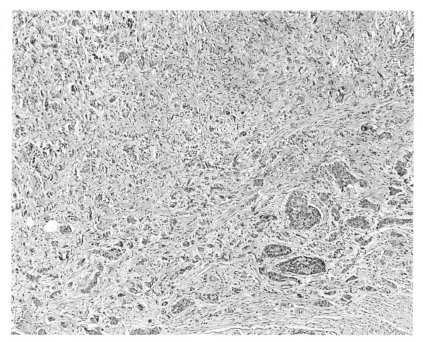

hemicolectomy is sometimes performed for these lesions. Further metastasis is quite rare. It remains somewhat unclear what factors significantly increase the risk of such nodal metastasis. Studies have reported various size cutoffs,[54–56] as well as lymphovascular invasion,[55] as predictive of metastatic spread. Tumor grade may not significantly impact behavior.[57] A recent case series reported that appendiceal NETs can rarely be multifocal, although this does not appear to indicate aggressive behavior.[58] Our own research has shown that size ≥1.0 cm is linked to increased metastatic risk (Noor et al, 2019, unpublished data). As small appendix NETs are extremely unlikely to metastasize, they may perhaps clinically be more akin to subcentimeter "neuroendocrine microadenomas" as described in the pancreas, which metastasize only extremely rarely.[59]

Two histologic variants of appendiceal NET have been described; both tend to be small and indolent.[60] L-cell NET (**Fig. 22**) consists entirely of linear trabeculae, and tubular NET (**Fig. 23**) consists of small tubular structures, which may mimic adenocarcinoma to the unwary. The designation "carcinoid" has been removed from these NETs in the new WHO classification, as with virtually all gastrointestinal NETs.

The entity formerly known as "goblet cell carcinoid" has been renamed goblet cell adenocarcinoma in the latest edition of the WHO classification.[61] It has been separated out from

appendiceal NENs and therefore will not be discussed further here. See the Norman J Carr's article, "Updates in Appendix Pathology: The Precarious Cutting Edge," elsewhere in this issue, for more information.

COLORECTAL NEUROENDOCRINE TUMORS

Rectal NETs are relatively common and are discussed first. Many rectal NETs form incidentally discovered polyps that can be removed endoscopically (**Fig. 24**), with no consequence to the patient except the need for routine surveillance afterward. Less commonly, however, rectal NETs can grow large (**Fig. 25**), necessitating surgical resection and additional workup to exclude distant metastasis. Rectal NETs can form a variety of architectural patterns, including the L-cell type also described in the appendix, but the cells are always distinctly neuroendocrine. In addition to neuroendocrine markers, rectal NETs can also stain positive by immunohistochemistry for prostatic acid phosphatase, a classic pitfall likely dulled with the advent of newer markers for prostate adenocarcinoma (such as NKX3.1).

Colonic neuroendocrine tumors are quite rare; as with the esophagus, NECs are likely more common at this site.[62] Most colonic NETs manifest similarly to rectal NETs, namely as candidates for polypectomy. A proportion of them specifically arise in patients with inflammatory bowel disease.

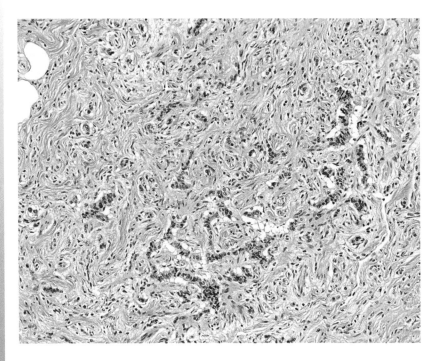

Fig. 22. A few histologic subtypes of appendiceal NETs have been described. This small L-cell NET is composed of linear cords and ribbons of neuroendocrine cells (hematoxylin-eosin, original magnification ×200).

It has been suggested that these actually represent an indolent form of neuroendocrine cell micronests, rather than "true NETs" (**Fig. 26**).[63] Regardless, prognosis overall appears excellent for colonic NETs as currently defined, unlike for colonic NECs. Older literature indicated a poor outcome for colonic NETs, possibly due to the inclusion of colonic NECs in those analyses.

Rarely, nests of bland neuroendocrine cells can be spotted in otherwise unremarkable tubulovillous adenomas (**Fig. 27**). This type of lesion was originally termed composite intestinal adenoma-

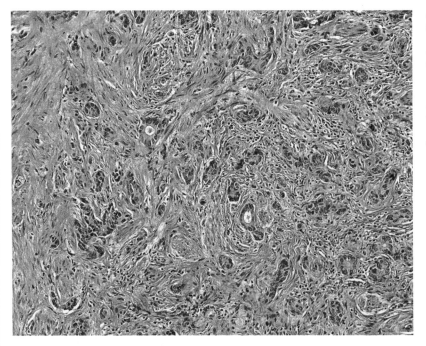

Fig. 23. A few histologic subtypes of appendiceal NETs have been described. This small tubular NET features neuroendocrine cells arranged in a glandular configuration, potentially mimicking an adenocarcinoma (hematoxylin-eosin, original magnification ×200).

Fig. 24. Rectal NETs commonly present as mucosal polyps easily retrieved during colonoscopy. They have a variety of potential histologic patterns, including the L-cell pattern also described in the appendix. This example shows the classic nested and trabecular architectural pattern (hematoxylin-eosin, original magnification ×40).

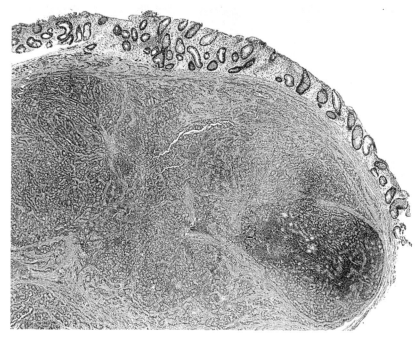

Fig. 25. If not caught early, rectal NETs can cause significant patient morbidity. This example penetrated into the muscularis propria and eventually metastasized to the liver (hematoxylin-eosin, original magnification ×20).

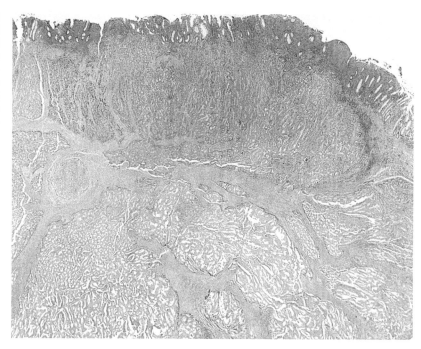

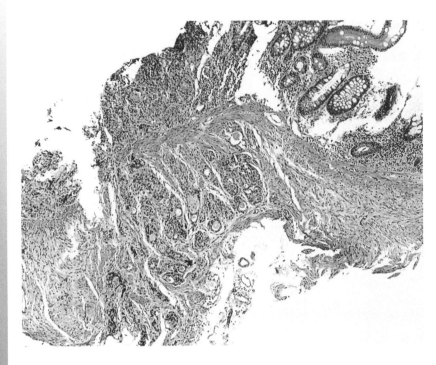

Fig. 26. Although colonic neuroendocrine tumors are rare, patients with inflammatory bowel disease sometimes develop "micronests" of neuroendocrine cells in the colon (hematoxylin-eosin, original magnification ×100).

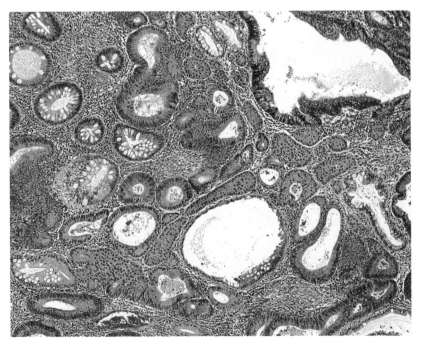

Fig. 27. Tiny nests of well-differentiated neuroendocrine cells rarely arise within tubular or tubulovillous adenomas in the colon. These are believed to represent composite lesions, rather than the adenoma serving as the precursor for a neuroendocrine neoplasm (hematoxylin-eosin, original magnification ×100).

microcarcinoid.[64] Although WHO does not specifically comment on this entity, the MiNEN-like term MANET (mixed adenoneuroendocrine tumor) has been proposed.[65,66] If adopted, this would eradicate the only remaining vestige of the word "carcinoid" applied to gastrointestinal NENs, with the exception of the clinical term "carcinoid syndrome."

DISCLOSURE

The authors have nothing to disclose.

REFERENCES

1. Amin MB, Edge SB, Greene FL, et al, editors. AJCC cancer staging manual. 8th edition. New York: Springer; 2017.

2. Klimstra DS, Klöppel G, La Rosa S, et al. Classification of neuroendocrine neoplasms of the digestive system. In: WHO Classification of Tumours Editorial Board, editor. WHO classification of tumours: digestive system tumours. 5th edition. Lyon (France): IARC; 2019. p. 16–9.

3. Rindi G, Klimstra DS, Abedi-Ardekani B, et al. A common classification framework for neuroendocrine neoplasms: an International Agency for Research on Cancer (IARC) and World Health Organization (WHO) expert consensus proposal. Mod Pathol 2018;31(12):1770–86.

4. Sorbye H, Welin S, Langer SW, et al. Predictive and prognostic factors for treatment and survival in 305 patients with advanced gastrointestinal neuroendocrine carcinoma (WHO G3): the NORDIC NEC study. Ann Oncol 2013;24(1):152–60.

5. Heetfeld M, Chougnet CN, Olsen IH, et al. Characteristics and treatment of patients with G3 gastroenteropancreatic neuroendocrine neoplasms. Endocr Relat Cancer 2015;22(4):657–64.

6. Tang LH, Untch BR, Reidy DL, et al. Well-differentiated neuroendocrine tumors with a morphologically apparent high-grade component: a pathway distinct from poorly differentiated neuroendocrine carcinomas. Clin Cancer Res 2016;22(4):1011–7.

7. Klöppel G, La Rosa S. Ki67 labeling index: assessment and prognostic role in gastroenteropancreatic neuroendocrine neoplasms. Virchows Arch 2018; 472(3):341–9.

8. Reid MD, Bagci P, Ohike N, et al. Calculation of the Ki67 index in pancreatic neuroendocrine tumors: a comparative analysis of four counting methodologies. Mod Pathol 2015;28:686–94.

9. Khan MS, Luong TV, Watkins J, et al. A comparison of Ki-67 and mitotic count as prognostic markers for metastatic pancreatic and midgut neuroendocrine neoplasms. Br J Cancer 2013;108(9): 1838–45.

10. Tang LH, Basturk O, Sue JJ, et al. A practical approach to the classification of WHO grade 3 (G3) well-differentiated neuroendocrine tumor (WD-NET) and poorly differentiated neuroendocrine carcinoma (PD-NEC) of the pancreas. Am J Surg Pathol 2016;40(9):1192–202.

11. La Rosa S, Sessa F, Uccella S. Mixed neuroendocrine-nonneuroendocrine neoplasms (MiNENs): unifying the concept of a heterogeneous group of neoplasms. Endocr Pathol 2016;27(4):284–311.

12. de Mestier L, Cros J, Neuzillet C, et al. Digestive system mixed neuroendocrine-non-neuroendocrine neoplasms. Neuroendocrinology 2017;105(4): 412–25.

13. Dasari A, Shen C, Halperin D, et al. Trends in the incidence, prevalence, and survival outcomes in patients with neuroendocrine tumors in the United States. JAMA Oncol 2017;3(10):1335–42.

14. Di Domenico A, Wiedmer T, Marinoni I, et al. Genetic and epigenetic drivers of neuroendocrine tumours (NET). Endocr Relat Cancer 2017;24(9):R315–34.

15. Shia J, Tang LH, Weiser MR, et al. Is nonsmall cell type high-grade neuroendocrine carcinoma of the tubular gastrointestinal tract a distinct disease entity? Am J Surg Pathol 2008;32(5):719–31.

16. Burkart J, Owen D, Shah MH, et al. Targeting BRAF mutations in high-grade neuroendocrine carcinoma of the colon. J Natl Compr Canc Netw 2018;16(9): 1035–40.

17. Idrees K, Padmanabhan C, Liu E, et al. Frequent BRAF mutations suggest a novel oncogenic driver in colonic neuroendocrine carcinoma. J Surg Oncol 2018;117(2):284–9.

18. Sahnane N, Furlan D, Monti M, et al. Microsatellite unstable gastrointestinal neuroendocrine carcinomas: a new clinicopathologic entity. Endocr Relat Cancer 2015;22(1):35–45.

19. Strosberg JR, Coppola D, Klimstra DS, et al. The NANETS consensus guidelines for the diagnosis and management of poorly differentiated (high-grade) extrapulmonary neuroendocrine carcinomas. Pancreas 2010;39(6):799–800.

20. Pellat A, Dreyer C, Couffignal C, et al. Clinical and biomarker evaluations of sunitinib in patients with grade 3 digestive neuroendocrine neoplasms. Neuroendocrinology 2018;107(1):24–31.

21. Weber MM, Fottner C. Immune checkpoint inhibitors in the treatment of patients with neuroendocrine neoplasia. Oncol Res Treat 2018;41(5):306–12.

22. Roberts JA, Gonzalez RS, Das S, et al. Expression of PD-1 and PD-L1 in poorly differentiated neuroendocrine carcinomas of the digestive system: a potential target for anti-PD-1/PD-L1 therapy. Hum Pathol 2017;70:49–54.

23. Hoang MP, Hobbs CM, Sobin LH, et al. Carcinoid tumor of the esophagus: a clinicopathologic study of four cases. Am J Surg Pathol 2002;26(4):517–22.

24. La Rosa S, Inzani F, Vanoli A, et al. Histologic characterization and improved prognostic evaluation of 209 gastric neuroendocrine neoplasms. Hum Pathol 2011;42(10):1373–84.

25. Delle Fave G, O'Toole D, Sundin A, et al. ENETS consensus guidelines update for gastroduodenal neuroendocrine neoplasms. Neuroendocrinology 2016;103(2):119–24.

26. Shi C, Adsay V, Bergsland EK, et al. Protocol for the examination of specimens from patients with neuroendocrine tumors (carcinoid tumors) of the stomach. Available at: https://documents.cap.org/protocols/cp-stomach-net-17protocol-4001.pdf. Accessed May 18, 2020.

27. Solcia E, Bordi C, Creutzfeldt W, et al. Histopathological classification of nonantral gastric endocrine growths in man. Digestion 1988;41(4):185–200.

28. Chai SM, Brown IS, Kumarasinghe MP. Gastroenteropancreatic neuroendocrine neoplasms: selected pathology review and molecular updates. Histopathology 2018;72(1):153–67.

29. Abraham SC, Carney JA, Ooi A, et al. Achlorhydria, parietal cell hyperplasia, and multiple gastric carcinoids: a new disorder. Am J Surg Pathol 2005; 29(7):969–75.

30. Garbrecht N, Anlauf M, Schmitt A, et al. Somatostatin-producing neuroendocrine tumors of the duodenum and pancreas: incidence, types, biological behavior, association with inherited syndromes, and functional activity. Endocr Relat Cancer 2008; 15(1):229–41.

31. Vanoli A, La Rosa S, Klersy C, et al. Four neuroendocrine tumor types and neuroendocrine carcinoma of the duodenum: analysis of 203 cases. Neuroendocrinology 2017;104(2):112–25.

32. Okubo Y, Wakayama M, Nemoto T, et al. Literature survey on epidemiology and pathology of gangliocytic paraganglioma. BMC Cancer 2011;11:187.

33. Zhuang Z, Yang C, Ryska A, et al. HIF2A gain-of-function mutations detected in duodenal gangliocytic paraganglioma. Endocr Relat Cancer 2016; 23(5):L13–6.

34. Anlauf M, Enosawa T, Henopp T, et al. Primary lymph node gastrinoma or occult duodenal microgastrinoma with lymph node metastases in a MEN1 patient: the need for a systematic search for the primary tumor. Am J Surg Pathol 2008;32(7):1101–5.

35. Bilimoria KY, Bentrem DJ, Wayne JD, et al. Small bowel cancer in the United States: changes in epidemiology, treatment, and survival over the last 20 years. Ann Surg 2009;249(1):63–71.

36. Landau M, Wisniewski S, Davison J. Jejunoileal neuroendocrine tumors complicated by intestinal ischemic necrosis are associated with worse overall survival. Arch Pathol Lab Med 2016;140(5):461–6.

37. Yantiss RK, Odze RD, Farraye FA, et al. Solitary versus multiple carcinoid tumors of the ileum: a clinical and pathologic review of 68 cases. Am J Surg Pathol 2003;27(6):811–7.

38. Numbere N, Huber AR, Shi C, et al. Should Ki67 immunohistochemistry be performed on all lesions in multifocal small intestinal neuroendocrine tumours? Histopathology 2019;74(3):424–9.

39. Strosberg JR, Weber JM, Feldman M, et al. Prognostic validity of the American Joint Committee on Cancer staging classification for midgut neuroendocrine tumors. J Clin Oncol 2013;31(4):420–5.

40. Sun Y, Lohse C, Smyrk T, et al. The influence of tumor stage on the prognostic value of Ki-67 index and mitotic count in small intestinal neuroendocrine tumors. Am J Surg Pathol 2018;42(2):247–55.

41. Klimstra DS. Hepatic neuroendocrine neoplasms. In: WHO Classification of Tumours Editorial Board, editor. WHO classification of tumours: digestive system tumours. 5th edition. Lyon (France): IARC; 2019. p. 263–4.

42. Gonzalez RS, Liu EH, Alvarez JR, et al. Should mesenteric tumor deposits be included in staging of well-differentiated small intestine neuroendocrine tumors? Mod Pathol 2014;27(9):1288–95.

43. Fata CR, Gonzalez RS, Liu E, et al. Mesenteric tumor deposits in midgut small intestinal neuroendocrine tumors are a stronger indicator than lymph node metastasis for liver metastasis and poor prognosis. Am J Surg Pathol 2017;41(1):128–33.

44. Woltering EA, Bergsland EK, Beyer DT, et al. Neuroendocrine tumors of the jejunum and ileum. In: Amin MB, Edge SB, Greene FL, et al, editors. AJCC cancer staging manual. 8th edition. New York: Springer; 2017. p. 375–87.

45. Gonzalez RS, Cates JMM, Shi C. Number, not size, of mesenteric tumor deposits affects prognosis of small intestinal well-differentiated neuroendocrine tumors. Mod Pathol 2018;31(10):1560–6.

46. Zaidi MY, Lopez-Aguiar AG, Dillhoff M, et al. Prognostic role of lymph node positivity and number of lymph nodes needed for accurately staging small-bowel neuroendocrine tumors. JAMA Surg 2019; 154(2):134–40.

47. Wright MF, Cates J, Gonzalez RS, et al. Impact of peritoneal metastasis on survival of patients with small intestinal neuroendocrine tumor. Am J Surg Pathol 2019;43(4):559–63.

48. Karpathakis A, Dibra H, Pipinikas C, et al. Prognostic impact of novel molecular subtypes of small intestinal neuroendocrine tumor. Clin Cancer Res 2016;22(1):250–8.

49. Ejaz A, Reames BN, Maithel S, et al. Cytoreductive debulking surgery among patients with neuroendocrine liver metastasis: a multi-institutional analysis. HPB (Oxford) 2018;20(3):277–84.

50. Shi C, Gonzalez RS, Zhao Z, et al. Liver metastases of small intestine neuroendocrine tumors: Ki-67 heterogeneity and World Health Organization grade

discordance with primary tumors. Am J Clin Pathol 2015;143(3):398–404.

51. Strosberg JR, Halfdanarson TR, Bellizzi AM, et al. The North American neuroendocrine tumor society consensus guidelines for surveillance and medical management of midgut neuroendocrine tumors. Pancreas 2017;46(6):707–14.

52. Dash A, Chakraborty S, Pillai MR, et al. Peptide receptor radionuclide therapy: an overview. Cancer Biother Radiopharm 2015;30(2):47–71.

53. Strosberg J, El-Haddad G, Wolin E, et al. Phase 3 trial of 177Lu-dotatate for midgut neuroendocrine tumors. N Engl J Med 2017;376(2):125–35.

54. Brighi N, La Rosa S, Rossi G, et al. Morphological factors related to nodal metastases in neuroendocrine tumors of the appendix: a multicentric retrospective study. Ann Surg 2020;271(3):527–33.

55. Groth SS, Virnig BA, Al-Refaie WB, et al. Appendiceal carcinoid tumors: predictors of lymph node metastasis and the impact of right hemicolectomy on survival. J Surg Oncol 2011;103(1):39–45.

56. Mehrvarz Sarshekeh A, Advani S, Halperin DM, et al. Regional lymph node involvement and outcomes in appendiceal neuroendocrine tumors: a SEER database analysis. Oncotarget 2017;8(59):99541–51.

57. Volante M, Daniele L, Asioli S, et al. Tumor staging but not grading is associated with adverse clinical outcome in neuroendocrine tumors of the appendix: a retrospective clinical pathologic analysis of 138 cases. Am J Surg Pathol 2013;37(4):606–12.

58. Mahajan H, Gosselink MP, Di Re AM, et al. A multifocal pattern of neuroendocrine neoplasms along the appendix: a series of six cases. Int J Surg Pathol 2019;27(6):613–8.

59. Kwon JH, Kim HJ, Park DH, et al. Incidentally detected pancreatic neuroendocrine microadenoma with lymph node metastasis. Virchows Arch 2018;473(5):649–53.

60. Carr NJ, Sobin LH. Neuroendocrine tumors of the appendix. Semin Diagn Pathol 2004;21(2):108–19.

61. Misdraji J, Carr NJ, Pai RK. Appendiceal goblet cell adenocarcinoma. In: WHO Classification of Tumours Editorial Board, editor. WHO classification of tumours: digestive system tumours. 5th edition. Lyon (France): IARC; 2019. p. 149–51.

62. Ramage JK, De Herder WW, Delle Fave G, et al. ENETS consensus guidelines update for colorectal neuroendocrine neoplasms. Neuroendocrinology 2016;103(2):139–43.

63. Wong M, Larson BK, Dhall D. Neuroendocrine proliferations in inflammatory bowel disease: differentiating neuroendocrine tumours from neuroendocrine cell micronests. Histopathology 2019;74(3):415–23.

64. Lin J, Goldblum JR, Bennett AE, et al. Composite intestinal adenoma-microcarcinoid. Am J Surg Pathol 2012;36(2):292–5.

65. La Rosa S, Marando A, Sessa F, et al. Mixed adeno-neuroendocrine carcinomas (MANECs) of the gastrointestinal tract: an update. Cancers (Basel) 2012;4(1):11–30.

66. La Rosa S, Uccella S, Molinari F, et al. Mixed adenoma well-differentiated neuroendocrine tumor (MANET) of the digestive system: an indolent subtype of mixed neuroendocrine-nonneuroendocrine neoplasm (MiNEN). Am J Surg Pathol 2018;42(11):1503–12.

Daily Dilemmas in Pediatric Gastrointestinal Pathology

Juan Putra, MD[a,b], Jeffrey D. Goldsmith, MD[c],*

KEYWORDS

- Mucosal eosinophilia • Eosinophilic esophagitis • Duodenal intraepithelial lymphocytosis
- Celiac disease • Terminal ileitis • Crohn disease • Ulcerative colitis • Backwash ileitis

Key points

- Eosinophilic esophagitis is the only primary eosinophilic gastrointestinal disorder with consensus diagnostic criteria; extraesophageal mucosal eosinophilia should be reported with a differential diagnosis as clinical correlation is mandatory.

- Duodenal intraepithelial lymphocytosis with preserved villous architecture may be identified in various conditions including symptomatic, asymptomatic, and treated celiac disease.

- In the setting of absent or negative serologic testing, duodenal intraepithelial lymphocytosis with preserved villous architecture should be reported descriptively with a differential diagnosis.

- Ileal inflammation in the setting of inflammatory bowel disease may be seen in ulcerative colitis and Crohn disease.

- "Backwash ileitis" usually shows mild acute inflammation without ulceration or chronic mucosal injury, whereas Crohn's disease-associated ileitis is often characterized by more pronounced chronic active ileitis.

ABSTRACT

The evaluation of gastrointestinal pathology in children often requires a different approach from that in adults. In this concise review, the authors outline 3 diagnostic challenges that are often encountered in daily practice; these include eosinophilic diseases, duodenal intraepithelial lymphocytosis with preserved villous architecture, and terminal ileal inflammation in the setting of idiopathic inflammatory bowel disease.

with adults. This review focuses on 3 areas of pediatric GI pathology that frequently cause diagnostic difficulty in the interpretation of endoscopically obtained mucosal biopsies, namely, mucosal eosinophilia, duodenal intraepithelial lymphocytosis with preserved villous architecture, and terminal ileal inflammation in inflammatory bowel disease. The article is intended as a practical resource for daily practice. Detailed information on each entity is beyond the scope of this review.

OVERVIEW

The interpretation of endoscopically obtained mucosal biopsies of the pediatric gastrointestinal (GI) tract often poses distinct challenges compared

EOSINOPHILIA OF THE GASTROINTESTINAL TRACT

OVERVIEW

Eosinophilia of the GI tract may represent a primary eosinophilic GI disorder or an inflammatory

[a] Department of Laboratory Medicine and Pathobiology, University of Toronto, 555 University Avenue, Toronto, Ontario M5G1X8, Canada; [b] Division of Pathology, Department of Paediatric Laboratory Medicine, The Hospital for Sick Children, 555 University Avenue, Toronto, Ontario M5G1X8, Canada; [c] Department of Pathology, Boston Children's Hospital, Harvard Medical School, 300 Longwood Avenue, Boston, MA 02115, USA
* Corresponding author.
E-mail address: Jeffrey.goldsmith@childrens.harvard.edu

Surgical Pathology 13 (2020) 399–411
https://doi.org/10.1016/j.path.2020.05.002
1875-9181/20/© 2020 Elsevier Inc. All rights reserved.

response to other conditions.[1] Eosinophilic esophagitis (EoE) is the most common eosinophilic GI disorder, with approximately one-fourth of the cases affecting patients aged 18 years or younger[2]; the diagnosis of EoE has relatively well-defined consensus criteria.[3] Other eosinophilic GI disorders, such as eosinophilic gastroenteritis, are uncommon and lack precise diagnostic criteria. One of the main reasons for this diagnostic difficulty is the lack of a consensus regarding normal numbers of mucosal eosinophils in areas outside of the esophagus. In addition, eosinophilic GI disorders can be difficult to distinguish from secondary causes of tissue eosinophilia on a histologic basis alone.

THE NUMBER AND DISTRIBUTION OF EOSINOPHILS IN THE NORMAL GASTROINTESTINAL TRACT

Eosinophils are normally absent in the esophagus; thus, any number of intraepithelial eosinophils at this anatomic site is generally considered abnormal. As a normal constituent of the stomach and intestines, eosinophils play an important role in the mucosal immunologic response. Several publications have attempted to describe the normal eosinophil counts in the GI tract of pediatric population[4–7]; however, these results have yet to be universally accepted, and consensus criteria have not been adopted. These data may not be accurate, because these studies evaluated pediatric patients who presented for endoscopic procedures owing to GI-associated symptoms.[4–7] Patients with functional abdominal pain, whose final clinical and pathologic diagnoses did not involve the GI system, are not necessarily representative of asymptomatic, healthy children.[8] Moreover, in a study by Chernetsova and colleagues,[6] the authors used hematoxylin-phloxine-saffron and Giemsa stains for eosinophil detection; therefore, they reported significantly higher eosinophilic counts compared with the other studies.

Owing to the lack of quantitative criteria for normal mucosal eosinophils in the stomach and intestines, the use of qualitative criteria is a reasonable approach. In the stomach, eosinophils are normally distributed singly in the lamina propria of the deep mucosa.[4–6] The small intestine tends to have lower numbers of lamina propria eosinophils compared with the colon[5,6]; rare single intraepithelial eosinophils are a part of the normal inflammatory milieu of the intestines. Eosinophil density in the large intestine decreases gradually from the cecum to the rectum.

In practice, increased eosinophils are detected by screening at low and medium magnifications. If sheets of eosinophils are detected in the lamina propria or intraepithelial clusters are seen, this finding should be considered pathologic. Extensive degranulation and associated epithelial injury can also be helpful findings in equivocal cases. Similarly, if greater numbers of eosinophils are seen in the left colon compared with the right colon, this finding is likely abnormal. As noted, we do not recommend counting eosinophils owing to the fact that normal numbers of mucosal eosinophils have not been definitively determined and likely vary by geographic location and season of the year.[8,9] Diagnosing eosinophilia in borderline cases is often subjective, and determining its clinical significance can be challenging. Increased eosinophils as part of a mixed inflammatory infiltrate should be interpreted carefully, because eosinophils are a normal component of an acute inflammatory response.[10]

EOSINOPHILIC ESOPHAGITIS

EoE is a T helper type 2–mediated esophageal disease often triggered by food allergens and characterized by clinical symptoms related to esophageal dysfunction, histologic evidence of eosinophil-predominant inflammation, and exclusion of other conditions to explain esophageal eosinophilia.[3] A recent meta-analysis of studies performed in developed countries reported an increasing prevalence and incidence of EoE in children.[11] The entity has a known male predominance with a male to female ratio of 3 to 1.[3,11]

The most common presenting symptoms in younger children and infants include reflux-like symptoms, vomiting, abdominal pain, food refusal, and failure to thrive. Meanwhile, older children and adults usually present with dysphagia, solid food impaction, and chest pain.[3,12,13] Endoscopic findings of EoE include esophageal rings, longitudinal furrows, exudates, edema, strictures, narrow-caliber esophagus, mucosal trachealization, and normal endoscopic appearances.[14] Obtaining multiple biopsy specimens from 2 or more esophageal levels is advised to increase the diagnostic yield and assists in the separation of EoE and reflux esophagitis.[15]

In addition to increased intraepithelial eosinophils, pathologic characteristics of EoE include basal cell hyperplasia, dilated intercellular spaces, papillary elongation, and lamina propria fibrosis. Intraepithelial eosinophils in EoE often demonstrate degranulation, superficial layering, microabscess formation, and superficial exudates (**Fig. 1**A,

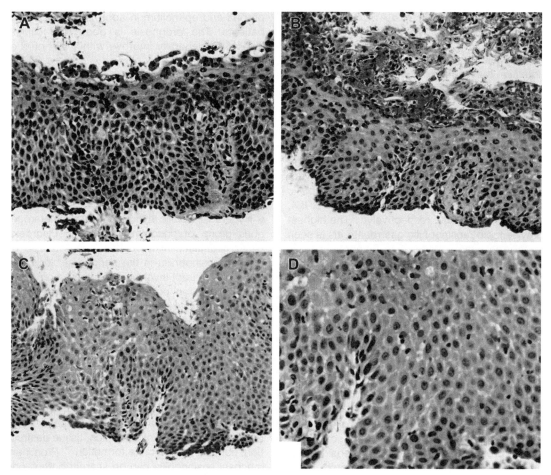

Fig. 1. EoE is characterized by (*A*) superficial layering of intraepithelial eosinophils, basal cell hyperplasia, and spongiosis (H&E, 10x). (*B*) Eosinophilic exudate is uncommonly identified in the superficial squamous epithelium and corresponds to the white exudates seen endoscopically (H&E, 10x). GERD (*C*) uncommonly shows greater than 15 eosinophils per high-power field, usually without superficial layering or microabscess formation (H&E, 10x). High-power view (*D*) shows scattered intraepithelial eosinophils with associated basal cell hyperplasia and dilated intercellular spaces (H&E 20x).

B).[16] The primary diagnosis of EoE requires histologic evidence of 15 or more intraepithelial eosinophils per high power field.[3] This number is somewhat arbitrary, and clinical judgment is required to interpret the significance of borderline counts.

Effective treatments to induce and maintain histologic and clinical remission include proton pump inhibitor therapy, topical steroids, and dietary modification; in addition to symptomatic response, peak eosinophil counts are often used to measure response to therapy.[17,18]

Gastroesophageal reflux disease (GERD) is the most common differential diagnosis of EoE and is common in the pediatric population. Distinguishing GERD from EoE can be challenging because both entities demonstrate overlapping clinical, endoscopic, and pathologic findings.

Rendering the diagnosis of EoE solely based on histologic criterion of 15 or more intraepithelial eosinophils per high power field would result in false-positive diagnoses. The inclusion of more proximal biopsies is helpful, because eosinophil counts of greater than 15 per high power field in the proximal and mid esophagus are less likely to be caused by reflux esophagitis alone.[1] In addition, eosinophilic microabscesses are rarely encountered in GERD (**Fig.** 1C, D).[19] EoE and GERD are thought to share a complex relationship; EoE may lead to secondary reflux owing to decreased esophageal compliance and dysmotility, whereas GERD can result in decreased epithelial barrier integrity, allowing antigen exposure and subsequent eosinophilia.[20]

PRIMARY EXTRAESOPHAGEAL EOSINOPHILIC GASTROINTESTINAL DISORDERS

Eosinophilic gastroenteritis is a poorly defined condition that is diagnosed on the basis of recurrent GI symptoms, histologic evidence of GI tract eosinophilia, and an absence of other known causes of eosinophilia.[21] Eosinophilic gastroenteritis can be subcategorized based on the site of involvement; however, the etiologic differences between gastric, small intestinal, and colonic involvement have not been observed. The reported prevalence rates of eosinophilic gastritis, gastroenteritis, and colitis are 6.3, 8.4, and 3.3 per 100,000, respectively.[22] The highest prevalence of eosinophilic gastroenteritis is seen in children aged younger than 5 years, whereas eosinophilic gastritis is more prevalent among older age groups. In contrast with EoE, these entities do not show a male predominance.[22] Coexisting atopic conditions and eosinophilia involving more than 1 site are common.[23] As noted elsewhere in this article, counting eosinophils outside of the esophagus is not recommended. The findings of eosinophil degranulation, abnormal distribution of eosinophils, sheets of lamina propria eosinophils, clusters of intraepithelial eosinophils, and involvement of submucosa without histologic evidence of chronic mucosal injury/crypt architecture distortion should prompt the consideration of eosinophilic GI disorders.[24] The pathologist should avoid rendering a definitive diagnosis of eosinophilic GI disorders based on histologic examination alone. The diagnosis should be made together with the clinician after other possible causes of eosinophilia have been excluded. Similar to EoE, the majority of patients treated with diet elimination and corticosteroids demonstrate clinical, endoscopic, and histologic improvements.[23] Additionally, anti-tumor necrosis factor biological drugs, such as infliximab and adalimumab, have been reported to be helpful in refractory cases.[25]

(Food protein-induced) allergic proctocolitis is a form of eosinophilic colitis that typically manifests as blood-streaked stool in well-appearing neonates.[26] The condition is transient and secondary to immune-mediated reactions to food allergen (cow's milk and soy proteins) via non–IgE-mediated pathways. Because of the characteristic clinical manifestations, colonoscopy and biopsy are only performed when there is diagnostic difficulty or a lack of response to dietary modification. Colonoscopy usually shows patchy areas of erythema, friable mucosa, erosions, and nodularity.[26] Patchy eosinophilia with normal crypt architecture is identified in the lamina propria and epithelium in approximately 89% of patients. The prognosis is good and clinical symptoms generally improve within 72 hours of food elimination.[27]

SECONDARY CAUSES OF GASTROINTESTINAL TRACT EOSINOPHILIA

Table 1 highlights pertinent clinical and/or pathologic findings that may be helpful to make the diagnosis of secondary causes of eosinophilia in the GI tract.[1,28–33] Selected entities are described. Fig. 2 demonstrates various conditions associated with GI tract eosinophilia.

Hypereosinophilic syndromes are a heterogenous group of uncommon systemic disorders, either neoplastic or idiopathic, characterized by marked eosinophilia in the peripheral blood and tissues.[29] GI tract involvement is more commonly seen in children compared with adults.[34] After exclusion of other causes of eosinophilia, the diagnostic evaluation includes morphologic review of the blood and bone marrow, standard cytogenetics, fluorescence in situ-hybridization, flow immunophenotyping, and T-cell clonality assessment to detect evidence for an acute or chronic hematolymphoid neoplasm.[35]

Eosinophils play proinflammatory and promotility roles in inflammatory bowel disease (IBD), resulting in diarrhea, inflammation, tissue destruction, fibrosis, and stricture formation.[36] Prominent mucosal eosinophilia can be seen in both Crohn disease (CD) and ulcerative colitis (UC), either in the active or quiescent phases.[1,37] Cases of IBD with mucosal eosinophilia seem to behave similarly to cases without significant eosinophilia.[38]

Infections may be characterized by mucosal eosinophilia.[39] GI tract eosinophilia in helminthic infections can be patchy or diffuse, and it may occur in any layer of the intestine, mimicking eosinophilic GI disorders.[1] Organisms are not always identified in the biopsy specimens, and the diagnosis is often made on the basis of stool and serologic tests. Fungal infections are usually associated with neutrophilic and granulomatous inflammation. However, a subset of fungal organisms such as *Basidiobolus ranarum* may elicit an eosinophilic response.[1] Moreover, mild eosinophilia has been observed in *Helicobacter pylori* gastritis, which usually resolves after therapy.[1]

DUODENAL LYMPHOCYTOSIS WITH PRESERVED VILLOUS ARCHITECTURE

Intraepithelial lymphocytes (IELs) are normally identified in the intestinal epithelium; they play active roles in the mucosal immune system.[40]

Table 1
Clinical and histologic clues for secondary causes of eosinophilia in the GI tract

Conditions	Clinical/Histologic Characteristics
GERD	Eosinophils are usually concentrated distally Eosinophilic abscesses and superficial layering are rare
Hypereosinophilic syndrome	Peripheral eosinophilia (>1.5 × 10^9/L) associated with evidence of eosinophil-induced tissue/organ damage No identified causes for eosinophilia May be neoplastic or idiopathic
Inflammatory bowel disease	Eosinophilia may be seen in active and quiescent phases Chronic mucosal injury (basal plasmacytosis and crypt loss) Active disease shows neutrophilic inflammation Non-necrotizing granulomas in Crohn disease
Infections	Mild eosinophilia in *Helicobacter pylori*-associated gastritis Fungal infection is usually associated with neutrophilic/granulomatous inflammation (*Basidiobolus ranarum* is associated with eosinophilia) Parasites associated with eosinophilia in the stomach and small intestine: *Ancylostoma caninum*, *Necator americanus*, *Enterobius vermicularis*, *Eustoma rotundatum*, *Ascaris lumbricoides*, *Trichuris trichiura*, *Anisakis sp.*, and *Schistosoma sp.* Parasites associated with eosinophilia in the large intestine: *T trichiura*, *Schistosoma sp.*, *Angiostrongylus costaricencis*, *Gnathostoma doloresi*, *Ascaris sp.*, and *E vermicularis*
Connective tissue disorders	Associated conditions include systemic lupus erythematous, rheumatoid arthritis, systemic sclerosis, dermatomyositis, polymyositis, and Sjogren syndrome
Autoimmune disorders and vasculitides	Eosinophilic granulomatosis with polyangiitis may show vasculitis and/or ischemic changes
Medication effects	Colonic involvement is more common compared with the upper GI tract Variable temporal association between the start of treatment and onset of symptoms
Graft-versus-host disease	History of hematopoietic stem cell transplantation Increased basal crypt epithelial apoptotic bodies Crypt loss and associated inflammation
Collagenous gastritis and colitis	Subepithelial collagen band (>10 μm) Eosinophilic infiltrate adjacent to collagen bands Increased intraepithelial lymphocytes may be present

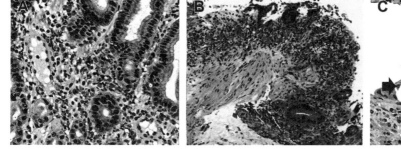
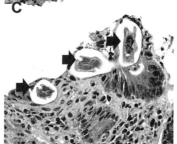

Fig. 2. Secondary causes of GI tract eosinophilia include tacrolimus-associated *gastric eosinophilia* (*A*) in a pediatric patient status-post liver transplant (H&E, 20x). Duodenal biopsy of a patient with Strongyloides stercoralis infection shows (*B*) marked eosinophilia in the lamina propria with associated reactive epithelial atypia (H&E, 10x), the organisms (*C, arrows*) are identified in an adjacent tissue fragment (H&E, 20x).

Duodenal intraepithelial lymphocytosis with associated villous blunting and reduction in the normal duodenal villous height-to-crypt depth ratio of 3 to 5:1 are the histologic hallmarks of gluten-sensitive enteropathy/celiac disease. However, the findings of duodenal lymphocytosis with preserved villous architecture are not specific and may be identified in various conditions (**Box 1**).[41]

In normal patients, duodenal IELs generally number less than 4 IELs per 20 epithelial cells, or 20 IELs/100 epithelial cells.[42] Hayat and colleagues[43] counted IELs in the distal duodenal biopsies of 20 healthy adult patients and found an average of 11 ± 6.8 IELs/100 enterocytes (range, 1.8–26 IELs/100 enterocytes). They proposed that 25 IELs per 100 enterocytes (mean ±2 standard deviations) would represent the upper limit of normal duodenal IEL as assessed on hematoxylin and eosin-stained tissue sections. Other studies showed similar results, and most pathologists consider 25 IELs per 100 enterocytes on hematoxylin and eosin to represent the upper limit of normal in duodenal biopsies.[44,45] Camarero and colleagues[46] used flow cytometry to identify the proportion of IELs in the duodenum of healthy children and adults and found that there was no significant difference between the 2 groups.

DIFFERENTIAL DIAGNOSIS OF DUODENAL INTRAEPITHELIAL LYMPHOCYTOSIS AND NORMAL VILLOUS ARCHITECTURE

Celiac Disease

Celiac disease is a common immune-mediated disorder triggered by sensitivity to gluten and related prolamins present in wheat, rye, and barley occurring in individuals with the HLA-DQ2 and/or HLA-DQ8 haplotypes.[47] The characteristic symptoms and signs of celiac disease include abdominal pain and distension with diarrhea or steatorrhea, whereas extraintestinal celiac disease symptoms, such as iron-deficiency anemia, growth failure, and dermatitis herpetiformis, are

---

Box 1
Differential diagnosis of duodenal intraepithelial lymphocytosis with preserved villous architecture

Celiac disease

   Infections
   - *H pylori* gastritis
   - Giardiasis
   - Tropical sprue
   - Cryptosporidium
   - Small intestinal bacterial overgrowth
   - Postviral enteritis

   Hypersensitivity to nongluten alimentary proteins
   - Cow's milk
   - Cereal
   - Soy product
   - Others (fish, rice, and chicken)

   Medications
   - Nonsteroidal anti-inflammatory drugs
   - Omelsartan (adults)

IBD

Autoimmune enteropathy (rare pattern)

Others
   - Lactase deficiency
   - Fructose malabsorption
   - IgA deficiency

more commonly identified in older children.[47,48] Treatment is lifelong exclusion of dietary gluten.

The IgA tissue transglutaminase antibody is the most reliable serologic test to identify patients who may have celiac disease (approximately 95% sensitivity and 95% specificity).[47,49] Histologic confirmation of celiac disease remains the diagnostic gold standard in the United States, because tissue transglutaminase has been shown to be somewhat less specific for celiac disease in the pediatric population.[50] The endoscopic findings, such as reduction or loss of duodenal folds, mosaic pattern, and scalloped folds, are moderately sensitive (approximately 60%) and highly specific (approximately 93%) for the diagnosis of celiac disease.[51,52] The recommended number of biopsies is at least 4 specimens from the postbulbar duodenum and 2 specimens from the duodenal bulb because celiac disease may show patchy histologic changes limited to the duodenal bulb.[53]

The histologic spectrum of celiac disease was described by Marsh[54] and subsequently modified by Oberhuber and colleagues,[55] who classified the small intestinal changes into type 1 (normal villous architecture with increased IELs), type 2 (crypt hyperplasia without villous flattening), and type 3 (crypt hyperplasia and villous flattening).[53]

In their pediatric cohort, Shmidt and colleagues[56] reported that increased IELs with normal villous architecture were identified in 4.3% of 1290 duodenal biopsies. The findings were more commonly seen in Caucasian females with an average age of 7.8 years who presented with abdominal pain. Approximately 9% of these cases represented new cases of celiac disease, whereas other patients were subsequently diagnosed with IBD, *H pylori* infection, medication-related injury, autoimmune disorders, lactase deficiency, fructose malabsorption, and selective IgA deficiency; a correlation between celiac disease diagnosis and higher IEL counts was not observed.[55] Moreover, the causes of duodenal lymphocytosis with preserved villous architecture remained unknown in a subset of children (39%) despite extensive clinical workup.[55]

Singh and colleagues[57] reported that children and adults (median age, 10.6 years; range, 3.0–62.5 years) with positive celiac serology and Marsh type 1 lesions demonstrate clinical and serologic improvements from gluten-free diet. Similarly, Kakar and colleagues[58] reported that 9.3% of patients, which included both adults and children, with duodenal IELs and normal mucosal architecture represent gluten sensitivity cases on the basis of favorable response to gluten-free diet. Therefore, celiac serology testing should be routinely performed in patients whose duodenal biopsies show normal villous architecture with increased IELs.

In patients with celiac disease with duodenal architectural abnormalities, the IEL counts are generally greater than 40 per 100 enterocytes.[53] IELs in celiac disease are often more prominent in the villous tips (**Fig. 3**).[59] Meanwhile, normal IELs are distributed along the lateral aspects of villi, with decreasing numbers of lymphocytes toward the villous tips. An IEL count should not be performed in the mucosa overlying lymphoid

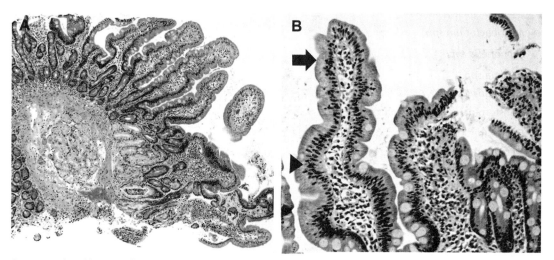

Fig. 3. Duodenal biopsy of a patient with confirmed an elevated tissue transglutaminase IgA level shows (*A*) small intestinal mucosa with preserved villous architecture (H&E, 4x) with (*B*) increased IELs (H&E, 10x); note that lymphocytosis is more prominent at villous tip (*arrow*) compared with the base (*arrowhead*), consistent with celiac disease, Marsh type 1.

aggregates, where IELs are normally increased. In addition, there is currently insufficient evidence to support the role of T-cell immunohistochemistry in increasing the detection of celiac disease.[60]

H pylori gastritis is identified in 6% to 14% of patients with duodenal biopsies showing increased IELs with normal villous architecture.[56,61,62] The duodenal lymphocytosis usually resolves after eradication of *Helicobacter* infection.[56,63]

The biopsies of most patients with giardiasis show preserved villous architecture.[64,65] Zylberberg and colleagues[64] reported that duodenal lymphocytosis with normal villous architecture was present in a small subset of patients (3%), whereas partial and total villous atrophy was present in 0.7% and 0.22% of patients, respectively. Other infections associated with duodenal lymphocytosis include tropical sprue, *Cryptosporidium*, small intestine bacterial overgrowth (associated with either hypochlorhydria or intestinal dysmotility), and postviral enteritis.[62,66]

Hypersensitivity to nonglutinous alimentary proteins such as cow's milk, cereal, soy products, fish, rice, and chicken is also associated with increased IELs, although variable degrees of villous atrophy and crypt hyperplasia are usually observed.[62,67]

Nonsteroidal anti-inflammatory drugs, including aspirin and cyclooxygenase-2 inhibitors, have been associated with duodenal lymphocytosis.[56] In adults, these histologic findings have also been seen in patients taking olmesartan (angiotensin II receptor antagonist), which is usually accompanied by villous blunting.[68]

Duodenal mucosa with normal villous architecture and increased IELs may also be identified in patients with IBD, particularly CD.[69,70] Coexisting focally enhanced gastritis is often seen in patients with IBD with duodenal lymphocytosis.

Box 2
Differential diagnosis of terminal ileitis

Idiopathic IBD
- UC
- CD

Infectious disease
- *Actinomyces israelii*
- *Anisakis simplex*
- *Clostridium difficile*
- *Cryptococcus neoformans*
- Cytomegalovirus
- *Histoplasma capsulatum*
- *Mycobacterium spp.*
- *Salmonella spp.*
- *Yersinia spp.*

Medications
- Nonsteroidal anti-inflammatory drugs
- Others (antihypertensives, potassium chloride, diuretics, etc)

Others
- Vasculitides (Behçet's disease, systemic lupus erythematosus, Henoch-Schonlein purpura, etc)
- Ischemia
- Spondyloarthropathies (ankylosing spondylitis, reactive arthritis, psoriasis, etc)
- Sarcoidosis
- Eosinophilic enteritis
- Radiation enteritis
- Malignancy

TERMINAL ILEITIS IN INFLAMMATORY BOWEL DISEASE

The classification of pediatric IBD at initial presentation is often challenging and differentiation of CD and UC is essential for surgical management and prognostication. Proper diagnosis and classification of patients with IBD requires integration of clinical, endoscopic, and histologic findings.[71] Histologically, non-necrotizing granulomas unassociated with crypt inflammation, seen in up to 60% of pediatric patients with CD at initial presentation,[72] remains one of the last remaining histologic findings on endoscopically obtained mucosal biopsies that distinguish CD from UC. In addition, the presence, extent, and nature of terminal ileal inflammation can also be used to help separate UC from CD in many cases. Of note, pathologists should also consider other causes of terminal ileitis before rendering the diagnosis of IBD (Box 2).

Backwash ileitis in UC is generally defined as mildly active, nonulcerative inflammation of the ileum in a contiguous pattern from the cecum in patients with extensive colonic disease (Fig. 4A, B).[73,74] The term has also been used to describe an abnormal appearance of the terminal ileum either endoscopically or radiologically. It is likely that backwash ileitis is a part of the disease spectrum in a subset of patients with UC; the hypothesis that ileal inflammation in UC is due to a backwash of toxic luminal contents through an incompetent ileocecal valve has never been proven.[74,75]

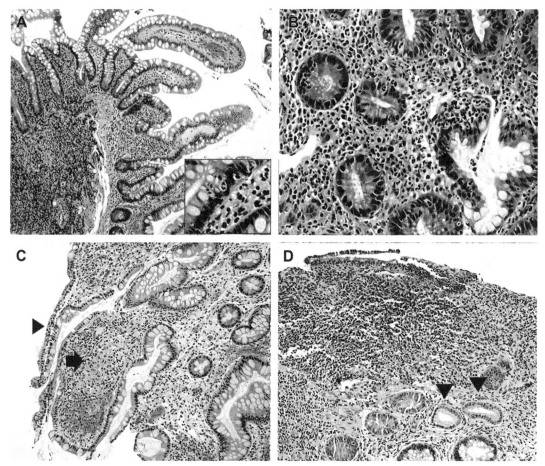

Fig. 4. *'Backwash ileitis' in a patient with UC.* Ileal biopsy shows (*A*) preserved villous architecture without evidence of chronic mucosal injury (H&E, 4x); inset shows focal active inflammation involving crypt epithelium (H&E, 20x). The adjacent cecum (*B*) demonstrates chronic active colitis with a focal neutrophilic crypt abscess (*arrow*) (H&E, 10x). *Terminal ileitis in a patient with CD* (*C*) is characterized by a non-necrotizing granuloma (*arrow*) with active (neutrophilic) inflammation involving the superficial epithelium (*arrowhead*) (H&E, 4x); (*D*) chronic mucosal injury is characterized by crypt dropout, increased mononuclear cell infiltrate in the lamina propria, and pyloric gland metaplasia (*arrowheads*) (H&E, 4x).

Table 2
Characteristics of terminal ileitis in Crohn disease and ulcerative colitis with backwash ileitis

	Crohn Disease-Associated Ileitis	Ulcerative Colitis with Backwash Ileitis
Frequency	~50% of pediatric Crohn disease	10%–20% of childhood ulcerative colitis
Endoscopy	Patchy ulceration of the ileocecal valve, skip lesions, deep linear ulcers, cobblestoned mucosa	Pancolitis with occasional macroscopic ileitis (mild erythema, mild granularity; no deep ulcers)
Histology	Non-necrotizing granulomas Pyloric gland metaplasia Mucosal erosion or ulceration.	Scattered areas of neutrophilic cryptitis; neutrophilic crypt abscesses uncommon Superficial erosions rarely seen Pyloric gland metaplasia and non-necrotizing granulomas unassociated with crypt inflammation absent.

In pediatric UC cases, backwash ileitis is generally identified in the setting of either endoscopic or microscopic pancolitis.[76,77] Children with ileitis and histologically unremarkable cecum and right colon are more likely to represent CD patients.[76] Unlike in adults, Najarian and colleagues[77] reported a lack of association between the presence of ileitis and the histologic severity of colitis.

Ileal disease in CD is endoscopically characterized by noncontiguous, aphthous or deep, linear ulcers showing chronic active inflammation, with or without non-necrotizing granulomas.[71] Ileocolonic involvement is seen in up to two-thirds of cases, with a small proportion of children showing isolated ileal disease.[78] Histologic features that are often identified in CD ileitis include evidence of non-necrotizing granulomas and chronic mucosal injury, including pyloric gland metaplasia, lamina propria expansion, active inflammation, and erosions or ulcers (**Fig. 4**C, D).[76] **Table 2** compares the clinicopathologic findings of CD-associated terminal ileitis and UC with backwash ileitis.

OTHER CAUSES OF TERMINAL ILEITIS

Terminal ileitis may also be seen in other conditions, such as infections, medication intake (nonsteroidal anti-inflammatory drugs), vasculitides, ischemia, spondyloarthropathies, sarcoidosis, eosinophilic enteritis, and others.[79–81] **Box 2** summarizes causes of terminal ileitis, and selected entities are discussed.

Yersinia enterocolitica and *Yersinia pseudotuberculosis* are usually acquired by ingestion of contaminated food and water.[79,81,82] The infection predominantly occurs in the distal ileum and cecum. Endoscopically, *Yersinia* infection shows mostly uniform aphthoid ulcers without evidence of fibrotic stenosis or fistula. It is also characterized by mucosal ulceration, neutrophil invasion, and a thickened ileal wall. The main clinical manifestations include small bowel obstruction and a tender abdominal mass. The diagnosis is made by stool culture and/or colonoscopy with biopsy.[79,83]

The typical features of NSAID-induced injury include endoscopic findings of discrete ulcerations with otherwise normal mucosa. Mucosal scarring and webs are occasionally noted. Microscopically, the active and chronic inflammation is usually superficial and multifocal. Pyloric gland metaplasia may be identified; however, fissuring ulcerations and granulomas are absent.[84]

SUMMARY

In this brief review, we have covered 3 of the most vexing problems in pediatric GI pathology, including eosinophilic diseases of the GI tract, duodenal intraepithelial lymphocytosis with normal villous architecture, and terminal ileal inflammation in IBD. It is our hope that this review assists the practicing pathologist during their daily signout.

DISCLOSURE

The authors have nothing to disclose.

REFERENCES

1. Conner JR, Kirsch R. The pathology and causes of tissue eosinophilia in the gastrointestinal tract. Histopathology 2017;71:177–99.

2. Dellon ES, Jensen ET, Martin CF, et al. Prevalence of eosinophilic esophagitis in the United States. Clin Gastroenterol Hepatol 2014;12:589–96.e1.

3. Dellon ES, Liacouras CA, Molina-Infante J, et al. Updated International Consensus Diagnostic Criteria for Eosinophilic Esophagitis: proceedings of the AGREE conference. Gastroenterology 2018;155:1022–33.

4. Silva J, Canao P, Espinheira MC, et al. Eosinophils in the gastrointestinal tract: how much is normal? Virchows Arch 2018;473:313–20.

5. DeBrosse CW, Case JW, Putnam PE, et al. Quantity and distribution of eosinophils in the gastrointestinal tract of children. Pediatr Dev Pathol 2006;9:210–8.

6. Chernetsova E, Sullivan K, de Nanassy J, et al. Histologic analysis of eosinophils and mast cells of the gastrointestinal tract in healthy Canadian children. Hum Pathol 2016;54:55–63.

7. Saad AG. Normal quantity and distribution of mast cells and eosinophils in the pediatric colon. Pediatr Dev Pathol 2011;14:294–300.

8. Kiss Z, Tel B, Farkas N, et al. Eosinophil counts in the small intestine and colon of children without apparent gastrointestinal disease: a meta-analysis. J Pediatr Gastroenterol Nutr 2018;67:6–12.

9. Pascal RR, Gramlich TL, Parker KM, et al. Geographic variations in eosinophil concentration in normal colonic mucosa. Mod Pathol 1997;10:363–5.

10. Yantiss RK. Eosinophils in the GI tract: how many is too many and what do they mean? Mod Pathol 2015;28:s7–21.

11. Navarro P, Arias A, Arias-Gonzalez L, et al. Systematic review with meta-analysis: the growing incidence and prevalence of eosinophilic oesophagitis in children and adults in population-based studies. Aliment Pharmacol Ther 2019;49:1116–25.

12. Chehade M, Jones SM, Pesek RD, et al. Phenotypical characterization of eosinophilic esophagitis in a large multicenter patient population from the consortium for food allergy research. J Allergy Clin Immunol Pract 2018;6:1534–44.

13. Lucendo AJ, Sanchez-Cazalilla M. Adult versus pediatric eosinophilic esophagitis: important differences and similarities for the clinician to understand. Expert Rev Clin Immunol 2012;8:733–45.

14. Liacouras CA, Spergel JM, Ruchelli E, et al. Eosinophilic esophagitis: a 10-year experience in 381 children. Clin Gastroenterol Hepatol 2005;3:1198–206.

15. Liacouras CA, Furuta GT, Hirano I, et al. Eosinophilic esophagitis: updated consensus recommendations for children and adults. J Allergy Clin Immunol 2011;128:3–20.e6.

16. Collins MH. Histopathology of eosinophilic esophagitis. Dig Dis 2014;32:68–73.

17. Munoz-Persy M, Lucendo AJ. Treatment of eosinophilic esophagitis in the pediatric patient: an evidence-based approach. Eur J Pediatr 2018;177:649–63.

18. Warners MJ, Ambarus CA, Bredenoord AJ, et al. Reliability of histologic assessment in patients with eosinophilic oesophagitis. Aliment Pharmacol Ther 2018;47:940–50.

19. Ngo P, Furuta GT, Antonioli DA, et al. Eosinophils in the esophagus— peptic or allergic eosinophilic esophagitis? Case series of three patients with esophageal eosinophilia. Am J Gastroenterol 2006;101:1666–70.

20. Spechler SJ, Genta RM, Souza RF. Thoughts on the complex relationship between gastroesophageal reflux disease and eosinophilic esophagitis. Am J Gastroenterol 2007;102:1301–6.

21. Furuta GT, Forbes D, Boey C, et al. Eosinophilic gastrointestinal diseases (EGIDs). J Pediatr Gastroenterol Nutr 2008;47:234–8.

22. Jensen ET, Martin CF, Kappelman MD, et al. Prevalence of eosinophilic gastritis, gastroenteritis, and colitis: estimates from a national administrative database. J Pediatr Gastroenterol Nutr 2016;62:36–42.

23. Pesek RD, Reed CC, Muir AB, et al. Increasing rates of diagnosis, substantial co-occurrence, and variable treatment patterns of eosinophilic gastritis, gastroenteritis, and colitis based on 10-year data across a multicenter consortium. Am J Gastroenterol 2019;114:984–94.

24. Collins MH. Histopathologic features of eosinophilic esophagitis and eosinophilic gastrointestinal diseases. Gastroenterol Clin North Am 2014;43:257–68.

25. Turner D, Wolters VM, Russell RK, et al. Anti-TNF, infliximab, and adalimumab can be effective in eosinophilic bowel disease. J Pediatr Gastroenterol Nutr 2013;56:492–7.

26. Feuille E, Nowak-Wegrzyn A. Food protein-induced enterocolitis syndrome, allergic proctocolitis, and enteropathy. Curr Allergy Asthma Rep 2015;15:50.

27. Lake AM. Food-induced eosinophilic proctocolitis. J Pediatr Gastroenterol Nutr 2000;30(Suppl):S58–60.

28. Collins MH, Capocelli K, Yang GY. Eosinophilic gastrointestinal disorders pathology. Front Med (Lausanne) 2018;4:261.

29. Klion AD, Bochner BS, Gleich GJ, et al. Approaches to the treatment of hypereosinophilic syndromes: a workshop summary report. J Allergy Clin Immunol 2006;117:1292–302.

30. Mouthon L, Dunogue B, Guillevin L. Diagnosis and classification of eosinophilic granulomatosis with polyangiitis (formerly named Churg-Strauss syndrome. J Autoimmun 2014;48-49:99–103.

31. Salomao M, Dorritie K, Mapara MY, et al. Histopathology of graft-vs-host disease of gastrointestinal

tract and liver: an update. Am J Clin Pathol 2015;5: 591–603.

32. Arnason T, Brown IS, Goldsmith JD, et al. Collagenous gastritis: a morphologic and immunohistochemical study of 40 patients. Mod Pathol 2015; 28:533–44.

33. Levy AM, Yamazaki K, Van Keulen VP, et al. Increased eosinophil infiltration and degranulation in colonic tissue from patients with collagenous colitis. Am J Gastroenterol 2001;96:1522–8.

34. Williams KW, Ware J, Abiodun A, et al. Hypereosinophilia in children and adults: a retrospective comparison. J Allergy Clin Immunol Pract 2016;4: 941–7.

35. Shomali W, Gotlib J. World Health Organization-defined eosinophilic disorders: 2019 update on diagnosis, risk stratification, and management. Am J Hematol 2019;94:1149–67.

36. Lampinen M, Ronnblom A, Amin K, et al. Eosinophil granulocytes are activated during the remission phase of ulcerative colitis. Gut 2005;54: 1714–20.

37. Bischoff SC, Wedemeyer J, Herrmann A, et al. Quantitative assessment of intestinal eosinophils and mast cells in inflammatory bowel disease. Histopathology 1996;28:1–13.

38. Boyle B, Collins MH, Wang Z, et al. Histologic correlates of clinical and endoscopic severity in children newly diagnosed with ulcerative colitis. Am J Surg Pathol 2017;41:1491–8.

39. Dixon H, Blanchard C, Deschoolmeester ML, et al. The role of Th2 cytokines, chemokines and parasite products in eosinophil recruitment to the gastrointestinal mucosa during helminth infection. Eur J Immunol 2006;36:1753–63.

40. Mahadeva S, Wyatt JI, Howdle PD. Is a raised intraepithelial lymphocyte count with normal duodenal villous architecture clinically relevant? J Clin Pathol 2012;55:424–8.

41. Rostami K, Aldulaimi D, Holmes G, et al. Microscopic enteritis: Bucharest consensus. World J Gastroenterol 2015;21:2593–604.

42. Hammer ST, Greenson JK. The clinical significance of duodenal lymphocytosis with normal villus architecture. Arch Pathol Lab Med 2013;137:1216–9.

43. Hayat M, Cairns A, Dixon MF, et al. Quantitation of intraepithelial lymphocytes in human duodenum: what is normal? J Clin Pathol 2002;55:393–4.

44. Veress B, Franzen L, Bodin L, et al. Duodenal intraepithelial lymphocyte-count revisited. Scand J Gastroenterol 2004;39:138–44.

45. Rostami K, Marsh MN, Johnson MW, et al. ROC-king onwards: intraepithelial lymphocyte counts, distribution & role in coeliac disease and mucosal interpretation. Gut 2017;66:2080–6.

46. Camarero C, Leon F, Sanchez L, et al. Age-related variation of intraepithelial lymphocytes subsets in normal human duodenal mucosa. Dig Dis Sci 2007;52:685–91.

47. Hill ID, Fasano A, Guandalini S, et al. NASPGHAN clinical report on the diagnosis and treatment of gluten-related disorders. J Pediatr Gastroenterol Nutr 2016;63:156–65.

48. Garampazzi A, Rapa A, Mura S, et al. Clinical pattern of celiac disease is still changing. J Pediatr Gastroenterol Nutr 2007;45:611–4.

49. Lewis NR, Scott BB. Meta-analysis: deamidated gliadin peptide antibody and tissue transglutaminase antibody compared as screening tests for coeliac disease. Aliment Pharmacol Ther 2010;31: 73–81.

50. Guandalini S, Newland C. Can we really skip the biopsy in diagnosing symptomatic children with celiac disease? J Pediatr Gastroenterol Nutr 2013;57:e24.

51. Pellegrino S, Furfaro F, Tortora A, et al. The importance of disease prevalence in assessing the diagnostic value of a test: endoscopic markers in celiac disease. Digestion 2013;87:254–61.

52. Sheiko MA, Feinstein JA, Capocelli KE, et al. The concordance of endoscopic and histologic findings of 1000 pediatric EGDs. Gastrointest Endosc 2015; 81:1385–91.

53. Robert ME, Crowe SE, Burgart L, et al. Statement on best practices in the use of pathology as a diagnostic tool for celiac disease: a guide for clinicians and pathologists. Am J Surg Pathol 2018;42:e44–58.

54. Marsh MN. Gluten, major histocompatibility complex, and the small intestine. A molecular and immunobiologic approach to the spectrum of gluten sensitivity ('celiac sprue'). Gastroenterology 1992; 102:330–54.

55. Oberhuber G, Granditsch G, Vogelsang H. The histopathology of coeliac disease: time for a standardized report scheme for pathologists. Eur J Gastroenterol Hepatol 1999;11:1185–94.

56. Shmidt E, Smyrk TC, Faubion WA, et al. Duodenal intraepithelial lymphocytosis with normal villous architecture in pediatric patients: Mayo Clinic experience, 2000-2009. J Pediatr Gastroenterol Nutr 2013;56:51–5.

57. Singh P, Lauwers GY, Garber JJ. Outcomes of seropositive patients with Marsh 1 histology in clinical practice. J Clin Gastroenterol 2016;50:619–23.

58. Kakar S, Nehra V, Murray JA, et al. Significance of intraepithelial lymphocytosis in small bowel biopsy samples with normal mucosal architecture. Am J Gastroenterol 2003;98:2027–33.

59. Mino M, Lauwers GY. Role of lymphocytic immunophenotyping in the diagnosis of gluten-sensitive enteropathy with preserved villous architecture. Am J Surg Pathol 2003;27:1237–42.

60. Serra S, Jani PA. An approach to duodenal biopsies. J Clin Pathol 2006;59:1133–50.

61. Aziz I, Evans KE, Hooper AD, et al. A prospective study into the etiology of lymphocytic duodenosis. Aliment Pharmacol Ther 2010;32:1392–7.

62. Lauwers GY, Fasano A, Brown IS. Duodenal lymphocytosis with no or minimal enteropathy: much ado about nothing? Mod Pathol 2015;28:S22–9.

63. Memeo L, Jhang J, Hibshoosh H, et al. Duodenal intraepithelial lymphocytosis with normal villous architecture: common occurrence in H. pylori gastritis. Mod Pathol 2005;18:1134–44.

64. Zylberberg HM, Green PHR, Turner KO, et al. Prevalence and predictors of giardia in the United States. Dig Dis Sci 2017;62:432–40.

65. Oberhuber G, Kastner N, Stolte M. Giardiasis: a histologic analysis of 567 cases. Scand J Gastroenterol 1997;32:48–51.

66. Brown IS, Bettington A, Bettington M, et al. tropical sprue: revisiting an underrecognized disease. Am J Surg Pathol 2014;38:666–72.

67. Brown I, Mino-Kenudson M, Deshpande V, et al. Intraepithelial lymphocytosis in architecturally preserved proximal small intestinal mucosa. Arch Pathol Lab Med 2006;130:1020–5.

68. Rubio-Tapia A, Herman ML, Ludvigsson JF, et al. Severe spruelike enteropathy associated with olmesartan. Mayo Clin Proc 2012;87:732–8.

69. Patterson ER, Shmidt E, Oxentenko AS, et al. Normal villous architecture with increased intraepithelial lymphocytes: a duodenal manifestation of Crohn disease. Am J Clin Pathol 2015;143:445–50.

70. Lahdeaho ML, Kaukinen K, Collin P, et al. Celiac disease: from inflammation to atrophy: a long-term follow-up study. J Pediatr Gastroenterol Nutr 2005;41:44–8.

71. Levine A, Griffiths A, Markowitz J, et al. Pediatric modification of the Montreal classification of inflammatory bowel disease: the Paris classification. Inflamm Bowel Dis 2011;17:1314–21.

72. De Matos V, Russo PA, Cohen AB, et al. Frequency and clinical correlation of granulomas in children with Crohn disease. J Pediatr Gastroenterol Nutr 2008;46:392–8.

73. Goldstein N, Dulai M. Contemporary morphologic definition of backwash ileitis in ulcerative colitis and features that distinguish it from Crohn disease. Am J Clin Pathol 2006;126:365–76.

74. Haskell H, Andrews CW Jr, Reddy SI, et al. Pathologic features and clinical significance of "backwash" ileitis in ulcerative colitis. Am J Surg Pathol 2005;29:1472–81.

75. Patil DT, Odze RD. Backwash is hogwash: the clinical significance of ileitis in ulcerative colitis. Am J Surg Pathol 2017;112:1211–4.

76. Sahn B, De Matos V, Stein R, et al. Histological features of ileitis differentiating pediatric Crohn disease from ulcerative colitis with backwash ileitis. Dig Liver Dis 2018;50:147–53.

77. Najarian RM, Ashworth LA, Wang HH, et al. Microscopic/"backwash" ileitis and its association with colonic disease in new onset pediatric ulcerative colitis. J Pediatr Gastroenterol Nutr 2019;68:835–40.

78. Meinzer U, Idestrom M, Alberti C, et al. Ileal involvement is age dependent in pediatric Crohn's disease. Inflamm Bowel Dis 2005;11:639–44.

79. Bojic D, Markovic S. Terminal ileitis is not always Crohn's disease. Ann Gastroenterol 2011;24:2715.

80. DiLauro S, Crum-Cianflone NF. Ileitis: when it is not Crohn's disease. Curr Gastroenterol Rep 2010;12:249–58.

81. Goulart RA, Barbalho SM, Gasparini RG, et al. Facing terminal ileitis: going beyond Crohn's disease. Gastroenterology Res 2016;9:1–9.

82. Naddei R, Martinelli M, Strisciuglio C, et al. Yersinia enterocolitica ileitis mimicking pediatric Crohn's disease. Inflamm Bowel Dis 2017;23:E15–6.

83. Matsumoto T, Iida M, Matsui T, et al. Endoscopic findings in Yersinia enterocolita enterocolitis. Gastrointest Endosc 1990;36:583–7.

84. Lengeling RW, Mitros FA, Brennan JA, et al. Ulcerative ileitis encountered at ileo-colonoscopy: likely role of nonsteroidal agents. Clin Gastroenterol Hepatol 2003;1:160–9.

Upper Gastrointestinal Manifestations of Inflammatory Bowel Disease

Noam Harpaz, MD, PhD[a,b,*],
Alexandros D. Polydorides, MD, PhD[a,b]

KEYWORDS

• Inflammatory bowel disease • Upper gastrointestinal tract • Ulcerative colitis • Crohn disease
• Esophagitis • Gastritis • Duodenitis

Key points

- Upper gastrointestinal tract (UGI) manifestations of ulcerative colitis (UC) and Crohn disease (CD) are common but often clinically silent or overshadowed by lower gastrointestinal tract manifestations. Nevertheless, they occasionally cause serious complications, especially in patients with CD.

- UGI manifestations of UC and CD are usually diagnosed in patients with established ileal, large intestinal, or perianal disease.

- Pathologic recognition of UGI inflammation in IBD is challenging because of gross and microscopic overlap with other disorders, some of which are much more prevalent, but is aided by access to patients' clinical and endoscopic data.

- Some histologic manifestations of UGI inflammation in CD, particularly lymphocytic esophagitis and focally enhanced gastritis, are more common and diagnostically significant in children than in adults.

- The impression that symptomatic UGI involvement by CD per se is an adverse prognostic risk factor is unsettled, but modern therapeutic agents have proven effective in improving clinical outcomes in these patients.

ABSTRACT

Although the features of lower gastrointestinal tract inflammation associated with ulcerative colitis and Crohn disease are generally familiar to pathologists, there is less awareness of and familiarity with the manifestations of inflammatory bowel disease in the esophagus, stomach, and duodenum. Nonetheless, their diagnosis has therapeutic and possibly prognostic implications, potentially foretelling severe complications. The recognition that ulcerative colitis can affect gastrointestinal organs proximal to the large intestine and terminal ileum represents a revision of concepts ingrained among generations of physicians. This article reviews the pathologic features and clinical significance of esophagitis, gastritis, and duodenitis associated with inflammatory bowel disease.

OVERVIEW

Esophagitis, gastritis, and duodenitis are increasingly recognized manifestations of inflammatory bowel disease (IBD) (**Table 1**). Although usually

---

[a] Department of Pathology, Molecular and Cell-Based Medicine, Icahn School of Medicine at Mount Sinai, Annenberg Building Room 15-38, 1468 Madison Avenue, New York, NY 10029, USA; [b] Department of Medicine, Icahn School of Medicine at Mount Sinai, Annenberg Building Room 15-38, 1468 Madison Avenue, New York, NY 10029, USA
* Corresponding author. Department of Pathology, Molecular and Cell-Based Medicine, Icahn School of Medicine at Mount Sinai, Annenberg Building Room 15-38, 1468 Madison Avenue, New York, NY 10029.
E-mail address: noam.harpaz@mountsinai.org

Surgical Pathology 13 (2020) 413–430
https://doi.org/10.1016/j.path.2020.05.003
1875-9181/20/© 2020 Elsevier Inc. All rights reserved.

Table 1
Definitions of terms

IBD	Collective term for a group of idiopathic chronic inflammatory disorders of the GI tract with a typically relapsing and remitting clinical course and cumulative inflammatory damage. The cause is unknown, but thought to reflect a complex interplay of genetic, environmental, immunological and microbial factors.
UC	One of two main subtypes of IBD, characterized by mucosal-based inflammation that involves the distal rectum along with a variable length of contiguous large intestine.
CD	The other major category of IBD, manifested by segmental transmural chronic inflammation anywhere in the GI tract (mouth to anus), often with nonnecrotizing epithelioid cell granulomas.
IBD, indeterminate type	A term reserved for colectomy specimens with overlapping macroscopic and histologic features of UC and CD.
IBD, unclassified	IBD that defies definitive classification as UC or CD, either clinically or in mucosal biopsy specimens.

Abbreviations: CD, Crohn disease; GI, gastrointestinal; UC, ulcerative colitis.

clinically silent, overshadowed by lower gastrointestinal (GI) disease or imitated by more prevalent disorders, they can cause serious complications in some patients, and their recognition may be valuable during patient management.

Incidence data reported in individual studies are widely divergent because of variations in study design, target populations, diagnostic modalities, and variations in the definition of disease involvement. Symptomatic upper GI (UGI) disease in patients with IBD affects up to 5% of patients with IBD, but screening studies have reported prevalence rates up to 50% to 60% in patients with ulcerative colitis (UC) and up to 70% to 90% in patients with Crohn disease (CD),[1,2] with a recent meta-analysis reporting UGI involvement in 34% of patients with CD.[3]

Because the endoscopic and microscopic manifestations of UGI inflammation in the setting of IBD are frequently nonspecific and overlap with those of other common disorders, such as reflux esophagitis and peptic gastroduodenitis, authors have cautioned against using them to diagnose or subclassify IBD without a coalescence of compelling clinical, radiologic, endoscopic, and histologic evidence.[4–9] However, it is acknowledged that UGI tract biopsies may shed diagnostic light on cases of unclassified IBD or indeterminate colitis.[7]

The classical concept of UC as a disease of the large intestine only, albeit ingrained among generations of physicians, has undergone revision in recent years. Although UGI inflammation remains more common in CD than in UC overall, the mere presence of UGI inflammation in a patient with

otherwise unclassified IBD is no longer regarded as pathognomonic of CD.

CD of the UGI tract has the potential to cause severe complications including obstruction, fistulae, and perforation.[4] Historically, it has been considered a risk factor for adverse clinical outcomes, indicating the need for aggressive management.[1,10,11] However, a recent large study of patients with CD found no differences in disease course and rate of complications between patients with UGI tract involvement and those without.[12]

CD of the UGI tract is usually diagnosed following or concurrently with a diagnosis of lower GI tract disease but has been reported in up to 28% of newly diagnosed pediatric patients who lack evidence of ileitis or colitis.[13] Biopsy sampling of the UGI tract is diagnostically revealing in patients with otherwise unclassified lower GI tract IBD, especially children,[14,15] and is more likely to yield diagnostic granulomatous inflammation than biopsies of the ileum or colon.[16] Professional societies therefore recommend that endoscopic evaluation of the UGI tract be included in the initial evaluation of children with suspected IBD, regardless of UGI symptoms.[17,18] Whether this recommendation should be applied to adults is unsettled. The higher rates of UGI involvement that have been reported in young patients with CD compared with adults may result from higher rates of routine clinical UGI evaluation, since the differences between them diminish when examined prospectively.

In this review, esophagitis, gastritis, and duodenitis in IBD are treated separately with respect to their respective clinical, endoscopic (**Box 1**), and

Box 1
Endoscopic manifestations of upper gastrointestinal involvement in IBD

Ulcerative colitis and Crohn disease

  Erythema

  Edema

  Obscured vascular pattern

  Granularity

  Friability

  Aphthous erosions, superficial ulcers

Crohn disease–specific

  Deep ulcers (usually linear or serpiginous)

  Fissures, fistula openings

  Thickened folds

  Nodularity, cobblestoning

  Bamboo-joint-like notching (proximal stomach, duodenum)

  Fixed stricture

  Mural rigidity, indistensibility

  Mucosal bridges

  Filiform pseudopolyps

  Gastroduodenal junction (ram's horn) deformity

Table 2
Microscopic manifestations of upper gastrointestinal involvement in IBD

	Crohn disease	Ulcerative colitis
Esophagus	Erosions, ulcers, granulation tissue Lamina propria fibrosis Granulomas Lymphocytic esophagitis (pediatric patients) Transmural lymphoid aggregates	Unspecified/nonspecific
Stomach	Erosions, ulcers, granulation tissue Granulomas Superficial chronic gastritis Lymphocytic gastritis Focally enhanced gastritis (pediatric patients) Follicular gastritis	Nonspecific chronic gastritis Lymphocytic gastritis Focally enhanced gastritis (pediatric patients) Erosions/ulcers (uncommon)
Duodenum	Erosions, ulcers, granulation tissue Granulomas Intraepithelial lymphocytosis with normal mucosal architecture Extensive foveolar metaplasia	Diffuse chronic duodenitis with mucosal expansion Architectural distortion Intraepithelial lymphocytosis with normal mucosal architecture

microscopic features (**Table 2**), including emphasis on features that might distinguish between UC and CD or those that differ between adult and pediatric patients. However, published data are often uninformative regarding the anatomic distribution of inflammatory lesions; their endoscopic and microscopic features; and whether confounding disorders, such as reflux disease and *Helicobacter pylori* infection, have been accounted for. Indeed, the revised Montreal classification of IBD combines all patients with UGI CD under the L4 designation without explicitly defining the anatomic distribution or whether the diagnosis was endoscopic, histologic, or both.[19,20]

ESOPHAGITIS IN CROHN DISEASE

Crohn esophagitis, the least frequent UGI manifestation of CD, was first recognized in 1950,[21] nearly two decades after Crohn and colleagues' landmark description of ileal CD.[22] Localizing symptoms are frequently absent but may include heartburn, retrosternal pain, odynophagia, or dysphagia. Chart reviews from a referral center spanning a 35-year interval reported esophageal CD in only 0.2% of patients with CD.[23,24] In contrast, screening studies have reported esophageal lesions in 7% to 17% of pediatric patients, 33% to 43% of adolescents, and 3% to 7% of adults.[25–27] At least 80% of patients have prior or concomitant diagnoses of ileal, large intestinal, or perianal CD at the time of diagnosis[23,24]; 20% have gastroduodenal manifestations; and 33% have oral lesions.[23] Isolated CD esophagitis is extremely uncommon and the subject of case reports.[28]

GROSS AND ENDOSCOPIC FEATURES

Endoscopically, most lesions are localized in the mid- or distal esophagus, but diffuse inflammation may occur.[23] Typical findings include edema, erythema, granularity, aphthae, and superficial ulcers; less common are fissures, deep longitudinal ulcers, cobblestoning, and stenosis. Rare patients present with mucosal bridges; filiform inflammatory polyps; or tracheobronchial, mesenteric, or gastric fistulas (**Fig. 1**). Transmural disease may culminate in mural thickening and fixed stenotic lesions that require dilatation or surgery. Surgical resections, albeit infrequently performed, produce rigid, thick-walled specimens, which precisely mirror the ulcerating, fissuring, transmural, granulomatous inflammatory features of their ileal and colonic counterparts.[28]

MICROSCOPIC FEATURES

Biopsies may disclose chronic inflammation despite the absence of endoscopic changes.[14,27] The inflammation is usually morphologically nonspecific, comprising lymphoplasmacytic infiltrates, fibrosis, erosions, ulcers, or granulation tissue. Nonnecrotizing granulomas, reported in 10% to 20% of adults and 10% to 40% of children,[15] are highly characteristic if foreign body granulomas and systemic granulomatous diseases are excluded.[15,23,25,29,30] Lymphocytic esophagitis (LE) occurs in 12% to 28% of pediatric patients with CD but has a low positive predictive value in adults (see below).[29–34]

DIFFERENTIAL DIAGNOSIS

A diagnosis of Crohn esophagitis usually depends on consolidation of relevant clinical, endoscopic, and histologic findings because no histologic features are pathognomonic in isolation. Esophageal ulceration and/or stricturing are potential complications of diverse disorders. Common ones include reflux disease, medication-related injury, candidiasis, and viral esophagitis; less common are radiation esophagitis, vasculitis, desquamative and bullous dermatoses,[35] Behçet's disease,[36] graft-versus-host disease, and lichen planus (**Table 3**).[37] Certain endoscopic features are characteristic of CD, including serpiginous ulcers, cobblestoning, fistulous openings, or bamboo-joint lesions (see below) in the gastric cardia, despite nonspecific histologic findings. The presence of nonnecrotizing granulomas in otherwise nonspecific inflammatory surroundings, albeit highly characteristic of CD, could be accounted for by a foreign body reaction or a systemic disease, such as sarcoidosis, chronic granulomatous disease, or infection (**Table 4**).

Reflux esophagitis may occur alone or in conjunction with other disorders, the diagnosis sometimes depending on empirical antisecretory therapy or pH monitoring. Likewise, candidiasis may accompany other conditions and should be routinely excluded by staining biopsies with periodic acid–Schiff or silver stains. Other causes of esophagitis are frequently recognized clinically or in some cases histologically. Pill esophagitis may present with discrete ulcers on opposing esophageal surfaces (kissing ulcers) and microscopic particulate residue. Dermatoses may involve the skin or oral cavity and exhibit specific histologic changes and immunofluorescence staining patterns.[38] For example, esophageal lichen planus is usually accompanied by oral or cutaneous involvement and presents a characteristic microscopic constellation of intraepithelial and lamina propria lymphocytosis, basal cell degeneration, squamous apoptotic bodies, and nodular IgM deposition at the dermal-epidermal junction.[37,39,40]

LE is characterized by peripapillary lymphocytosis, spongiosis, and few if any granulocytes. The cutoff values for lymphocytosis are unsettled, ranging from 20 to 50 lymphocytes per high-power field or even higher among different studies, leading some authors to advocate a pattern-based diagnosis.[29,31,33,34,41] Besides pediatric CD, LE occurs in reflux disease, candidiasis, lichen planus, lichenoid esophagitis (defined by lichen-planus-like inflammation without confirmatory findings),[42] and autoimmune disorders[41,43] and sporadically in patients without predisposing conditions. In contrast with cytotoxic CD8+ T-lymphocyte predominance reported in CD, reflux disease, and other inflammatory disorders, patients with esophageal CD4+ T lymphocytosis may have primary esophageal dysmotility.[44,45]

ESOPHAGITIS IN ULCERATIVE COLITIS

Esophagitis has been described in pediatric patients with UC, but the endoscopic and histologic features have either been unspecified or nonspecific, and the contributions of unrelated conditions, such as reflux disease, medications, or *Candida*, are difficult to gauge.[15,27,46] Granulomas have not been reported. LE occurs in 7% of pediatric patients with UC but is not significantly more common than in non-IBD control subjects.[29]

GASTRITIS IN CROHN DISEASE

Gastritis is the most common manifestation of UGI CD, occurring in roughly 50% of patients with CD

Fig. 1. Pathologic features of esophagitis in Crohn disease. (*A*) Esophageal resection specimen featuring tracheobronchial fistula and filiform inflammatory pseudopolyps. *White arrow*, proximal stomach; *black arrow*, mid and distal esophagus; *asterisk*, tracheobronchial fistula. (*B*) Whole mount section of esophagus involved by Crohn disease featuring mural thickening and transmural lymphoid aggregates. (*C*) Esophageal mucosa and submucosa with superficial ulcer, massively thickened muscularis mucosae, lymphoid aggregates, and granulomas.

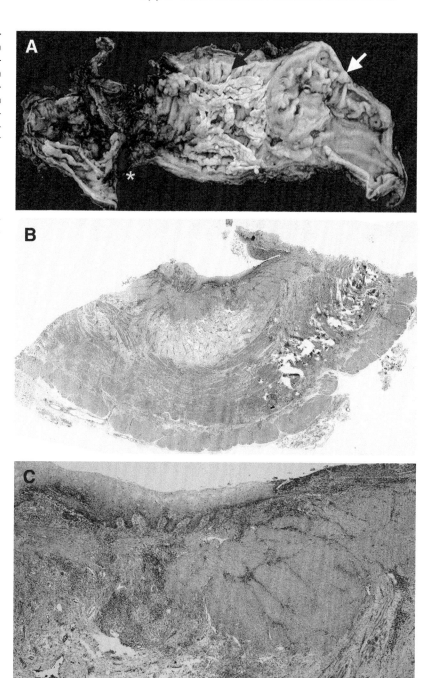

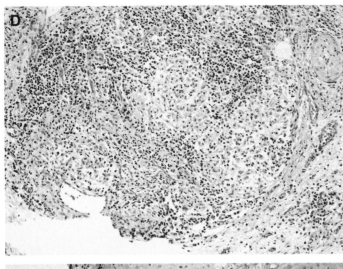

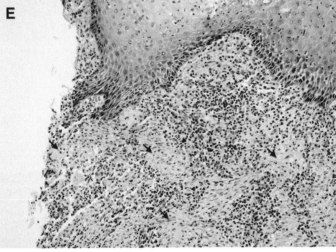

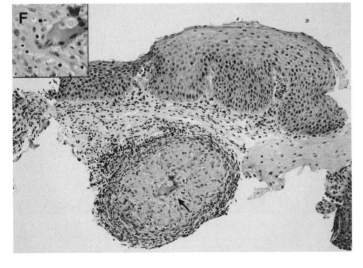

Fig. 1. (*continued*). (*D*) Lymphoid aggregates and granulomas at higher magnification. (*E*) Subepithelial epithelioid cell granulomas (*arrows*). (*F*) Esophageal biopsy with foreign body granuloma (*arrow*), seen at higher magnification in inset. (*G*) Lymphocytic esophagitis featuring dense peripapillary lymphocytosis and spongiosis. Granulocytes are absent. Hematoxylin-eosin, original magnification ×10 (*A*), ×40 (*B*), ×200 (*C–E*), ×100 (*F*), ×400 (*F, inset*), x400 (*G*).

Fig. 1.

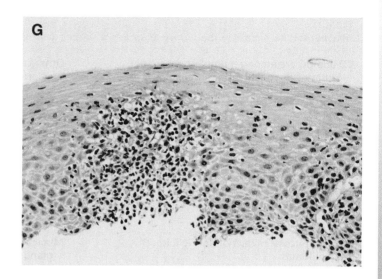

Table 3
Differential diagnosis of upper gastrointestinal manifestations of IBD

Esophagus	Gastroesophageal reflux disease Medication injury Infection (*Candida*, CMV, HSV) Vasculitis Behçet disease Lichen planus Other dermatoses (eg, epidermolysis bullosa, pemphigus, bullous pemphigoid) Radiation esophagitis Graft-versus-host disease
Stomach	*Helicobacter* gastritis Lymphocytic gastritis (eg, celiac disease, medications, HIV) Erosive gastritis, chemical gastropathy (eg, medications such as NSAIDs, alcohol, physiologic stress) Granulomatous gastritis (eg, foreign body reaction, sarcoidosis, syphilis, TB, histoplasmosis, chronic granulomatous disease) Radiation Collagenous gastritis Autoimmune atrophic gastritis Nonspecific chronic gastritis Eosinophilic gastritis
Duodenum	Peptic duodenitis Medication injury (eg, NSAIDs) Celiac disease Sarcoidosis Henoch-Schönlein purpura Behçet disease Infection (eg, CMV, TB)

Abbreviations: CMV, cytomegalovirus; HIV, human immunodeficiency virus; HSV, herpes simplex virus; NSAID, nonsteroidal anti-inflammatory drug; TB, tuberculosis.

Table 4
Histopathologic pitfalls in the biopsy diagnosis of upper gastrointestinal IBD

CD and UC are among multiple nonceliac causes of duodenal intraepithelial lymphocytosis with normal mucosal architecture	Other causes include gastric *Helicobacter pylori* infection, medications, viral enteritis, postinfectious states, connective tissue disorders, and common variable immunodeficiency.
Chronic active gastritis may be caused by *H pylori* infection despite the absence of organisms	Organisms may be absent because of low burden; persistence of inflammation after successful eradication; or proximal "migration" from the gastric antrum associated with antisecretory therapy, partial treatment, long-standing infection, or antral atrophy with intestinal metaplasia.
Beware mucosal mimics of epithelioid cell granulomas	Mimics may include tangentially sectioned glands, smooth muscle bundles of muscularis mucosae or blood vessels, foreign body reaction to ruptured glands, nerve bundles, ganglia, or germinal centers. Serial sections are helpful in resolving uncertainties.
Histologic clues to granulomatous mimics of CD	Mycobacterial granulomas tend to be >0.4 mm and confluent, with central necrosis. Acid-fast, silver, and spirochete stains should be done routinely. Inspect for suture fragments, antacids, iron, vegetable matter, and so forth, and use a polarized light source to identify foreign body granulomas. Yellow-pigmented granulomas occur in chronic granulomatous disease. Sarcoidosis does not generally elicit chronic inflammation, but exceptions occur.

(reported range, 24%–83%) and may be more common in pediatric patients than in adults.[10–12,14,47–58] The gastric antrum is most often involved, frequently together and contiguously with the duodenum. As a result, much of the data in the literature are based on patients with combined gastroduodenitis. Symptoms often mimic peptic ulcer disease, including nonradiating postprandial epigastric pain that is relieved by food, and manifestations of delayed gastric emptying or outlet obstruction including nausea, vomiting, melena, and weight loss.[7,11,59,60] Primary gastric fistulas are extremely rare compared with secondary fistulas originating in the ileum or colon.[61]

GROSS AND ENDOSCOPIC FEATURES

Macroscopic changes are seen in up to 30% to 40% of patients at initial diagnosis and up to 75% overall. They include erythema, obscured vasculature, friability, aphthous erosions, linear or serpiginous ulcers (which contrast with the more circular ulcers of peptic disease), thickened folds, nodules, strictures, and fistulas.[4,53] Bamboo-joint-like notching in the proximal stomach is considered characteristic of CD, occurring in 54% to 65% of patients with CD but only 5% of those with UC.[62] It is characterized by longitudinal, edematous gastric folds punctuated by linear perpendicular notches that correspond to erosions, furrows, fissures, and grooves **(Fig. 2)**.[1,4,62–67] Diffuse transmural gastric inflammation may result in mural rigidity, raising concern for diffuse malignancies, syphilis, and infiltrative diseases.[4,47]

MICROSCOPIC FEATURES

CD presents several distinct patterns of gastritis, alone or in combination; however, none are specific per se **(Fig. 3)**.[3,13,15,16,27,47,56,68–77] Chronic superficial gastritis (CSG) features a dense band of lymphocytes and plasma cells that occupy the

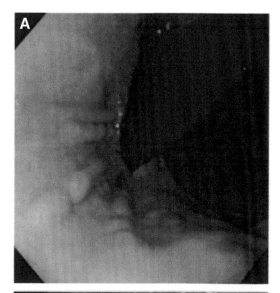

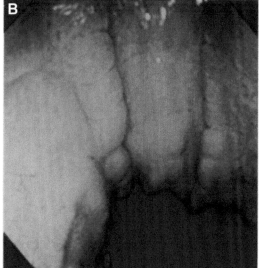

Fig. 2. (*A, B*) Endoscopic view of bamboo-joint-like notching in stomach involved by CD. (*From* Yokota K, Saito Y, Einami K, et al. A bamboo-joint-like appearance of the gastric body and cardia: possible association with Crohn's disease. *Gastrointest Endosc.* 1997;46(3):268-272; with permission.)

superficial lamina propria with or without neutrophil infiltration of the glands. Focally enhanced gastritis (FEG) is characterized by isolated small collections of lymphocytes, plasma cells, macrophages, and occasional neutrophils surrounding one or two foveolae or glands, typically in the antrum, within a background of normal or minimally inflamed mucosa. Acute erosive gastritis refers to disruption of the surface epithelium and replacement by necrosis and fibrinoinflammatory exudates. Granulomatous gastritis (GG) features

nonnecrotizing epithelioid cell granulomas within the lamina propria with or without accompanying lymphoplasmacytosis. Gastric granulomas are typically loose and range from collections up to 400 μm in diameter that may distort adjacent glands to inconspicuous clusters of five or fewer histiocytes (microgranulomas). Lymphocytic gastritis is characterized by foveolar surface intraepithelial lymphocytosis (IEL), defined as 25 or more intraepithelial lymphocytes per 100 epithelial cells and comprising mainly CD3[+] T lymphocytes. Both the antrum and body are typically involved, and accompanying lamina propria inflammation is variable. Finally, chronic gastritis not otherwise specified (CG-NOS) features scattered clusters of lamina propria plasma cells, often accompanied by lymphocytes or eosinophils. The term "follicular gastritis" is applied when lymphoid follicles are present in the deep mucosa.

DIFFERENTIAL DIAGNOSIS

The main differential diagnosis for CSG is *H pylori* infection, particularly if there is neutrophil infiltration of the isthmic region of the glands.[75,76] Immunoperoxidase-based or other conventional stains are essential when organisms are not evident in routine hematoxylin-eosin sections. Familiarity with the patient's recent clinical history is advisable, because a robust inflammatory infiltrate may persist up to 6 months following successful eradication of *H pylori*. Patients with CD may also have concurrent *H pylori* infection, although the incidence is reportedly lower than in the general population and in patients with UC.[74,78,79]

FEG is reported in 30% to 75% of patients with CD and 12% to 30% of patients with UC. It is most common in children, where it is considered specific for IBD, albeit not reliable in distinguishing CD from UC.[56,69,71,80–82] FEG in adults is not considered specific for IBD but may signal gastric involvement by CD in patients with isolated terminal ileitis.[70]

Acute erosive gastritis may be seen, besides in CD, with exposure to chemical insults (such as nonsteroidal anti-inflammatory medications, aspirin, bisphosphonates, iron, doxycycline, alcohol, and bile reflux) as well as with physiologic stress or radiation.[75]

GG occurs in 10% to 28% of gastric biopsies from patients with CD[63] and patients with sarcoidosis; congenital immune deficiencies; granulomatous infections, such as tuberculosis; syphilis; fungi and parasites; malignant tumors; foreign bodies; or unidentified causes. It is unsettled whether *H pylori* itself can cause GG.

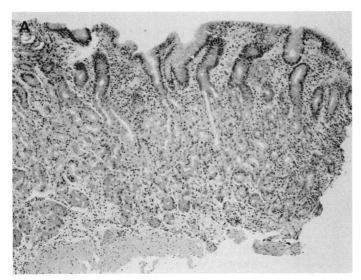

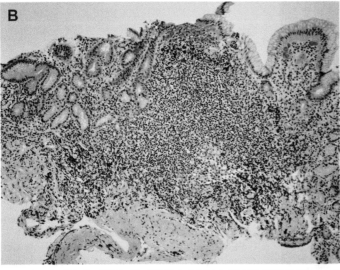

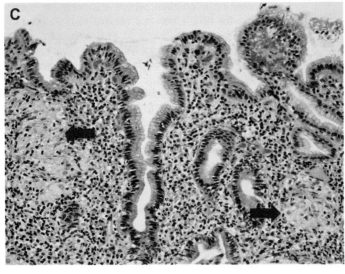

Fig. 3. Histopathologic patterns in Crohn disease–associated gastritis. (*A*) Chronic superficial gastritis featuring diffuse, mostly superficial infiltration of gastric body mucosa by lymphocytes and plasma cells. (*B*) Follicular gastritis with full-thickness involvement of antral mucosa. (*C*) Granulomatous gastritis. Antral mucosa with active chronic inflammation and non-necrotizing epithelioid cell granulomas (*arrows*) occupying the lamina propria. The granulomas are small and loose, contain occasional giant cells, and displace normal crypts.

Fig. 3. (*D*) Lymphocytic gastritis. Antral mucosal biopsy with more than 25 intraepithelial lymphocytes per 100 surface epithelial cells and involvement of the foveolae. (*E*) Acute erosive gastritis. Antral mucosa with surface erosion (*arrow*), fibrinoinflammatory exudate, and adjacent reactive mucin-depleted epithelium. (*F*) Focally enhanced gastritis. Antral mucosal biopsy with gland obscured by an aggregate of mononuclear cells and a few neutrophils (*arrow*). The background mucosa is normal. Hematoxylin-eosin, original magnification ×100 (*A*, *B*), ×200 (*C*–*F*).

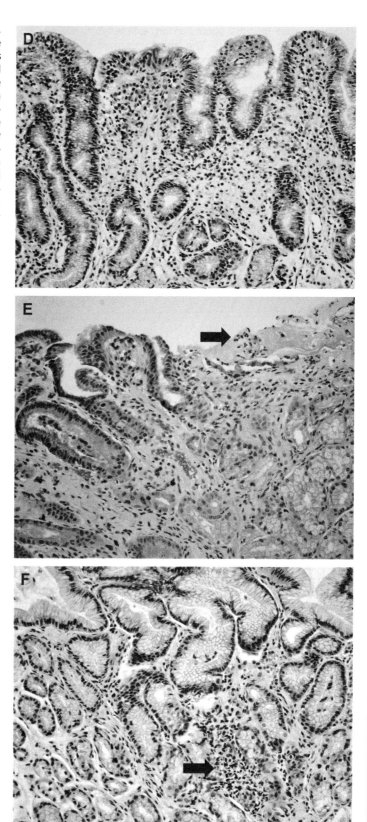

Lymphocytic gastritis occurs in an estimated 4% of gastric biopsies.[76] The most common causes besides CD are *H pylori* infection and celiac disease, the latter usually localizing in the antrum. Other associations include angiotensin II receptor blocking agents, immune checkpoint inhibitors, autoimmune disorders, infections (eg, human immunodeficiency virus and syphilis), collagenous gastritis, and some neoplasms; but an identifiable cause is absent in up to 20% of cases.

CG-NOS encompasses a diverse array of environmental or dietary causes that are difficult to confirm or exclude. Follicular gastritis occurs in CD but may indicate current or previous *H pylori* infection. Other *H pylori*–negative gastritides, such as corpus-predominant (autoimmune) atrophic gastritis and eosinophilic gastritis, have not been associated with CD.[83–85]

GASTRITIS IN ULCERATIVE COLITIS

Gastritis or gastroduodenitis is reported in 5% to 8% of patients with UC.[86–92] It is most common in postcolectomy patients with a long postoperative interval or in patients with extensive colitis or pancolitis. Most patients have either mild localizing symptoms or none at all, but severe gastritis or gastroduodenitis is described in patients with postcolectomy panenteritis[91] or ileoanal pouchitis.[86,90] Recent studies in children have reported that active inflammation in the stomach and/or duodenum may correlate with medically refractory UC, the intensity of gastric inflammation mirroring that seen in the colon and diminishing as the colitis is controlled.[92]

GROSS AND ENDOSCOPIC FEATURES

Gastritis in the setting of UC is manifested by diffuse mucosal granularity or friability, although aphthous lesions have been reported.[89,90]

MICROSCOPIC FEATURES

Compared with CD, the histologic features of gastritis in UC are less well defined. In their series, Lin and colleagues[87] described three patterns of inflammation: focal inflammation similar to FEG, CSG, and CG-NOS; erosions or ulcers were uncommon. Patchy or focal inflammation occurs less frequently in UC than in CD and only slightly more frequently than in patients without IBD.[74,87] Granulomas are invariably absent.

DIFFERENTIAL DIAGNOSIS

The presence of mild chronic antral gastritis with or without neutrophils in patients with UC is of doubtful specificity and may be related to environmental and dietary factors. Compared with UC, the inflammatory cell infiltration seen in *H pylori*–associated gastritis and in CSG associated with gastric CD is denser and more diffuse. Eosinophil-predominant inflammation is uncommon in IBD despite evidence that eosinophils can participate in the pathogenesis of IBD.[84,85]

DUODENITIS IN CROHN DISEASE

Primary Crohn duodenitis, first described in 1937,[93] can affect any portion or all of the duodenum. Proximal duodenitis is often contiguous with involvement of the gastric antrum and pylorus, whereas distal duodenitis is often contiguous with jejunitis.[8,94–96] A retrospective database review of patients with IBD who underwent UGI endoscopy for any indication reported duodenitis in 26% (40% in patients younger than 18)[97]; however, clinically significant duodenitis is reported in only 4% of patients with CD.[7,94]

Symptoms are usually attributable to obstruction or to ulceration, and may include upper abdominal pain, early satiety, nausea and vomiting, weight loss, and overt or occult bleeding. In most cases, duodenitis is diagnosed concurrently with or following the diagnosis of ileal, large intestinal, or perianal CD.[8,98] When isolated duodenitis is encountered, involvement of other organs by CD usually ensues within several years.[95,96]

GROSS AND ENDOSCOPIC FEATURES

Endoscopic lesions occur in approximately 14% of patients when sought prospectively.[63] They range from edema, patchy erythema, friability, granularity, or aphthous ulcers at one extreme to linear or serpiginous ulcers, cobblestoning, bamboo-joint notching, stenosis, indistensibility, and fistula tracts at the other.[4] Contiguous involvement of the distal stomach and proximal duodenum may produce radiologically distinctive tapering referred to as a "ram's horn" deformity.[99,100] Primary duodenal fistulas may involve the abdominal wall or stomach, whereas secondary fistulas can originate from other intestinal sites, especially from prior anastomotic sites.[98]

MICROSCOPIC FEATURES

Duodenal biopsy findings are usually nonspecific, including active chronic inflammation, villous blunting, aphthae, ulcers, mucosal scarring, and foveolar metaplasia, which tends to be extensive.[101–103] IEL, defined as greater than 25 to 30 lymphocytes per 100 epithelial cells, occurs in conjunction with normal villous architecture. One pediatric study reported IEL in 4 of 27 patients with CD (15%) and 4 of 13 patients (31%) with UC compared with 0 of 22 patients with suspected gastroesophageal reflux.[15] In another study, 74 (6.4%) of 1161 patients with IEL had IBD, 70 adults and four children, of whom 58 (including all four children) (78%) had CD, 13 had UC, and three had unclassified IBD.[104] The lymphocytes tend to be distributed evenly along the sides of the villi, in contrast with celiac disease, where they concentrate near the villous tips.

Granulomatous duodenitis (Fig. 4A) is characteristic of CD, occurring in 4% to 12% of cases,[63,102] but is mimicked by other disorders and by foreign body granulomas including reactions to mucin released from ruptured Brunner glands.

DIFFERENTIAL DIAGNOSIS

The differential diagnosis of duodenitis in CD is broad, including peptic disease associated with H pylori and hypersecretory states; medication-associated duodenitis; celiac disease; sarcoidosis; congenital or acquired immunodeficiency states; Behçet's disease; Henoch-Schönlein purpura and other vasculitides; and infections, such as cytomegalovirus, parasitoses, and tuberculosis. Particularly helpful features are the presence of established extraduodenal CD and endoscopic or radiologic studies revealing bamboo-joint lesions, fistulas, or scarring and effacement of the pyloric valve. Microscopically, granulomatous duodenitis should always be evaluated with acid-fast and silver stains, an infectious cause being most likely when granulomas are large (>0.4 mm), confluent, or centrally necrotizing. IEL should elicit serologic evaluation for celiac disease despite preserved villous architecture, especially when lymphocytes are concentrated near the villous tips. Biopsy tissues should be carefully screened for parasites and for absence of plasma cells as seen in common variable immunodeficiency. Behçet's disease is difficult to distinguish histologically from CD in the absence of granulomas, but is reportedly much less likely to elicit foveolar metaplasia.[101]

DUODENITIS IN ULCERATIVE COLITIS

Chronic duodenitis in the setting of UC was first reported in 1960[105] and has been documented subsequently in several series and case reports[86,89,90,106–113]; however, it remains uncommon. A retrospective database review of patients with UC undergoing UGI endoscopy for any cause reported a prevalence of only 3% overall and 0% in younger patients.[97] The most common symptom referable to duodenitis is dyspepsia, but it is often overshadowed by symptoms of colitis.[88] In some series, most patients with symptomatic duodenitis have had severe colitis requiring colectomy; interestingly, some patients with a continent ileoanal pouch have experienced concomitant pouchitis.[88,90]

GROSS AND ENDOSCOPIC FEATURES

The endoscopic findings in symptomatic patients, reviewed by Choi and colleagues,[112] include diffuse edema, granularity, friability, ulceration, luminal narrowing, and inflammatory pseudopolyps.

MICROSCOPIC FEATURES

The microscopic features of duodenitis attributed to UC resemble the classical features of colonic UC including mucosal expansion, diffuse mononuclear inflammatory cell infiltration, neutrophilic inflammation, and distortion of glands and erosions or ulcers (Fig. 4B).[106] Additionally, a subset of pediatric patients may have IEL.[15,104]

DIFFERENTIAL DIAGNOSIS

UC-related duodenitis is rarely diagnosed because of its nonspecific gross and microscopic characteristics and the overlap with peptic duodenitis, celiac disease and medication-associated duodenitis. Nonetheless, awareness of the entity should be maintained in the clinical setting of established UC, particularly when colectomy has been previously performed for extensive severe colitis and if the patient is experiencing concurrent pouchitis or enteritis.

MANAGEMENT AND PROGNOSIS

Medical therapy is usually successful in treating symptomatic UGI involvement by IBD but has a high rate of failure in treating obstructive symptoms and fistulas associated with CD. Many patients are on maintenance therapy for distal disease when diagnosed with UGI CD but may receive additional therapy with antacids, antisecretory drugs, aminosalicylates, and eradication of H pylori if present. Patients with isolated, disproportionate, or refractory symptoms are treated with immunosuppressive agents including steroids and/or antimetabolites followed by

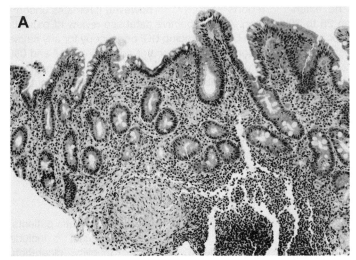

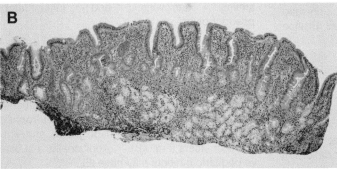

Fig. 4. Histology of duodenitis in IBD. (*A*) Duodenal biopsy in a patient with Crohn duodenitis featuring submucosal nonnecrotizing granuloma. (*B*) Duodenal biopsy in patient with ulcerative colitis. Note the villous blunting, mucosal expansion, and full-thickness lymphoplasmacytosis. Hematoxylin-eosin, original magnification ×100 (*A*), ×40 (*B*).

escalation to biologics if needed to achieve control.[11,23] The results reported for different therapeutic regimens have generally been favorable albeit based on small series,[23,114,115] and the role of individual therapeutic agents, such as steroids and infliximab, is debated.[11] Treatment of UGI strictures related to CD by means of endoscopic intervention including stenting and balloon dilation can obviate surgery in some cases. Recent studies have reported short-term efficacy in 87% of patients undergoing pneumatic balloon dilatation but short-term symptom recurrence in most, redilation performed in more than half, and surgery ultimately performed in nearly one-third.[116,117] Surgery is generally reserved for patients with fistulizing disease or refractory strictures.[118]

CONCLUSION

The UGI manifestations of IBD are less common and often less distinctive than its intestinal features and therefore pose a continuing diagnostic challenge. Given the growing clinical emphasis on achieving deep remission of IBD as a therapeutic goal, which is predicated on accurate patient staging and subclassification, the role of the practicing pathologist in meeting this challenge assumes increasing importance.

DISCLOSURE

The authors have nothing to disclose.

REFERENCES

1. Dabkowski K, Graca-Pakulska K, Zawada I, et al. Clinical significance of endoscopic findings in the upper gastrointestinal tract in Crohn's disease. Scand J Gastroenterol 2019;54(9):1075–80.
2. Turner D, Griffiths AM. Esophageal, gastric, and duodenal manifestations of IBD and the role of upper endoscopy in IBD diagnosis. Curr Gastroenterol Rep 2007;9(6):475–8.
3. Diaz L, Hernandez-Oquet RE, Deshpande AR, et al. Upper gastrointestinal involvement in Crohn disease: histopathologic and endoscopic findings. South Med J 2015;108(11):695–700.
4. Kefalas CH. Gastroduodenal Crohn's disease. Proc (Bayl Univ Med Cent) 2003;16(2):147–51.

5. Wagtmans MJ, van Hogezand RA, Griffioen G, et al. Crohn's disease of the upper gastrointestinal tract. Neth J Med 1997;50(2):S2–7.

6. Aggarwal SN, Cavanagh Y, Wang L, et al. Upper gastrointestinal Crohn's disease: literature review and case presentation. Case Rep Gastrointest Med 2019;2019:2708909.

7. Isaacs KL. Upper gastrointestinal tract endoscopy in inflammatory bowel disease. Gastrointest Endosc Clin N Am 2002;12(3):451–62, vii.

8. Nugent FW, Roy MA. Duodenal Crohn's disease: an analysis of 89 cases. Am J Gastroenterol 1989; 84(3):249–54.

9. Feakins RM, British Society of G. Inflammatory bowel disease biopsies: updated British Society of Gastroenterology reporting guidelines. J Clin Pathol 2013;66(12):1005–26.

10. Sakuraba A, Iwao Y, Matsuoka K, et al. Endoscopic and pathologic changes of the upper gastrointestinal tract in Crohn's disease. Biomed Res Int 2014;2014:610767.

11. Schwartzberg DM, Brandstetter S, Grucela AL. Crohn's disease of the esophagus, duodenum, and stomach. Clin Colon Rectal Surg 2019;32(4): 231–42.

12. Greuter T, Piller A, Fournier N, et al. Upper gastrointestinal tract involvement in Crohn's disease: frequency, risk factors, and disease course. J Crohns Colitis 2018;12(12):1399–409.

13. North American Society for Pediatric Gastroenterology, Hepatology, and Nutrition, Colitis Foundation of America, Bousvaros A, et al. Differentiating ulcerative colitis from Crohn disease in children and young adults: report of a working group of the North American Society for Pediatric Gastroenterology, Hepatology, and Nutrition and the Crohn's and Colitis Foundation of America. J Pediatr Gastroenterol Nutr 2007;44(5):653–74.

14. Castellaneta SP, Afzal NA, Greenberg M, et al. Diagnostic role of upper gastrointestinal endoscopy in pediatric inflammatory bowel disease. J Pediatr Gastroenterol Nutr 2004;39(3):257–61.

15. Tobin JM, Sinha B, Ramani P, et al. Upper gastrointestinal mucosal disease in pediatric Crohn disease and ulcerative colitis: a blinded, controlled study. J Pediatr Gastroenterol Nutr 2001;32(4): 443–8.

16. Abdullah BA, Gupta SK, Croffie JM, et al. The role of esophagogastroduodenoscopy in the initial evaluation of childhood inflammatory bowel disease: a 7-year study. J Pediatr Gastroenterol Nutr 2002; 35(5):636–40.

17. American Society for Gastrointestinal Endoscopy Standards of Practice Committee, Shergill AK, Lightdale JR, et al. The role of endoscopy in inflammatory bowel disease. Gastrointest Endosc 2015; 81(5):1101–21.e1-113.

18. Levine A, Koletzko S, Turner D, et al. ESPGHAN revised porto criteria for the diagnosis of inflammatory bowel disease in children and adolescents. J Pediatr Gastroenterol Nutr 2014;58(6): 795–806.

19. Silverberg MS, Satsangi J, Ahmad T, et al. Toward an integrated clinical, molecular and serological classification of inflammatory bowel disease: report of a Working Party of the 2005 Montreal World Congress of Gastroenterology. Can J Gastroenterol 2005;19(Suppl A):5A–36A.

20. Satsangi J, Silverberg MS, Vermeire S, et al. The Montreal classification of inflammatory bowel disease: controversies, consensus, and implications. Gut 2006;55(6):749–53.

21. Franklin RH, Taylor S. Nonspecific granulomatous (regional) esophagitis. J Thorac Surg 1950;19(2): 292–7.

22. Crohn BB, Ginzburg L, Oppenheimer GD. Landmark article Oct 15, 1932. Regional ileitis. A pathological and clinical entity. By Burril B. Crohn, Leon Ginzburg, and Gordon D. Oppenheimer. JAMA 1984;251(1):73–9.

23. De Felice KM, Katzka DA, Raffals LE. Crohn's disease of the esophagus: clinical features and treatment outcomes in the biologic Era. Inflamm Bowel Dis 2015;21(9):2106–13.

24. Decker GA, Loftus EV Jr, Pasha TM, et al. Crohn's disease of the esophagus: clinical features and outcomes. Inflamm Bowel Dis 2001;7(2):113–9.

25. Geboes K, Janssens J, Rutgeerts P, et al. Crohn's disease of the esophagus. J Clin Gastroenterol 1986;8(1):31–7.

26. Mashako MN, Cezard JP, Navarro J, et al. Crohn's disease lesions in the upper gastrointestinal tract: correlation between clinical, radiological, endoscopic, and histological features in adolescents and children. J Pediatr Gastroenterol Nutr 1989; 8(4):442–6.

27. Ruuska T, Vaajalahti P, Arajarvi P, et al. Prospective evaluation of upper gastrointestinal mucosal lesions in children with ulcerative colitis and Crohn's disease. J Pediatr Gastroenterol Nutr 1994;19(2):181–6.

28. Wang W, Ni Y, Ke C, et al. Isolated Crohn's disease of the esophagus with esophago-mediastinal fistula formation. World J Surg Oncol 2012;10:208.

29. Ebach DR, Vanderheyden AD, Ellison JM, et al. Lymphocytic esophagitis: a possible manifestation of pediatric upper gastrointestinal Crohn's disease. Inflamm Bowel Dis 2011;17(1):45–9.

30. Rubio CA, Sjodahl K, Lagergren J. Lymphocytic esophagitis: a histologic subset of chronic esophagitis. Am J Clin Pathol 2006;125(3):432–7.

31. Habbal M, Scaffidi MA, Rumman A, et al. Clinical, endoscopic, and histologic characteristics of lymphocytic esophagitis: a systematic review. Esophagus 2019;16(2):123–32.

32. Sutton LM, Heintz DD, Patel AS, et al. Lymphocytic esophagitis in children. Inflamm Bowel Dis 2014; 20(8):1324–8.

33. Patil DT, Hammer S, Langer R, et al. Lymphocytic esophagitis: an update on histologic diagnosis, endoscopic findings, and natural history. Ann N Y Acad Sci 2018;1434(1):185–91.

34. Haque S, Genta RM. Lymphocytic oesophagitis: clinicopathological aspects of an emerging condition. Gut 2012;61(8):1108–14.

35. Chen WC, Krishna M, Jeffers KB, et al. Desquamative esophagitis: a refractory mucosal injury pattern. Dis Esophagus 2017;30(8):1–5.

36. Mori S, Yoshihira A, Kawamura H, et al. Esophageal involvement in Behcet's disease. Am J Gastroenterol 1983;78(9):548–53.

37. Abraham SC, Ravich WJ, Anhalt GJ, et al. Esophageal lichen planus: case report and review of the literature. Am J Surg Pathol 2000;24(12):1678–82.

38. Kridin K, Bergman R. The usefulness of indirect immunofluorescence in pemphigus and the natural history of patients with initial false-positive results: a retrospective cohort study. Front Med (Lausanne) 2018;5:266.

39. Katzka DA, Smyrk TC, Bruce AJ, et al. Variations in presentations of esophageal involvement in lichen planus. Clin Gastroenterol Hepatol 2010;8(9): 777–82.

40. Harewood GC, Murray JA, Cameron AJ. Esophageal lichen planus: the Mayo Clinic experience. Dis Esophagus 1999;12(4):309–11.

41. Pittman ME, Hissong E, Katz PO, et al. Lymphocyte-predominant esophagitis: a distinct and likely immune-mediated disorder encompassing lymphocytic and lichenoid esophagitis. Am J Surg Pathol 2020;44(2):198–205.

42. Salaria SN, Abu Alfa AK, Cruise MW, et al. Lichenoid esophagitis: clinicopathologic overlap with established esophageal lichen planus. Am J Surg Pathol 2013;37(12):1889–94.

43. Rouphael C, Gordon IO, Thota PN. Lymphocytic esophagitis: still an enigma a decade later. World J Gastroenterol 2017;23(6):949–56.

44. Resnick MB, Finkelstein Y, Weissler A, et al. Assessment and diagnostic utility of the cytotoxic T-lymphocyte phenotype using the specific markers granzyme-B and TIA-1 in esophageal mucosal biopsies. Hum Pathol 1999;30(4):397–402.

45. Xue Y, Suriawinata A, Liu X, et al. Lymphocytic esophagitis with CD4 T-cell-predominant intraepithelial lymphocytes and primary esophageal motility abnormalities: a potential novel clinicopathologic entity. Am J Surg Pathol 2015;39(11): 1558–67.

46. Ashton JJ, Bonduelle Q, Mossotto E, et al. Endoscopic and histological assessment of paediatric inflammatory bowel disease over a 3-year follow-up period. J Pediatr Gastroenterol Nutr 2018; 66(3):402–9.

47. Alcantara M, Rodriguez R, Potenciano JL, et al. Endoscopic and bioptic findings in the upper gastrointestinal tract in patients with Crohn's disease. Endoscopy 1993;25(4):282–6.

48. Annunziata ML, Caviglia R, Papparella LG, et al. Upper gastrointestinal involvement of Crohn's disease: a prospective study on the role of upper endoscopy in the diagnostic work-up. Dig Dis Sci 2012;57(6):1618–23.

49. Glickman JN, Antonioli DA. Gastritis. Gastrointest Endosc Clin N Am 2001;11(4):717–40, vii.

50. Kuriyama M, Kato J, Morimoto N, et al. Specific gastroduodenoscopic findings in Crohn's disease: comparison with findings in patients with ulcerative colitis and gastroesophageal reflux disease. Dig Liver Dis 2008;40(6):468–75.

51. Lauwers GY, Fujita H, Nagata K, et al. Pathology of non-*Helicobacter pylori* gastritis: extending the histopathologic horizons. J Gastroenterol 2010;45(2): 131–45.

52. Oberhuber G, Hirsch M, Stolte M. High incidence of upper gastrointestinal tract involvement in Crohn's disease. Virchows Arch 1998;432(1): 49–52.

53. Rutgeerts P, Onette E, Vantrappen G, et al. Crohn's disease of the stomach and duodenum: a clinical study with emphasis on the value of endoscopy and endoscopic biopsies. Endoscopy 1980;12(6): 288–94.

54. Srivastava A, Lauwers GY. Pathology of non-infective gastritis. Histopathology 2007;50(1): 15–29.

55. Weinstein WM. Emerging gastritides. Curr Gastroenterol Rep 2001;3(6):523–7.

56. Wright CL, Riddell RH. Histology of the stomach and duodenum in Crohn's disease. Am J Surg Pathol 1998;22(4):383–90.

57. Abuquteish D, Putra J. Upper gastrointestinal tract involvement of pediatric inflammatory bowel disease: a pathological review. World J Gastroenterol 2019;25(16):1928–35.

58. Hummel TZ, ten Kate FJ, Reitsma JB, et al. Additional value of upper GI tract endoscopy in the diagnostic assessment of childhood IBD. J Pediatr Gastroenterol Nutr 2012;54(6):753–7.

59. Inayat F, Ullah W, Hussain Q, et al. Crohn's disease presenting as gastric outlet obstruction: a therapeutic challenge? BMJ Case Rep 2017;2017.

60. Zhi XT, Hong JG, Li T, et al. Gastric Crohn's disease: a rare cause of intermittent abdominal pain and vomiting. Am J Med 2017;130(5):e181–5.

61. Greenstein AJ, Present DH, Sachar DB, et al. Gastric fistulas in Crohn's disease. Report of cases. Dis Colon Rectum 1989;32(10):888–92.

62. Yokota K, Saito Y, Einami K, et al. A bamboo joint-like appearance of the gastric body and cardia: possible association with Crohn's disease. Gastrointest Endosc 1997;46(3):268–72.

63. Horjus Talabur Horje CS, Meijer J, Rovers L, et al. Prevalence of upper gastrointestinal lesions at primary diagnosis in adults with inflammatory bowel disease. Inflamm Bowel Dis 2016;22(8):1896–901.

64. Laube R, Liu K, Schifter M, et al. Oral and upper gastrointestinal Crohn's disease. J Gastroenterol Hepatol 2018;33(2):355–64.

65. Long MD, Barnes E, Isaacs K, et al. Impact of capsule endoscopy on management of inflammatory bowel disease: a single tertiary care center experience. Inflamm Bowel Dis 2011;17(9):1855–62.

66. Nomura Y, Moriichi K, Fujiya M, et al. The endoscopic findings of the upper gastrointestinal tract in patients with Crohn's disease. Clin J Gastroenterol 2017;10(4):289–96.

67. Tanabe H, Yokota K, Nomura Y, et al. The clinical importance of "bamboo joint-like appearance" on upper gastrointestinal endoscopy for the diagnosis of Crohn's disease. Nihon Shokakibyo Gakkai Zasshi 2016;113(7):1208–15.

68. Meining A, Bayerdorffer E, Bastlein E, et al. Focal inflammatory infiltrations in gastric biopsy specimens are suggestive of Crohn's disease. Crohn's Disease Study Group, Germany. Scand J Gastroenterol 1997;32(8):813–8.

69. Oberhuber G, Puspok A, Oesterreicher C, et al. Focally enhanced gastritis: a frequent type of gastritis in patients with Crohn's disease. Gastroenterology 1997;112(3):698–706.

70. Petrolla AA, Katz JA, Xin W. The clinical significance of focal enhanced gastritis in adults with isolated ileitis of the terminal ileum. J Gastroenterol 2008;43(7):524–30.

71. Sharif F, McDermott M, Dillon M, et al. Focally enhanced gastritis in children with Crohn's disease and ulcerative colitis. Am J Gastroenterol 2002;97(6):1415–20.

72. Xin W, Greenson JK. The clinical significance of focally enhanced gastritis. Am J Surg Pathol 2004;28(10):1347–51.

73. Yardley JH, Hendrix TR. Gastroduodenal Crohn's disease: the focus is on focality. Gastroenterology 1997;112(3):1031–3.

74. Parente F, Cucino C, Bollani S, et al. Focal gastric inflammatory infiltrates in inflammatory bowel diseases: prevalence, immunohistochemical characteristics, and diagnostic role. Am J Gastroenterol 2000;95(3):705–11.

75. El-Zimaity H, Choi WT, Lauwers GY, et al. The differential diagnosis of *Helicobacter pylori* negative gastritis. Virchows Arch 2018;473(5):533–50.

76. Polydorides AD. Pathology and differential diagnosis of chronic, noninfectious gastritis. Semin Diagn Pathol 2014;31(2):114–23.

77. Goldstein NS, Amin M. Upper gastrointestinal tract in inflammatory bowel disease. Surg Pathol Clin 2010;3(2):349–59.

78. Parente F, Molteni P, Bollani S, et al. Prevalence of *Helicobacter pylori* infection and related upper gastrointestinal lesions in patients with inflammatory bowel diseases. A cross-sectional study with matching. Scand J Gastroenterol 1997;32(11):1140–6.

79. Roka K, Roubani A, Stefanaki K, et al. The prevalence of *Helicobacter pylori* gastritis in newly diagnosed children with inflammatory bowel disease. Helicobacter 2014;19(5):400–5.

80. Roka K, Roma E, Stefanaki K, et al. The value of focally enhanced gastritis in the diagnosis of pediatric inflammatory bowel diseases. J Crohns Colitis 2013;7(10):797–802.

81. McHugh JB, Gopal P, Greenson JK. The clinical significance of focally enhanced gastritis in children. Am J Surg Pathol 2013;37(2):295–9.

82. Ushiku T, Moran CJ, Lauwers GY. Focally enhanced gastritis in newly diagnosed pediatric inflammatory bowel disease. Am J Surg Pathol 2013;37(12):1882–8.

83. Lwin T, Melton SD, Genta RM. Eosinophilic gastritis: histopathological characterization and quantification of the normal gastric eosinophil content. Mod Pathol 2011;24(4):556–63.

84. Filippone RT, Sahakian L, Apostolopoulos V, et al. Eosinophils in inflammatory bowel disease. Inflamm Bowel Dis 2019;25(7):1140–51.

85. Woodruff SA, Masterson JC, Fillon S, et al. Role of eosinophils in inflammatory bowel and gastrointestinal diseases. J Pediatr Gastroenterol Nutr 2011;52(6):650–61.

86. Hisabe T, Matsui T, Miyaoka M, et al. Diagnosis and clinical course of ulcerative gastroduodenal lesion associated with ulcerative colitis: possible relationship with pouchitis. Dig Endosc 2010;22(4):268–74.

87. Lin J, McKenna BJ, Appelman HD. Morphologic findings in upper gastrointestinal biopsies of patients with ulcerative colitis: a controlled study. Am J Surg Pathol 2010;34(11):1672–7.

88. Shen B, Wu H, Remzi F, et al. Diagnostic value of esophagogastroduodenoscopy in patients with ileal pouch-anal anastomosis. Inflamm Bowel Dis 2009;15(3):395–401.

89. Hori K, Ikeuchi H, Nakano H, et al. Gastroduodenitis associated with ulcerative colitis. J Gastroenterol 2008;43(3):193–201.

90. Ikeuchi H, Hori K, Nishigami T, et al. Diffuse gastroduodenitis and pouchitis associated with ulcerative colitis. World J Gastroenterol 2006;12(36):5913–5.

91. Hoentjen F, Hanauer SB, Hart J, et al. Long-term treatment of patients with a history of ulcerative

colitis who develop gastritis and pan-enteritis after colectomy. J Clin Gastroenterol 2013;47(1):52–7.

92. Sullivan KJ, Wei M, Chernetsova E, et al. Value of upper endoscopic biopsies in predicting medical refractoriness in pediatric patients with ulcerative colitis. Hum Pathol 2017;66:167–76.

93. Gottlieb D, Alpert S. Regional jejunitis. Am J Roentgenol 1937;38:881–3.

94. Reynolds HL Jr, Stellato TA. Crohn's disease of the foregut. Surg Clin North Am 2001;81(1):117–35, viii.

95. Nugent FW, Richmond M, Park SK. Crohn's disease of the duodenum. Gut 1977;18(2):115–20.

96. Farmer RG, Hawk WA, Turnbull RB Jr. Crohn's disease of the duodenum (transmural duodenitis): clinical manifestations. Report of 11 cases. Am J Dig Dis 1972;17(3):191–8.

97. Sonnenberg A, Melton SD, Genta RM. Frequent occurrence of gastritis and duodenitis in patients with inflammatory bowel disease. Inflamm Bowel Dis 2011;17(1):39–44.

98. Yamamoto T, Bain IM, Connolly AB, et al. Gastroduodenal fistulas in Crohn's disease: clinical features and management. Dis Colon Rectum 1998;41(10): 1287–92.

99. Xiang H, Han J, Ridley WE, et al. Ram's horn sign: gastric antrum in Crohn's disease. J Med Imaging Radiat Oncol 2018;62(Suppl 1):101.

100. Farman J, Faegenburg D, Dallemand S, et al. Crohn's disease of the stomach: the "ram's horn" sign. Am J Roentgenol Radium Ther Nucl Med 1975;123(2):242–51.

101. Akemoto Y, Sakuraba H, Tanaka M, et al. Gastric focal neutrophil infiltration and wide duodenal gastric foveolar metaplasia are histologic discriminative markers for Crohn's disease and Behcet's disease. Digestion 2019;100(3):210–9.

102. Jaskiewicz K, Lemmer E. Histological findings in gastroduodenal mucosa in patients with Crohn's disease. Any diagnostic significance? Pol J Pathol 1996;47(3):115–8.

103. Schuffler MD, Chaffee RG. Small intestinal biopsy in a patient with Crohn's disease of the duodenum. The spectrum of abnormal findings in the absence of granulomas. Gastroenterology 1979;76(5 Pt 1):1009–14.

104. Patterson ER, Shmidt E, Oxentenko AS, et al. Normal villous architecture with increased intraepithelial lymphocytes: a duodenal manifestation of Crohn disease. Am J Clin Pathol 2015;143(3):445–50.

105. Thompson JW 3rd, Bargen JA. Ulcerative duodenitis and chronic ulcerative colitis: report of two cases. Gastroenterology 1960;38:452–5.

106. Valdez R, Appelman HD, Bronner MP, et al. Diffuse duodenitis associated with ulcerative colitis. Am J Surg Pathol 2000;24(10):1407–13.

107. Terashima S, Hoshino Y, Kanzaki N, et al. Ulcerative duodenitis accompanying ulcerative colitis. J Clin Gastroenterol 2001;32(2):172–5.

108. Rubenstein J, Sherif A, Appelman H, et al. Ulcerative colitis associated enteritis: is ulcerative colitis always confined to the colon? J Clin Gastroenterol 2004;38(1):46–51.

109. Kawai K, Watanabe T, Nakayama H, et al. Images of interest. Gastrointestinal: small bowel inflammation and ulcerative colitis. J Gastroenterol Hepatol 2005;20(11):1791.

110. Akitake R, Nakase H, Tamaoki M, et al. Modulation of Th1/Th2 balance by infliximab rescues postoperative occurrence of small-intestinal inflammation associated with ulcerative colitis. Dig Dis Sci 2010;55(6):1781–4.

111. Chiba M, Ono I, Wakamatsu H, et al. Diffuse gastroduodenitis associated with ulcerative colitis: treatment by infliximab. Dig Endosc 2013;25(6): 622–5.

112. Choi YS, Kim JK, Kim WJ, et al. Remission of diffuse ulcerative duodenitis in a patient with ulcerative colitis after infliximab therapy: a case study and review of the literature. Intest Res 2019;17(2): 273–7.

113. Willington AJ, Taylor G, White J, et al. Gastrointestinal: ulcerative colitis-associated duodenitis. J Gastroenterol Hepatol 2018;33(5):973.

114. D'Haens G, Rutgeerts P, Geboes K, et al. The natural history of esophageal Crohn's disease: three patterns of evolution. Gastrointest Endosc 1994; 40(3):296–300.

115. Korelitz BI, Adler DJ, Mendelsohn RA, et al. Long-term experience with 6-mercaptopurine in the treatment of Crohn's disease. Am J Gastroenterol 1993; 88(8):1198–205.

116. Bettenworth D, Mucke MM, Lopez R, et al. Efficacy of endoscopic dilation of gastroduodenal Crohn's disease strictures: a systematic review and meta-analysis of individual patient data. Clin Gastroenterol Hepatol 2019;17(12):2514–22.e8.

117. Singh A, Agrawal N, Kurada S, et al. Efficacy, safety, and long-term outcome of serial endoscopic balloon dilation for upper gastrointestinal Crohn's disease-associated strictures: a cohort study. J Crohns Colitis 2017;11(9):1044–51.

118. Davis KG. Crohn's disease of the foregut. Surg Clin North Am 2015;95(6):1183–93, vi.

Gastric Epithelial Polyps
When to Ponder, When to Panic

Shoko Vos, MD, PhD[a], Rachel S. van der Post, MD, PhD[a], Lodewijk A.A. Brosens, MD, PhD[a,b,*]

KEYWORDS
- Stomach • Gastric • Polyp • Polyposis • Hereditary • Dysplasia

---

Key points

- Gastric epithelial polyps comprise a wide spectrum of lesions with different cause, histology, malignant potential, and sometimes associations with tumor predisposition syndromes.

- Most gastric polyps are sporadic with no malignant potential, but clinical correlation is necessary, and pathologists should be familiar with the morphologic characteristics of gastric polyps as an indication for a search for an underlying genetic syndrome, such as familial adenomatous polyposis, Peutz-Jeghers syndrome, or juvenile polyposis syndrome.

- In the presence of a gastric polyp, preferably biopsies of background mucosa are taken of at least the antrum and corpus. Evaluation of the background nonpolypoid mucosa is essential in reaching a diagnosis that can characterize the condition in which the polyp developed and may have therapeutic consequences.

ABSTRACT

This review provides an overview of different types of gastric epithelial polyps. The polyps are classified based on their cell or epithelial compartment of origin. Some of these polyps can be considered reactive or nonneoplastic, whereas others are neoplastic in origin, are sometimes associated with a hereditary polyposis/cancer syndrome, and may have malignant potential. The aim of this review is to provide a pragmatic overview for the practicing pathologist about how to correctly diagnose and deal with gastric epithelial polyps and when (not) to ponder, and when (not) to panic.

OVERVIEW

Gastric polyps comprise a wide spectrum of lesions arising from different cell or epithelial compartments in the stomach and with different causes, histology, malignant potential, and association with different tumor predisposition syndromes. Gastric polyps can be defined as lesions projecting above the plane of the surrounding gastric mucosa.[1] In about 1% to 6% of gastroscopies, polyps are found in the stomach.[2,3] Most polyps are of epithelial origin and asymptomatic.[2] Less frequently found subepithelial lesions presenting as gastric polyps include neuroendocrine tumors, pancreatic heterotopia, mesenchymal polyps (eg, inflammatory fibroid polyp, gastrointestinal stromal tumor, leiomyoma, schwannoma, inflammatory myofibroblastic tumor) as well as lymphomas.[4]

Large geographic differences have been observed in the occurrence of gastric polyps, mainly caused by differences in *Helicobacter pylori* (H pylori) infection rate.[5] In areas with high rates of *H pylori* infection, hyperplastic polyps (HPs), with or without dysplasia, are most prevalent. In contrast, fundic gland polyps (FGPs) are the most frequently encountered type of polyps

Funded by: VSNU2020.
[a] Department of Pathology, Radboud University Medical Center, Geert Grooteplein Zuid 10, Nijmegen 6525 GA, The Netherlands; [b] Department of Pathology, University Medical Center Utrecht, Utrecht University, Heidelberglaan 100, Utrecht 3584 CX, The Netherlands
* Corresponding author. Department of Pathology, University Medical Center Utrecht, Utrecht University, Heidelberglaan 100, Utrecht 3584 CX, The Netherlands.
E-mail address: l.a.a.brosens@umcutrecht.nl

Surgical Pathology 13 (2020) 431–452
https://doi.org/10.1016/j.path.2020.05.004

in areas with a low prevalence of *H pylori* infection as well as high use of proton-pump inhibitory therapy, for example, western countries.[3,4] Gastric polyps often arise in association with an inflammatory background or a polyposis syndrome. Careful attention to the background mucosa and awareness of syndromic gastric polyps are therefore important for correct interpretation and diagnosis of gastric polyps.

Gastric polyps can be classified based on their cell or epithelial compartment of origin (**Table 1**). The stomach consists of the following anatomic regions: cardia, fundus, body, antrum, and pylorus. These areas have variable histologic appearances, which reflect differences in physiologic functions. Gastric pits or foveolae, lined by mucus-secreting foveolar cells, comprise the whole luminal surface of the stomach. Underneath these pits, the mucous neck cells as well as deep gastric glands are located, of which the cellular composition is region-dependent. The glands in the fundus and body consist of parietal cells, chief cells, and enterochromaffin-like cells. In the cardia, antrum, and pylorus, mainly mucus cells with

Table 1
Overview of gastric epithelial polyps classified by cell or epithelial compartment of origin

Origin	Nonneoplastic	Neoplastic	
Foveolar layer	*Hyperplastic polyp*	*Foveolar-type adenoma*	*Intestinal-type adenoma*
Characteristics	Polyp consisting of dilated, branched, and elongated glands in edematous stroma Background of chronic gastritis	Polyp with atypical foveolar cells (at least low-grade dysplasia) No background of inflammation, atrophy, or metaplasia Expression of MUC5AC; usually no expression of MUC2	Polyp with intestinal-type columnar epithelium containing absorptive cells, goblet cells, endocrine cells, and/or Paneth cells with at least low-grade dysplasia Background of intestinal metaplasia and/or inflammation or atrophy. Variable expression of MUC2; no or slight expression of MUC5AC and MUC6
Of note	Histopathologically indistinguishable from hamartomatous polyp/hamartomatous polyposis syndrome Reasonable risk of malignancy (background)	Association with FAP Low risk of malignant transformation	Association with FAP (although rare) Relatively high risk of malignant transformation
Glandular layer	*Fundic gland polyp*	*Pyloric gland adenoma*	*Oxyntic gland adenoma*
Characteristics	Polyp consisting of dilated glands with parietal and chief cells and some mucous cells	Polyp with atypical pyloric-type glands (at least low-grade dysplasia) No background of inflammation, atrophy, or metaplasia Expression of MUC6; usually no expression of MUC2	Polyp with atypical oxyntic glands, consisting of chief cells or combination of chief and parietal cells (at least low-grade dysplasia) In general, no background of inflammation, atrophy, or metaplasia
Of note	Sporadic (association with PPI therapy) or in the context of FAP Low risk of malignant transformation	Association with several polyposis/tumor predisposition syndromes Relatively high risk of malignant transformation	Low risk of malignant transformation

clear cytoplasm line the deep glands with a small mixture of neuroendocrine cells. In the transitional zones, small numbers of parietal and chief cells are present. Familiarity with these histologic features will aid in gastric polyp recognition and diagnosis.

FUNDIC GLAND POLYP

INTRODUCTION

FGPs are the most common type of gastric polyp, comprising almost 80% of all gastric polyps, and seem to be more common in areas with low *H pylori* infection rates.[3,4] Sporadic FGPs are strongly related to the use of proton-pump inhibitors (PPIs). Long-term use leads especially to increased risk of developing FGPs. PPI therapy gives acid suppression, which elevates serum gastrin, a growth factor for oxyntic mucosa and a downstream target of Wnt signaling. Patients on PPI therapy have hyperplasia and protrusions of parietal cells in their gastric biopsy, which is thought to be an initial step in the development of an FGP. After this, there is development of small and subsequently larger fundic gland cysts. The glands dilate because of increased intraglandular pressure, probably because of the parietal cell hyperplasia that gives increased outflow resistance.

In younger patients with multiple FGPs (>20), that is, fundic gland polyposis, or FGPs with dysplasia, an underlying familial adenomatous polyposis (FAP) syndrome (owing to a germline mutation in the *Adenomatous Polyposis Coli* [*APC*] gene) or *MUTYH* polyposis should be considered, and colonoscopy is advised, in particular if there are also duodenal adenomas.

GROSS FEATURES

FGPs are typically less than 5 mm and have a smooth surface. Sporadic FGPs are usually solitary or few in number (**Fig. 1**). However, FGPs can be numerous in patients using PPIs and in patients with familial polyposis syndrome (**Fig. 2**).[5,6]

MICROSCOPIC FEATURES

FGPs are characterized by cystically dilated oxyntic glands mainly lined by parietal and chief cells and variable numbers of mucous neck cells (**Fig. 3**). The overlying foveolar surface is usually normal. Surface erosion can be present with resulting reactive changes of the foveolar epithelium, which may be misinterpreted as dysplasia. Sporadic single FGPs rarely show dysplasia; however, in some FGPs, dysplasia of the overlying foveolar epithelium is observed. Dysplasia in FGPs is of foveolar type, characterized by low columnar cells resembling foveolar cells with round to oval nuclei (**Fig. 4**). The cytoplasm contains a MUC5AC-positive mucin cap. The surrounding mucosa of FGPs is normal or shows signs of PPI use. There is no background of atrophy or intestinal metaplasia.

(DIFFERENTIAL) DIAGNOSIS

In general, FGPs are straightforward to diagnose both endoscopically and microscopically. Some FGPs can be difficult to differentiate from pyloric or oxyntic gland adenomas (OGAs), depending on the degree of cystic changes and pyloric or oxyntic differentiation, respectively. *GNAS* mutations are often present in pyloric gland adenomas

Fig. 1. Sporadic FGP: gross features. Several sporadic FGPs in the cardiac region of the stomach.

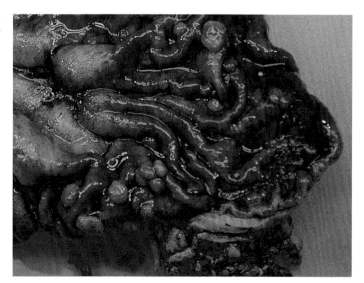

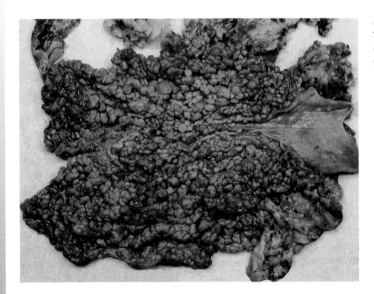

Fig. 2. FAP-associated FGP: gross features. Numerous FGPs and foveolar adenomas throughout the stomach of a patient with FAP syndrome.

(PGAs) and absent in FGPs, and this may be used to differentiate between PGA and FGP.[7] Very large FGPs can pose a differential diagnosis with HPs. The key difference between FGPs and HPs is that the cystically dilated glands in FGPs are lined by a mixture of cell types, including parietal and foveolar cells, whereas in HPs, the glands are lined by hyperplastic foveolar epithelium. FGPs with

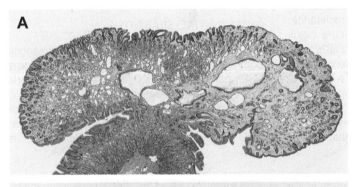

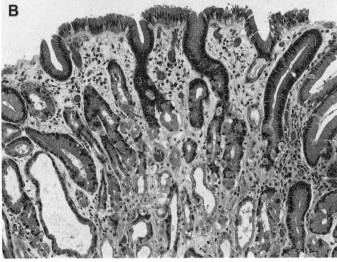

Fig. 3. FGP: microscopic features. (*A*) Low-power view of an FGP, consisting of cystically dilated glands lined by parietal and chief cells and variable numbers of mucous neck cells. (*B*) High-power view of the same polyp. The polyp is lined by nondysplastic foveolar epithelium at the surface.

Fig. 4. FGP with high-grade dysplasia. (*A*) This FGP from a patient with FAP shows a focus of high-grade dysplasia of the overlying foveolar epithelium, characterized by columnar cells showing severe nuclear atypia with round to oval, vesicular nuclei with prominent nucleoli and loss of polarity as well as some architectural atypia with crowding and branching of glands. (*B*) The dysplastic cells show p53 overexpression.

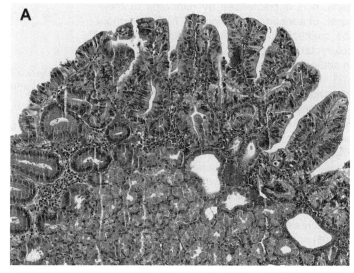

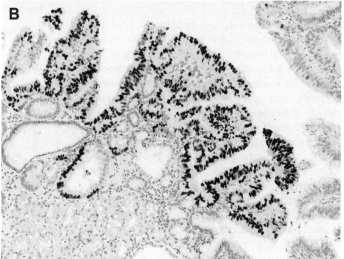

dysplasia can be difficult to distinguish from foveolar-type adenomas with low-grade dysplasia, but this is of little clinical significance because both lesions carry a low risk of neoplastic progression.[8]

PROGNOSIS, WHEN TO PONDER, WHEN TO PANIC

FGPs are generally regarded as nonneoplastic lesions, either hamartomatous or hyperplastic/functional in nature, because they are retention cysts caused by corpus gland secretion impairment. However, the frequent finding of mutations in the Wnt pathway (*APC* and *CTNNB1* genes) indicates that FGPs are neoplastic growths as well. Most (60%–90%) sporadic FGPs without dysplasia

have somatic *CTNNB1* mutations.[9,10] Dysplastic sporadic FGPs may have a somatic *APC* mutation without *CTNNB1* (β-catenin) mutation.[9] In contrast, FGPs in FAP show somatic second-hit inactivation of the *APC* gene that precedes dysplasia, but lacks *CTNNB1* mutations.[11] The type of second-hit *APC* mutation may play a role in the chance of progression to high-grade dysplasia in FAP-associated FGPs.[12]

Dysplasia in sporadic FGPs is extremely rare and has an indolent nature.[13–17] In general, sporadic FGPs do not progress to cancer and tend to regress when PPI therapy is stopped. Presence of FGPs is inversely correlated with *H pylori* infection, active gastritis, and gastric neoplasia.[18]

FAP is an autosomal-dominant polyposis syndrome caused by a germline mutation in the *APC* gene. It is characterized by hundreds to thousands of adenomatous polyps (≥100) throughout the colorectum and inevitable development of colorectal cancer if left untreated by colectomy. In addition, FAP patients develop several benign and malignant extracolonic lesions. In the stomach, most patients with FAP have multiple FGPs (polyposis). Low-grade dysplasia is often seen in FGPs in FAP, but the risk of malignant progression is low.[5,19] Based on older literature, western FAP patients are considered not to carry an increased risk of gastric cancer compared with the general population,[20] whereas a 3 to 4 times increased risk of gastric cancer was reported in FAP patients from South Korea and Japan.[21,22] The increased risk of gastric cancer in Asian populations likely results from higher prevalence of *H pylori* infection and associated atrophic gastritis and intestinal metaplasia in these populations.

However, several recent reports of FAP patients with gastric cancer suggest an increased incidence of gastric cancer in western patients.[23,24] Interestingly, these gastric cancers are almost exclusively located in the proximal stomach and are associated with extensive carpeting fundic gland polyposis, and a large size (>20 mm) of polyps and dysplasia.[25] One study reported an association between gastric cancer and desmoid tumors in FAP patients, suggesting a genotype-phenotype correlation for gastric cancer.[23] In addition, gastric adenocarcinoma and proximal polyposis of the stomach (GAPPS) is characterized by carpeting proximal fundic gland polyposis of the stomach with antral sparing, increased risk of gastric cancer, and no or a small number of duodenal and colorectal adenomas. Because it is caused by a point mutation in exon 1B of *APC*, it is now considered a variant of FAP with a unique gastric phenotype, further supporting that gastric cancer risk may depend on the genotype.[26–28] GAPPS patients with gastric cancer more often have gastric adenomas, FGPs, and PGAs with high-grade dysplasia.[25] Thus, although low-grade gastric foveolar-type dysplasia is not very alarming in FAP patients, extensive proximal gastric polyposis and possibly also the presence of PGAs (see later discussion) may be markers of an increased risk of proximal gastric cancer in FAP. In addition, it remains important to detect FAP patients with *H pylori* infection, gastric atrophy, and intestinal-type adenomas because these patients seem to be at increased risk for distal intestinal-type adenocarcinomas.[29]

Pathologic Key Features

- Cystically dilated oxyntic glands lined by parietal and chief cells
- Lined by nondysplastic foveolar epithelium
- Rarely foveolar-type dysplasia (mainly in FAP)

Differential Diagnosis

- Pyloric or oxyntic gland adenomas
- Large FGPs can be difficult to distinguish from HPs
- FGPs with dysplasia versus foveolar-type adenomas

Pitfall

! Multiple FGPs (fundic gland polyposis) are associated with FAP and GAPPS.

HYPERPLASTIC POLYP/INFLAMMATORY POLYP/HAMARTOMATOUS POLYP

INTRODUCTION

Gastric HPs are among the most common epithelial polyps of the stomach; incidences vary among populations and range between 15% and 75% of all gastric polyps.[30] HPs are localized, nonneoplastic mucosal expansions consisting of elongated, tortuous, and cystically dilated foveolae supported by an edematous lamina propria with distended vessels. In contrast to colonic HPs, which are neoplastic polyps, gastric HPs are reactive lesions resulting from reparative and regenerative responses to mucosal injury. First, there is an ongoing healing and reparative response in the form of foveolar hyperplasia after mucosal injury and erosion. This hyperplastic reaction can end or persist and progress with the formation of an

HP. Mostly the initial inflammation is caused by *H pylori* or autoimmune gastritis, although any agent causing chronic gastritis or mucosal erosion may lead to the formation of an HP. In addition, mucosal prolapse can result in HPs.[31] HPs can be multiple, which is the case in 20% of patients.[30] Gastric "inflammatory polyp" is a commonly used misnomer for an HP and should not be used in the stomach to avoid confusion with an inflammatory fibroid polyp. Hamartoma defines an overgrowth of normal tissue elements in their own native location. Hamartomatous gastric polyps are rare in the stomach and are, from a histopathological point of view, indistinguishable from HPs because they share the same morphology. Hamartomatous gastric polyps occur in the context of Peutz-Jeghers syndrome (PJS), juvenile polyposis syndrome (JPS), and Cowden (*PTEN* hamartoma tumor) syndrome.[32]

GROSS FEATURES

HPs are mostly small, generally less than 2 cm, although sizes of up to 12 cm are reported. The polyps are usually solitary, smooth or lobulated, and can be sessile or pedunculated. There is often surface erosion. HPs cannot reliably be distinguished from small adenomas endoscopically. HPs are most common in the antrum (60%), but may arise throughout the stomach, including the cardia and gastroesophageal area.[30,33]

MICROSCOPIC FEATURES

HPs have a polypoid form and show elongated, branching, and cystically dilated foveolar glands (Fig. 5). The foveolar cells have a hyperplastic appearance with abundant mucinous cytoplasm. The glands may contain prominent globoid cells. There is crowding of foveolar cells, and glands may be tortuous or have a corkscrew appearance. The lamina propria can be edematous and moderately to heavily infiltrated by immune cells. In other cases, the lamina propria is more fibrotic with or without chronic inflammatory infiltrate. The surface of the polyp can be eroded and have a regenerative appearance with nuclear enlargement and depletion of cytoplasmic mucin.[30] Small lesions may be best addressed as polypoid foveolar hyperplasia.[31]

(DIFFERENTIAL) DIAGNOSIS

HPs have an overlapping morphology with polyps arising in juvenile polyposis, Peutz-Jeghers (PJ) polyposis, and Cowden/*PTEN* hamartoma tumor syndrome (see Overview).[32] Many of the hamartomatous syndrome polyps lack specific histology,

and to distinguish them from each other and from sporadic HPs based on only histology is unreliable. Therefore, one should think of the possibility of an underlying hamartomatous polyposis syndrome in the case of multiple gastric hyperplastic-type polyps but at the same time be cautious to establish a diagnosis of a polyposis syndrome based on gastric polyp pathologic condition alone.[5,32] The syndromes in which they can occur are now briefly discussed.

PJS is an autosomal-dominant inherited disorder caused by a germline mutation in *LKB1* (*STK11*). Intestinal PJ polyps have characteristic features with an arborizing pattern of smooth muscle proliferating between mucosal epithelial components.[34] However, this is less pronounced in gastric PJ polyps (Fig. 6). Thus, in gastric polyps, there are mostly only foveolar hyperplastic features without the characteristic arborizing smooth muscle fibers. Therefore, clinical correlation and information on previous gastrointestinal polyps are necessary.[35] A classic clinical feature of PJS is perioral hyperpigmentation, and patients also are at high risk of developing malignancies in the gastrointestinal tract, pancreas, lung, breast, and gynecologic tract.[36] Diagnostic criteria for PJS are as follows: (1) 3 or more morphologically defined PJ polyps; (2) a personal diagnosis in combination with a family history of PJ polyps; and (3) characteristic mucocutaneous hyperpigmentation with a personal or family history of PJ polyps. Gastric cancer risk is increased with a cumulative lifetime risk of 29% from age 15 to 64 years.[36] Interestingly, polyps in PJS are likely not the obligate precursor lesion in PJS, but an epiphenomenon owing to mucosal prolapse. In this regard, it interesting to note that mucosal prolapse also plays a role in the pathogenesis of a subset of sporadic gastric HPs.[31] Dysplasia is rare in gastric PJ polyps.[5,37]

JPS is caused by germline mutation in *SMAD4* or *BMPR1A* and characterized by a few to multiple juvenile polyps throughout the gastrointestinal tract. Because germline mutations are only found in 50% to 60% of JPS patients, the diagnosis is made when a patient fulfills any of the following criteria: (1) 3 or more colorectal juvenile polyps; (2) juvenile polyps throughout the gastrointestinal tract; or (3) any number of juvenile polyps in combination with a family history of juvenile polyposis.[38,39] Gastric juvenile polyposis may be quite extensive, in particular, in patients with *SMAD4* germline mutations, and can simulate Ménétrier disease. Polyps are described being more "stroma-rich" with elongated filiform projections, smooth outer surfaces, and prominent stroma with edema and mixed inflammation (Fig. 7).[40]

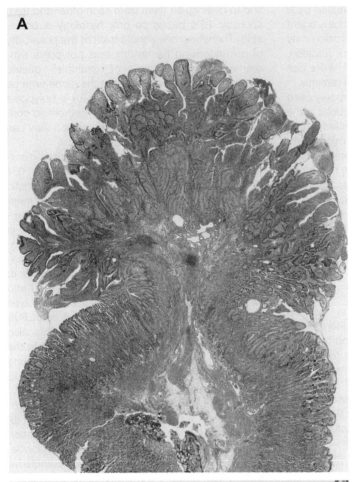

A

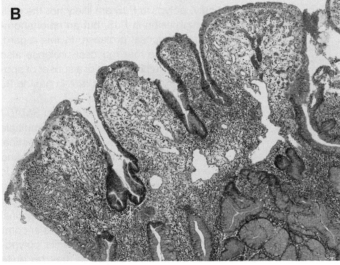

B

Fig. 5. HP. (*A*) Low-power view of an HP, showing elongated, branching, and cystically dilated foveolar glands with abundant mucinous cytoplasm. The lamina propria is edematous and infiltrated by immune cells. (*B*) High-power view of the same polyp.

On the other hand, "epithelium-rich" juvenile gastric polyps have little stromal edema, but tightly packed glands and surface epithelium with hyperplasia.[40] Immunohistochemistry for SMAD4 can be used because polyps from carriers of a *SMAD4* germline mutation can show decreased or absent staining compared with normal epithelium.[5,40,41] Massive gastric polyposis, associated

Fig. 6. PJ polyp (hamartomatous polyp). A PJ hamartomatous polyp showing an arborizing pattern of smooth muscle proliferation between the epithelial components. This characteristic arborization pattern is often less pronounced in gastric polyps compared with intestinal PJ polyps. Therefore, these polyps generally cannot be reliably distinguished from gastric HPs based on histopathological characteristics.

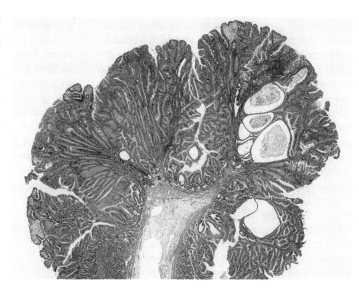

Fig. 7. Juvenile polyp (hamartomatous polyp). (*A*) Hamartomatous polyp in the context of JPS (juvenile polyp). Juvenile polyps are described as being more "stroma-rich" with smooth outer surfaces and prominent edematous and inflamed stroma. However, these polyps generally cannot be reliably distinguished from gastric HPs based on morphologic characteristics, although SMAD4 immunohistochemistry may be of help because juvenile polyps show decreased or absent staining compared with normal epithelium and (sporadic) HPs (*B*).

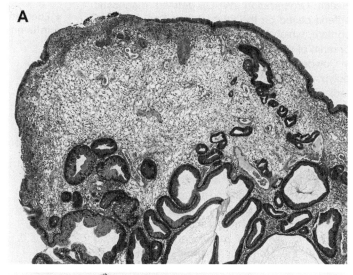

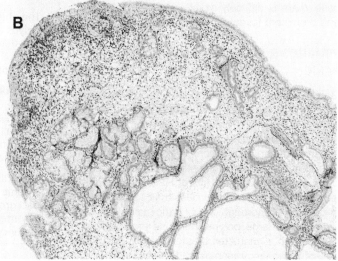

with *SMAD4* germline mutation, is often impossible to control endoscopically, and partial or complete gastrectomy is often necessary.[38] High-grade dysplasia and gastric cancer can develop in juvenile polyposis patients. Estimates of gastric cancer risk vary between 10% and 30%.[5,38,40]

Phosphatase and tensin homolog (PTEN) hamartoma tumor syndrome comprises a heterogeneous group of disorders, including Cowden (most cases), Bannayan-Riley-Ruvalcaba, and Proteus syndromes, all of which result from various germline mutations in *PTEN*. Clinical features of Cowden syndrome include mental retardation, macrocephaly, mucocutaneous lesions (facial trichilemmoma, acral keratoses, papillomatous papules), esophageal glycogenic acanthosis, thyroid lesions, fibrocystic disease, breast cancer, and a spectrum of gastrointestinal polyps, including hamartomatous polyps, adenomas, lipomas, and ganglioneuromas.[42,43] The World Health Organization (WHO) defined diagnostic criteria based on the International Cowden Consortium, which is based on the presence of one or more of the mentioned diseases that can occur in Cowden syndrome. Gastric Cowden syndrome polyps are multiple and small and simulate sporadic HPs.[44,45] Probably there is an increased gastric cancer risk, but no definite estimates are available.[43–45]

Biopsies in patients with Ménétrier disease show hyperplastic foveolar epithelium, which on biopsies may be impossible to differentiate from HPs. The clinical and endoscopic information and biopsies of surrounding mucosa are especially needed to distinguish HPs from the protein-losing gastropathy in Ménétrier disease. This condition typically involves the oxyntic area (fundus and body) of the stomach, whereas HPs are more commonly situated in the antrum. In Ménétrier disease, there is diffusely oxyntic glandular atrophy and prominent foveolar hyperplasia.[46]

PROGNOSIS, WHEN TO PONDER, WHEN TO PANIC

Gastric HPs were thought to be generally benign and banal polyps, but most HPs arise in a background of mucosal disease with a strong association with chronic gastritis with atrophy and intestinal metaplasia, which are the main risk factors of gastric cancer. Intestinal metaplasia can be observed in around 15% of HPs, dysplasia in less than 5%, and cancer in less than 1%.[30] There should be a thorough search and sampling for dysplasia in large polyps, because especially in polyps with a diameter greater than 2 cm, the risk of malignancy increases. Patients with HPs are at increased risk of gastric cancer, because of background of chronic (atrophic) gastritis in which HPs arise. Preferably, HPs are removed endoscopically in order to determine their nature and prove that the lesions are benign. Because HPs are important markers for an abnormal gastric mucosal background and are not isolated preneoplastic lesions, endoscopic evaluation with biopsies of the background mucosa is necessary to look for concomitant conditions like *H pylori* inflammation, intestinal metaplasia, atrophy, dysplasia, and malignancy.[47]

 Pathologic Key Features

- Elongated, branching, and dilated foveolar glands with a hyperplastic appearance with abundant mucinous cytoplasm
- Edematous stroma and chronic (active) inflammation

 Differential Diagnosis

- Syndromic hamartomatous polyps
- Ménétrier disease

 Pitfalls

! The histology of gastric hamartomatous polyps arising in the context of PJS, JPS, and Cowden syndrome is not specific, and reliable distinction between syndromic hamartomatous polyps and HPs is impossible.

! An underlying hamartomatous polyposis syndrome should be considered in the case of multiple gastric hyperplastic-type polyps. Clinical correlation is pivotal because these syndromes have typical clinical characteristics and a family history.

! Sporadic HPs are associated with *H pylori* chronic gastritis. Therefore, biopsies of the background mucosa are necessary to look for intestinal metaplasia, dysplasia, and malignancy.

GASTRIC FOVEOLAR-TYPE ADENOMA

INTRODUCTION

Gastric foveolar-type adenomas are epithelial polyps consisting of neoplastic foveolar epithelium.[39] Foveolar-type adenomas are rare and show an equal sex distribution.[8,48,49] The mean age of diagnosis is 44 years.[48,49] These adenomas can occur sporadically, but there is also an association with FAP and GAPPS.[8]

GROSS FEATURES

Gastric foveolar-type adenomas are typically solitary lesions, usually less than 1 cm in diameter, and occur more frequently in the body and fundus than in the antral region.[39,48,49] In patients with FAP or GAPPS, these polyps usually coexist with multiple FGPs (see above).[8]

MICROSCOPIC FEATURES

Gastric foveolar-type adenomas are composed of gastric epithelial mucin cells with a pink or pale apical mucin cap and show at least low-grade dysplasia (**Fig. 8**).[5,48,49] These polyps can be distinguished from the background mucosa by an abrupt transition from normal to atypical foveolar cells with hyperchromatic, crowded, and slightly disorganized nuclei, extending to the epithelial surface. Immunohistochemical expression for MUC5AC (gastric mucin marker) can confirm gastric differentiation, whereas expression of MUC6 (pyloric mucin marker), MUC2, and CDX2 (intestinal markers) are generally absent in these lesions.[48,49] Foveolar-type adenomas typically occur in normal gastric mucosa without metaplasia, atrophy, or inflammation.[5,48,49] Moreover, they rarely show high-grade dysplasia (characterized by severe nuclear atypia, loss of polarity, and/or architectural atypia) (**Fig. 9**) or carcinoma (**Fig. 10**).[5,48,49]

(DIFFERENTIAL) DIAGNOSIS

Differential diagnostic considerations include other types of gastric adenomas (intestinal-type adenomas and PGAs). The cytoplasmic feature of the foveolar cells as described above helps to distinguish foveolar-type adenomas from the other types, although distinction may become more challenging in high-grade dysplasia. Intestinal-type adenomas show at least focal goblet cell or Paneth cell differentiation. Gastric foveolar-type adenomas rarely show high-grade dysplasia or carcinoma, whereas this is more common in intestinal-type adenomas. Moreover, the background mucosa of intestinal-type adenomas typically shows inflammation, atrophy, and/or intestinal metaplasia, whereas the background mucosa of foveolar-type adenomas is normal.[48] No statistically significant differences in genetic mutations have been found between foveolar-type and intestinal-type adenomas.[50] Foveolar-type adenomas in the context of FAP show biallelic *APC* inactivation, whereas sporadic variants infrequently harbor *APC* or *KRAS* mutations.[39] PGAs are characterized by an apical neutral mucin cap, show expression for MUC6 rather than MUC5AC, and harbor *GNAS* mutations not found in gastric foveolar-type and intestinal-type adenomas (see later discussion).[51,52]

Fig. 8. Foveolar-type adenoma with low-grade dysplasia. High-power view of a foveolar-type adenoma with low-grade dysplasia, showing atypical foveolar cells at the surface with hyperchromatic, crowded, and slightly disorganized nuclei.

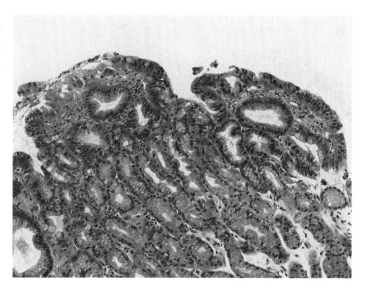

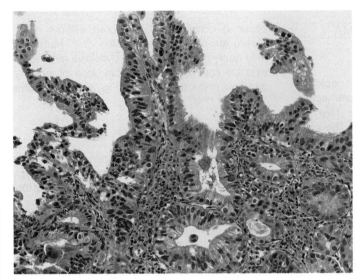

Fig. 9. Foveolar-type adenoma with high-grade dysplasia. High-power view of a foveolar-type adenoma with high-grade dysplasia, showing foveolar cells at the surface with more severe nuclear atypia as compared with **Fig. 8**, with round to oval, hyperchromatic nuclei with prominent nucleoli, loss of polarity, high nuclear-to-cytoplasmic ratio, and some architectural atypia with crowding and branching of glands. This case was from a patient with FAP syndrome.

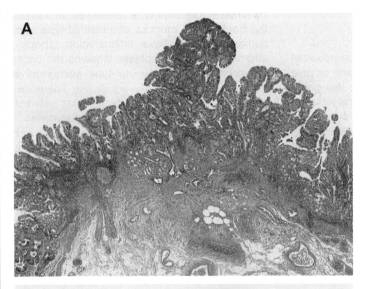

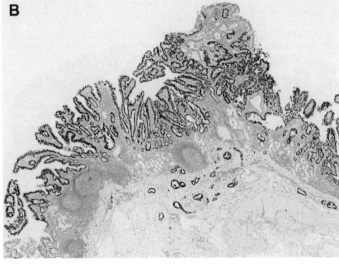

Fig. 10. Foveolar-type adenoma with invasive carcinoma. (*A*) This foveolar-type adenoma shows intramucosal and superficial submucosal invasion with atypical back-to-back glands. (*B*) The neoplastic and invasive glands can be easily detected in this p53 staining, as they show p53 overexpression.

PROGNOSIS, WHEN TO PONDER, WHEN TO PANIC

For foveolar-type adenomas, the rate of progression to high-grade dysplasia or cancer is exceedingly low (irrespective of sporadic or familial setting).[8,48] A genetic background of FAP syndrome can be found in 68% of foveolar-type adenomas.[8] Foveolar-type adenomas are the most frequent type of gastric adenomas in western FAP patients (85%). It should be noted, however, that distinguishing a gastric foveolar-type adenoma and an FGP with low-grade dysplasia can be difficult, but this is of little clinical significance because both lesions harbor a low risk of malignant transformation.[8] Similar to sporadic cases, the background mucosa of FAP patients with a foveolar-type adenoma is typically normal. Western FAP patients likely do not carry an increased risk of gastric cancer, although recently several cases of gastric cancer were reported in western patients with FAP and GAPPS[23,24,53] (see also above, Prognosis of fundic gland polyps).

Pathologic Key Features

- Lesion composed of foveolar cells with a clear or pale apical mucin cap

- Per definition, at least low-grade dysplasia

- Immunohistochemistry: expression of MUC5AC; negative for MUC2, CDX2, and MUC6

- In general, normal background gastric mucosa

Differential Diagnosis

- Intestinal-type adenoma (at least focal presence of goblet cells and/or Paneth cells, expression of MUC2, background gastric mucosa with inflammation, atrophy, and intestinal metaplasia)

- Pyloric gland adenoma (pyloric-type glands, expression of MUC6)

- FGP with dysplasia (cystically dilated glands lined by parietal and chief cells)

- Reactive atypia (more gradual gradient in atypia, background of inflammation/erosion)

Pitfall

! Association with FAP and GAPPS (low risk of malignant transformation)

GASTRIC INTESTINAL-TYPE ADENOMA

INTRODUCTION

Gastric intestinal-type adenomas are localized polypoid lesions composed of dysplastic intestinalized epithelium and are the most frequent type of all gastric adenomas.[39] They occur more commonly in men than women (ratio 3:1), and usually in patients 60 to 80 years of age.[48] Risk factors for developing this type of adenoma are any cause of gastric intestinal metaplasia (eg, *H pylori* infection, autoimmune atrophic gastritis).[39]

GROSS FEATURES

Gastric intestinal-type adenomas are usually single, well-circumscribed, sessile or pedunculated lesions, measuring less than 2 cm^3. They are mostly found in the antral and pyloric region (about 60%) where intestinal metaplasia is most prevalent.[50]

MICROSCOPIC FEATURES

Gastric intestinal-type adenomas show an intestinal-type columnar epithelium containing absorptive cells, goblet cells, endocrine cells, and/or Paneth cells (although they may be sparse) and show by definition at least low-grade dysplasia (**Fig. 11**). These lesions show columnar cells with hyperchromatic, elongated nuclei with pseudostratification and crowding, extending to the surface, similar to tubular adenomas in the colon and rectum. There is increased mitotic activity. Often, a distinct brush border is present that confirms intestinal differentiation in the dysplastic epithelium. Because of an abrupt transition from the background mucosa with striking hyperchromasia, these lesions can usually be easily detected at low power, although reactive epithelial changes in surrounding mucosa can cause diagnostic challenges. Architectural complexity (cribriform, branching, budding, or crowding glands) as well as severe cytologic atypia (rounded nuclei with loss of polarity, clumped chromatin, and prominent nucleoli) are features of high-grade dysplasia.

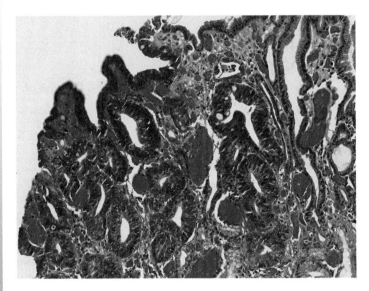

Fig. 11. Intestinal-type adenoma. High-power view of an intestinal-type adenoma with low-grade dysplasia, showing columnar cells with hyperchromatic, elongated nuclei and pseudostratification, extending to the surface. Several goblet cells and Paneth cells can be seen.

Almost all intestinal-type adenomas occur in background gastric mucosa with *H pylori* infection (42%), background gastritis and atrophy (environmental atrophic metaplastic gastritis [52%], autoimmune metaplastic atrophic gastritis [19%]), and/or intestinal metaplasia.[5,48] Intestinal-type adenomas show variable expression of intestinal markers MUC2 and CD10. There is no or slight expression for gastric mucins MUC5AC and MUC6.

(DIFFERENTIAL) DIAGNOSIS

Differential diagnostic considerations include other types of gastric adenomas (foveolar-type adenomas and PGAs; see Differential diagnosis section of Gastric foveolar-type adenomas). Another diagnostic difficulty can be caused by reactive epithelial changes due to inflammation or erosion, which is frequently present in chronic gastritis. In contrast to intestinal-type adenomas, reactive atypia is characterized by a gradual gradient in atypia from the background mucosa with slight hyperchromatic nuclei and no nuclear crowding.

PROGNOSIS, WHEN TO PONDER, WHEN TO PANIC

It is important to realize that intestinal-type adenomas have a reasonable risk of malignant transformation. Approximately 40% of lesions show high-grade dysplasia, and approximately 25% progress to adenocarcinoma.[48,50] Therefore, complete (endoscopic) excision is important, and the lesions should be processed entirely for microscopic examination to identify potential areas of high-grade dysplasia or carcinoma. Moreover, these adenomas are also associated with separate foci of intestinal metaplasia (97%), flat dysplasia (6%), and adenocarcinoma (16%) elsewhere in the stomach.[48] Therefore, biopsies of the background mucosa are crucial.

Intestinal-type adenomas are very rare in western FAP patients (1%–2% of gastric adenomas in FAP) but more common in Asian FAP patients, probably related to differences in prevalence of *H pylori* infection and atrophic gastritis.[8,54] FAP patients with intestinal-type adenomas with additional *H pylori* infection and gastric atrophy especially seem to have an increased risk of developing intestinal-type gastric adenocarcinoma.[29,54]

 Pathologic Key Features

- Localized lesion composed of dysplastic intestinalized epithelium with at least focal presence of goblet cells and/or Paneth cells

- Per definition, at least low-grade dysplasia

- Immunohistochemistry: expression of MUC2; negative for MUC5AC and MUC6

- Background gastric mucosa often shows inflammation, atrophy, and/or intestinal metaplasia

Differential Diagnosis

- Foveolar-type adenomas (foveolar-type cells with pale or clear mucin cap, no goblet cells or Paneth cells)

- Pyloric gland adenoma (pyloric-type glands, positive for MUC6)

- Reactive atypia (more gradual gradient in atypia)

! Pitfalls

! Reasonable risk of malignant transformation (high-grade dysplasia or carcinoma in same lesion, or presence of synchronous lesions with high-grade dysplasia or carcinoma)

! Association with FAP syndrome, especially in non-western populations

! FAP patients with intestinal-type adenoma together with *H pylori* infection and gastric atrophy are especially at risk for developing gastric adenocarcinoma

GASTRIC GLANDULAR ADENOMAS: PYLORIC GLAND ADENOMA AND OXYNTIC GLAND ADENOMA

INTRODUCTION

PGA and OGA are rare polyps. They are the most recently recognized gastric epithelial polyps, characterized by closely packed pyloric or oxyntic glands, respectively. Of these polyps, PGAs are the more common. Sporadic PGAs are found in patients with conditions resulting in pyloric metaplasia, such as autoimmune atrophic gastritis or chronic *H pylori* gastritis. More than 30% of PGAs arise in a background of autoimmune atrophic gastritis.[49,55] Nevertheless, PGAs remain a rare finding, even in patients with autoimmune atrophic gastritis, and most polyps in patients with autoimmune atrophic gastritis are HPs (80%), oxyntic mucosa pseudopolyps (10%), or intestinal adenomas (10%).[56] Of note, PGAs were recently also described in FAP patients, where

they arise in nonatrophic background mucosa.[8] PGAs have also been reported in Lynch syndrome, McCune-Albright syndrome, and JPS.[57–59] Various terms have been used in the literature for gastric neoplasms with oxyntic gland differentiation. Most such lesions are best addressed as OGA, whereas rare cases with atypia and submucosal invasion may be better addressed as gastric adenocarcinoma of fundic gland type (GA-FG).[60] Neoplasms with oxyntic gland differentiation are exceedingly rare, and most cases have been reported in Japanese literature. Gastric glandular adenoma has been suggested as an appropriate unifying diagnostic term for polyps arising from the glandular compartment, as opposed to gastric foveolar and intestinal type adenomas.[7]

GROSS FEATURES

Most PGAs form polypoid lesions or masses varying from a few millimeters to 10 cm, with an average of 2 cm. OGAs tend to be smaller in size (usually <1 cm), whereas GA-FG are larger (1.5–4 cm).

MICROSCOPIC FEATURES

Histologically, PGA is characterized by densely packed cuboidal to low columnar epithelium resembling pyloric gland cells (**Fig. 12**). Immunohistochemically, PGAs are positive for both MUC6 (strong) and MUC5AC (slight or partially). PGAs typically lack expression of intestinal markers MUC2 and CDX2, although MUC2 is sometimes positive in areas with transition to intestinal metaplasia.[61] High-grade dysplasia has been reported in about half of PGAs and is characterized by disturbed architecture and loss of nuclear polarity. Ki-67 immunohistochemistry can be helpful to identify high-grade dysplasia in PGAs (**Fig. 13**). Activating *GNAS* mutations are relatively specific for PGA because it is found in most PGAs but not in gastric foveolar-type or intestinal-type adenomas or FGPs.[7,51,52]

Gastric neoplasms with oxyntic gland differentiation are characterized by closely packed oxyntic gland with either a monotonous proliferation of chief cells or an admixture of chief cells and parietal cells resembling fundic glands (**Fig. 14**).[60,62] Most of these tumors have only very mild atypia and are restricted to the mucosa. These lesions are benign and best addressed as OGA. Some of these lesions show superficial submucosal involvement (<0,1 cm). Larger lesions (>1.5 cm) can show more aggressive histologic features with deeper submucosal invasion, atypical cellular differentiation (ie, mucus neck or foveolar

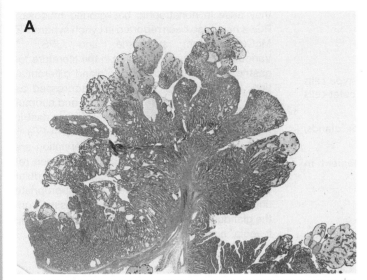

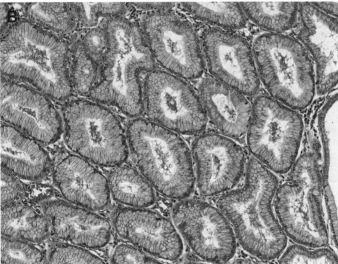

Fig. 12. PGA. (*A*) Low-power view of a PGA showing densely packed, sometimes cystically dilated, monotonous pyloric-type glands. (*B*) High-power view of the same polyp showing cells with ground-glass cytoplasm. PGAs show strong expression of MUC6 (not shown).

differentiation), and mild to moderate nuclear atypia and may be best addressed as GA-FG.[60] In contrast to PGA, OGAs arise in oxyntic mucosa without atrophy or pyloric metaplasia.[60]

(DIFFERENTIAL) DIAGNOSIS

The differential diagnosis is mainly with other gastric glandular polyps, such as FGP. In contrast to GA-FG, dysplastic changes in FGP are only present in the superficial foveolar layer, whereas the glandular part of the lesion lacks atypia and architectural complexity. Depending on the background mucosa, distinction between PGA and OGA can be challenging.[7] There is a morphologic continuum between OGA and GA-FG, if these are indeed considered as separate entities.[63]

PROGNOSIS, WHEN TO PONDER, WHEN TO PANIC

Up to half of PGAs harbor high-grade dysplasia, but submucosal invasion is rare (<10%).[49,64] Therefore, radical local excision is indicated. After radical resection, recurrence rate is low (<10%).[64] Although submucosal invasion is commonly found in OGA, these lesions have a very low malignant potential. Lymphovascular invasion has only been found in lesions fulfilling criteria of GA-FG. Even in those cases with invasion, lymph node metastasis is extremely rare, and complete (endoscopic) resection of GA-FG seems adequate treatment.[60,63,65]

In contrast to sporadic cases, PGAs in FAP patients develop in nonatrophic mucosa and show variable presence of parietal cells, making differentiation from OGA sometimes very difficult or even impossible. Based on these observations and the common *GNAS* mutations in OGA and PGA, it has been hypothesized that PGA and OGA are likely the same lesions within a spectrum with subtle histologic differences depending on the background mucosa in which they arise.[7]

Pathologic Key Features

- Pyloric gland adenoma: densely packed pyloric-type glands
- OGA: closely packed oxyntic glands (can be chief cell-predominant or an admixture of chief cells and parietal cells)

Differential Diagnosis

- FGPs
- Distinction between PGA and OGA can be difficult and may depend on type of background mucosa (eg, atrophic mucosa with pseudopyloric metaplasia or nonatrophic oxyntic mucosa)
- OGA versus GA-FG is a histologic continuum

HOW TO RECOGNIZE EARLY INVASION IN GASTRIC POLYPS (INTRAMUCOSAL CARCINOMA)

INTRODUCTION

Most gastric polyps, such as adenomas, HPs, FGPs, and PGAs, are sporadic with no significant malignant potential; however, it is important to search for areas of high-grade dysplasia and infiltrative growth. Early gastric cancer, defined as carcinoma confined to the mucosa or submucosa, may be encountered in endoscopically benign-appearing polyps.[65] Especially in the Japanese population, there is experience with the risks that intramucosal cancers exhibit. Patients with well-differentiated early gastric cancer

limited to the mucosa or the upper submucosa (SM1, up to a depth of 500 μm) and without lymphovascular invasion generally have a very low risk of lymph node metastases.[65,66] Therefore, surgery is not necessary in most early gastric cancers, and these may be treated effectively with endoscopic resection or endoscopic polypectomy.

MICROSCOPIC FEATURES

Polyps with low-grade dysplasia are characterized by mild to moderate nuclear atypia and crowding of nuclei with mild pseudostratification. There is no complex architecture. Features of high-grade dysplasia are cribriform architecture, marked glandular crowding, full-thickness nuclear stratification, and severe nuclear atypia. Intramucosal carcinomas are defined by invasion into the lamina propria. It is difficult to distinguish nuclear features of intramucosal carcinomas from high-grade dysplasia. Features in favor of carcinoma are syncytial growth pattern, effacement of normal architecture with back-to-back glands, and single cells infiltrating the lamina propria (see **Fig. 10**). Often there are cystic glands. Desmoplastic stroma is often lacking or difficult to detect in intramucosal cancer. Intramucosal cancer should be classified and graded. Classification is preferably according to the WHO classification scheme.[39] Grading applies only to tubular and papillary gastric cancers. A tumor can be designated as poorly differentiated if there are marked architecturally distorted glands and single cells are present. Tumors with signet ring cells or diffuse growth are classified as poorly cohesive cancers; these gastric cancers often have a higher stage with consequently a poor prognosis. Therefore, limited endoscopic resection is often inferior for the treatment of these tumors, especially in a western population. Assessing the extent of invasion into the mucosa and/or submucosa is essential to determine whether the patient requires a (partial) gastrectomy.[65] As for all gastric polyps, the nonneoplastic surrounding epithelium should be assessed for features predisposing to neoplasia, such as intestinal metaplasia, atrophic mucosa, and *H pylori* infection.

CONCLUDING REMARKS

In this review, the authors provide an overview of different types of gastric epithelial polyps, based

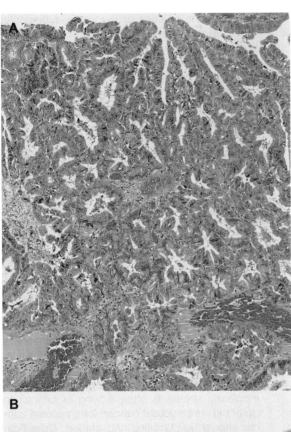

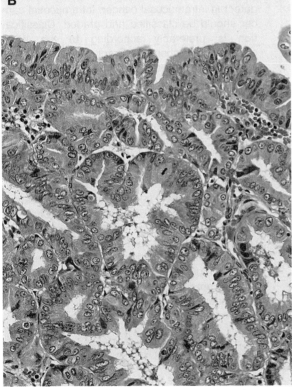

Fig. 13. High-grade dysplasia in a PGA. (*A*) High-grade dysplasia in a PGA characterized by complex architecture and loss of nuclear polarity. (*B*) High-power view showing loss of nuclear polarity and mitotic activity.

Fig. 13. (*continued*). (*C*) Increased Ki-67 immu-nolabeling in high-grade dysplasia in a PGA. Note Ki-67 negativity in the low-grade glands at the bottom.

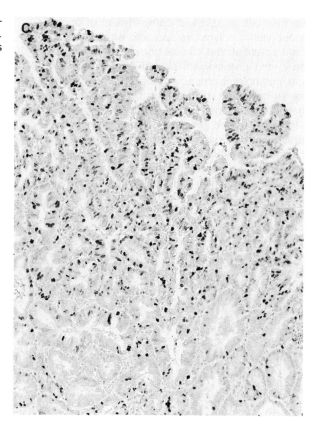

Fig. 14. OGA. High-power view of an OGA showing densely packed oxyntic glands with a monotonous prolifera-tion of parietal and chief cells.

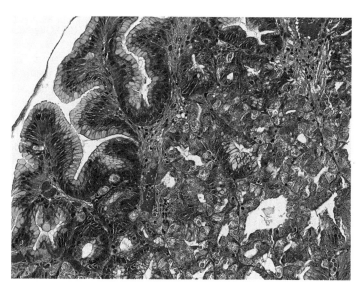

on their cell or epithelial compartment of origin. Most gastric polyps are sporadic with no malignant potential, but clinical correlation is necessary, and pathologists should be familiar with the morphologic characteristics of gastric polyps as an indication for a search for an underlying genetic syndrome, such as FAP, PJS, or JPS. Moreover, in the presence of a gastric polyp, preferably biopsies of background mucosa are taken of at least the antrum and corpus. Evaluation of the background nonpolypoid mucosa is essential in reaching a diagnosis that can characterize the condition in which the polyp developed, which may have therapeutic consequences.

ACKNOWLEDGMENTS

The authors thank Folkert Morsink for his help with the figures.

DISCLOSURE

The authors have nothing to disclose.

REFERENCES

1. Park DY, Lauwers GY. Gastric polyps: classification and management. Arch Pathol Lab Med 2008; 132(4):633–40.
2. Castro R, Pimentel-Nunes P, Dinis-Ribeiro M. Evaluation and management of gastric epithelial polyps. Best Pract Res Clin Gastroenterol 2017;31(4):381–7.
3. Carmack SW, Genta RM, Graham DY, et al. Management of gastric polyps: a pathology-based guide for gastroenterologists. Nat Rev Gastroenterol Hepatol 2009;6(6):331–41.
4. Carmack SW, Genta RM, Schuler CM, et al. The current spectrum of gastric polyps: a 1-year national study of over 120,000 patients. Am J Gastroenterol 2009;104(6):1524–32.
5. Brosens LAA, Wood LD, Offerhaus GJ, et al. Pathology and genetics of syndromic gastric polyps. Int J Surg Pathol 2016;24(3):185–99.
6. Vogt S, Jones N, Christian D, et al. Expanded extracolonic tumor spectrum in MUTYH-associated polyposis. Gastroenterology 2009;137(6):1976–85.e1-10.
7. Hackeng WM, Montgomery EA, Giardiello FM, et al. Morphology and genetics of pyloric gland adenomas in familial adenomatous polyposis. Histopathology 2017;70(4):549–57.
8. Wood LD, Salaria SN, Cruise MW, et al. Upper GI tract lesions in familial adenomatous polyposis (FAP). Am J Surg Pathol 2014;38(3):389–93.
9. Abraham SC, Park SJ, Mugartegui L, et al. Sporadic fundic gland polyps with epithelial dysplasia: evidence for preferential targeting for mutations in the adenomatous polyposis coli gene. Am J Pathol 2002;161(5):1735–42.
10. Sekine S, Shibata T, Yamauchi Y, et al. Beta-catenin mutations in sporadic fundic gland polyps. Virchows Arch 2002;440(4):381–6.
11. Abraham SC, Nobukawa B, Giardiello FM, et al. Fundic gland polyps in familial adenomatous polyposis. Am J Pathol 2000;157(3):747–54.
12. Sekine S, Shimoda T, Nimura S, et al. High-grade dysplasia associated with fundic gland polyposis in a familial adenomatous polyposis patient, with special reference to APC mutation profiles. Mod Pathol 2004;17(11):1421–6.
13. Straub SF, Drage MG, Gonzalez RS. Comparison of dysplastic fundic gland polyps in patients with and without familial adenomatous polyposis. Histopathology 2018;72(7):1172–9.
14. Levy MD, Bhattacharya B. Sporadic fundic gland polyps with low-grade dysplasia: a large case series evaluating pathologic and immunohistochemical findings and clinical behavior. Am J Clin Pathol 2015;144(4):592–600.
15. Abraham SC. Fundic gland polyps: common and occasionally problematic lesions. Gastroenterol Hepatol (N Y) 2010;6(1):48–51.
16. Burt RW. Gastric fundic gland polyps. Gastroenterology 2003;125(5):1462–9.
17. Torbenson M, Lee J-H, Cruz-Correa M, et al. Sporadic fundic gland polyposis: a clinical, histological, and molecular analysis. Mod Pathol 2002;15(7): 718–23.
18. Genta RM, Schuler CM, Robiou CI, et al. No association between gastric fundic gland polyps and gastrointestinal neoplasia in a study of over 100,000 patients. Clin Gastroenterol Hepatol 2009; 7(8):849–54.
19. Brosens LAA, Offerhaus GJA, Giardiello FM. Hereditary colorectal cancer: genetics and screening. Surg Clin North Am 2015;95(5):1067–80.
20. Offerhaus GJ, Giardiello FM, Krush AJ, et al. The risk of upper gastrointestinal cancer in familial adenomatous polyposis. Gastroenterology 1992;102(6): 1980–2.
21. Park J-G, Park KJ, Ahn Y-O, et al. Risk of gastric cancer among Korean familial adenomatous polyposis patients. Dis Colon Rectum 1992;35(10):996–8.
22. Iwama T, Mishima Y, Utsunomiya J. The impact of familial adenomatous polyposis on the tumorigenesis and mortality at the several organs. Its rational treatment. Ann Surg 1993;217(2):101–8.
23. Walton S-J, Frayling IM, Clark SK, et al. Gastric tumours in FAP. Fam Cancer 2017;16(3):363–9.
24. Mankaney G, Leone P, Cruise M, et al. Gastric cancer in FAP: a concerning rise in incidence. Fam Cancer 2017;16(3):371–6.
25. Leone PJ, Mankaney G, Sarvapelli S, et al. Endoscopic and histologic features associated with

gastric cancer in familial adenomatous polyposis. Gastrointest Endosc 2019;89(5):961–8.

26. Worthley DL, Phillips KD, Wayte N, et al. Gastric adenocarcinoma and proximal polyposis of the stomach (GAPPS): a new autosomal dominant syndrome. Gut 2012;61(5):774–9.

27. Li J, Woods SL, Healey S, et al. Point mutations in exon 1B of APC reveal gastric adenocarcinoma and proximal polyposis of the stomach as a familial adenomatous polyposis variant. Am J Hum Genet 2016;98(5):830–42.

28. van der Post RS, Carneiro F. Emerging concepts in gastric neoplasia: heritable gastric cancers and polyposis disorders. Surg Pathol Clin 2017;10(4): 931–45.

29. Leggett B. FAP: another indication to treat H pylori. Gut 2002;51(4):463–4.

30. Abraham SC, Singh VK, Yardley JH, et al. Hyperplastic polyps of the stomach: associations with histologic patterns of gastritis and gastric atrophy. Am J Surg Pathol 2001;25(4):500–7.

31. Gonzalez-Obeso E, Fujita H, Deshpande V, et al. Gastric hyperplastic polyps: a heterogeneous clinicopathologic group including a distinct subset best categorized as mucosal prolapse polyp. Am J Surg Pathol 2011;35(5):670–7.

32. Lam-Himlin D, Park JY, Cornish TC, et al. Morphologic characterization of syndromic gastric polyps. Am J Surg Pathol 2010;34(11):1656–62.

33. Abraham SC, Singh VK, Yardley JH, et al. Hyperplastic polyps of the esophagus and esophagogastric junction: histologic and clinicopathologic findings. Am J Surg Pathol 2001;25(9):1180–7.

34. Tse JY, Wu S, Shinagare SA, et al. Peutz-Jeghers syndrome: a critical look at colonic Peutz-Jeghers polyps. Mod Pathol 2013;26(9):1235–40.

35. Shaco-Levy R, Jasperson KW, Martin K, et al. Morphologic characterization of hamartomatous gastrointestinal polyps in Cowden syndrome, Peutz-Jeghers syndrome, and juvenile polyposis syndrome. Hum Pathol 2016;49:39–48.

36. Giardiello FM, Brensinger JD, Tersmette AC, et al. Very high risk of cancer in familial Peutz-Jeghers syndrome. Gastroenterology 2000;119(6): 1447–53.

37. Jansen M, de Leng WWJ, Baas AF, et al. Mucosal prolapse in the pathogenesis of Peutz-Jeghers polyposis. Gut 2006;55(1):1–5.

38. Syngal S, Brand RE, Church JM, et al. ACG clinical guideline: genetic testing and management of hereditary gastrointestinal cancer syndromes. Am J Gastroenterol 2015;110(2):223–62, [quiz: 263].

39. Lokuhetty D, White VA, Watanabe R, et al, WHO Classification of tumors 5th edition Digestive system. IARC 2019;76-80.

40. Gonzalez RS, Adsay V, Graham RP, et al. Massive gastric juvenile-type polyposis: a clinicopathological analysis of 22 cases. Histopathology 2017;70(6): 918–28.

41. Langeveld D, van Hattem WA, de Leng WWJ, et al. SMAD4 immunohistochemistry reflects genetic status in juvenile polyposis syndrome. Clin Cancer Res 2010;16(16):4126–34.

42. Shaco-Levy R, Jasperson KW, Martin K, et al. Gastrointestinal polyposis in Cowden syndrome. J Clin Gastroenterol 2017;51(7):e60–7.

43. Pilarski R, Burt R, Kohlman W, et al. Cowden syndrome and the PTEN hamartoma tumor syndrome: systematic review and revised diagnostic criteria. J Natl Cancer Inst 2013;105(21):1607–16.

44. Coriat R, Mozer M, Caux F, et al. Endoscopic findings in Cowden syndrome. Endoscopy 2011;43(8):723–6.

45. Levi Z, Baris HN, Kedar I, et al. Upper and lower gastrointestinal findings in PTEN mutation–positive Cowden syndrome patients participating in an active surveillance program. Clin Transl Gastroenterol 2011;2(11):e5.

46. Wolfsen HC, Carpenter HA, Talley NJ. Menetrier's disease: a form of hypertrophic gastropathy or gastritis? Gastroenterology 1993;104(5):1310–9.

47. Goddard AF, Badreldin R, Pritchard DM, et al, British Society of Gastroenterology. The management of gastric polyps. Gut 2010;59(9):1270–6.

48. Abraham SC, Montgomery EA, Singh VK, et al. Gastric adenomas. Am J Surg Pathol 2002;26(10): 1276–85.

49. Chen Z-M, Scudiere JR, Abraham SC, et al. Pyloric gland adenoma: an entity distinct from gastric foveolar type adenoma. Am J Surg Pathol 2009; 33(2):186–93.

50. Abraham SC, Park SJ, Lee J-H, et al. Genetic alterations in gastric adenomas of intestinal and foveolar phenotypes. Mod Pathol 2003;16(8):786–95.

51. Matsubara A, Sekine S, Kushima R, et al. Frequent GNAS and KRAS mutations in pyloric gland adenoma of the stomach and duodenum. J Pathol 2013;229(4):579–87.

52. Hashimoto T, Ogawa R, Matsubara A, et al. Familial adenomatous polyposis-associated and sporadic pyloric gland adenomas of the upper gastrointestinal tract share common genetic features. Histopathology 2015;67(5):689–98.

53. de Boer WB, Ee H, Kumarasinghe MP. Neoplastic lesions of gastric adenocarcinoma and proximal polyposis syndrome (GAPPS) are gastric phenotype. Am J Surg Pathol 2017;42(1):1.

54. Nakamura S, Matsumoto T, Kobori Y, et al. Impact of Helicobacter Pylori Infection and Mucosal Atrophy on Gastric Lesions in Patients With Familial Adenomatous Polyposis. Gut 2002;51(4):485–9. https://doi.org/10.1136/gut.51.4.485.

55. Vieth M, Kushima R, Borchard F, et al. Pyloric gland adenoma: a clinico-pathological analysis of 90 cases. Virchows Arch 2003;442(4):317–21.

56. Park JY, Cornish TC, Lam-Himlin D, et al. Gastric lesions in patients with autoimmune metaplastic atrophic gastritis (AMAG) in a tertiary care setting. Am J Surg Pathol 2010;34(11):1591–8.

57. Lee SE, Kang SY, Cho J, et al. Pyloric gland adenoma in Lynch syndrome. Am J Surg Pathol 2014; 38(6):784–92.

58. Ma C, Giardiello FM, Montgomery EA. Upper tract juvenile polyps in juvenile polyposis patients: dysplasia and malignancy are associated with foveolar, intestinal, and pyloric differentiation. Am J Surg Pathol 2014;38(12):1618–26.

59. Wood LD, Noë M, Hackeng W, et al. Patients with McCune-Albright syndrome have a broad spectrum of abnormalities in the gastrointestinal tract and pancreas. Virchows Arch 2017;470(4):391–400.

60. Ushiku T, Kunita A, Kuroda R, et al. Oxyntic gland neoplasm of the stomach: expanding the spectrum and proposal of terminology. Mod Pathol 2019. https://doi.org/10.1038/s41379-019-0338-1.

61. Vieth M, Kushima R, Mukaisho K, et al. Immunohistochemical analysis of pyloric gland adenomas using a series of Mucin 2, Mucin 5AC, Mucin 6, CD10, Ki67 and p53. Virchows Arch 2010;457(5): 529–36.

62. Singhi AD, Lazenby AJ, Montgomery EA. Gastric adenocarcinoma with chief cell differentiation. Am J Surg Pathol 2012;36(7):1030–5.

63. Benedict MA, Lauwers GY, Jain D. Gastric adenocarcinoma of the fundic gland type: update and literature review. Am J Clin Pathol 2018;149(6): 461–73.

64. Choi W-T, Brown I, Ushiku T, et al. Gastric pyloric gland adenoma: a multicentre clinicopathological study of 67 cases. Histopathology 2018;72(6): 1007–14.

65. Gannon BR, Riddell RH. Gastric polyps with intramucosal carcinoma. Pathol Case Rev 2008;13(5): 199–202.

66. Ishikawa S, Togashi A, Inoue M, et al. Indications for EMR/ESD in cases of early gastric cancer: relationship between histological type, depth of wall invasion, and lymph node metastasis. Gastric Cancer 2007;10(1):35–8.

Approaches to Biopsy and Resection Specimens from the Ampulla

Yue Xue, MD, PhD[a], Michelle D. Reid, MD, MS[b],*

KEYWORDS

- Ampulla • Ampullary • Duodenal adenoma • Ampullary carcinoma
- Intra-ampullary papillary-tubular neoplasm • IAPN

Key points

- The ampulla of Vater is a unique saclike transitional zone where multiple anatomic structures of divergent histology converge.
- Ampullary carcinoma is frequently a tubular-type adenocarcinoma (of intestinal, pancreatobiliary, or mixed [in 40%] lineage), but nontubular carcinoma may also occur.
- Ampullary carcinoma has a much better prognosis than pancreatic ductal adenocarcinoma, hence anatomic distinction is critical.
- Anatomic/site-specific classification of ampullary carcinoma has shown prognostic significance and is incorporated into the new College of American Pathologists synoptic protocols.
- Prognostic markers in ampullary carcinoma include location (or site-specific classification), histologic type (pancreatobiliary is worse than intestinal), pathologic stage, and MUC5AC expression.

ABSTRACT

The ampulla of Vater gives rise to a versatile group of cancers of mixed/hybrid histologic phenotype. Ampullary carcinomas (ACs) are most frequently intestinal or pancreatobiliary adenocarcinomas but other subtypes, such as medullary, mucinous, or signet ring/poorly cohesive cell carcinoma, may be encountered. Ampullary cancer can also be subclassified based on immunohistochemical features, however these classification systems fail to show robust prognostic reliability. More recently, the molecular landscape of AC has been uncovered, and has been shown to have prognostic and predictive significance. In this article, the site-specific, histologic, and genetic characteristics of ampullary carcinoma and its precursor lesions are discussed.

CARCINOMA OF THE AMPULLA OF VATER

The term ampulla describes a spherical or globular flask with 2 handles that was used by the ancient Greeks and Romans to transport ointments or wine. The ampulla of Vater is a complex saclike outpouching that represents the convergence of multiple anatomic and histologic structures. It consists of 4 compartments featuring 3 types of lining epithelium: (1) the distal common bile duct and pancreatic duct, which are lined by pancreatobiliary-type epithelium; (2) the mucosa of papilla of Vater (ie, the duodenal protuberance surrounding the ampullary orifice), which is covered by specialized epithelium resembling gastric-foveolar epithelium and has scattered goblet cells; (3) the duodenal surface of the papilla,

[a] Department of Pathology and Laboratory Medicine, Northwestern University, 251 East Huron Street, Room 7332, Chicago, IL 60611, USA; [b] Department of Pathology and Laboratory Medicine, Emory University Hospital, 1364 Clifton Road Northeast, Room H 180A, Atlanta, GA 30322, USA
* Corresponding author.
E-mail address: michelle.reid@emory.edu

Surgical Pathology 13 (2020) 453–467
https://doi.org/10.1016/j.path.2020.05.005
1875-9181/20/© 2020 Elsevier Inc. All rights reserved.

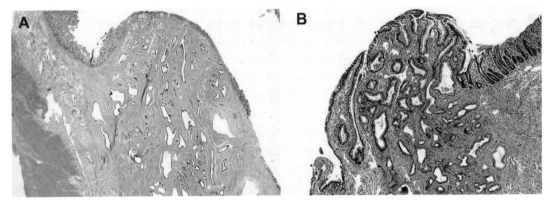

Fig. 1. The ampulla of Vater is a raised, dome-shaped mucosal elevation. (*A*) It consists of 4 compartments: (1) a roof of duodenal mucosa and (2) papilla of Vater, (3) a lateral wall of ductules and sphincter Oddi muscle, and (4) a floor consisting of distal common bile duct and pancreatic duct (PD) (hematoxylin-eosin, original magnification ×200). (*B*) It features 3 types of epithelium: (1) pancreatobiliary, which lines the common bile duct, PD, and ductules of the ampullary wall; (2) specialized gastric foveolar–like epithelium, which covers the papilla of Vater; and (3) small intestinal epithelium, which covers the duodenal surface of the papilla (hematoxylin-eosin, original magnification ×400).

which is lined by small intestinal epithelium; (4) the wall of the ampulla with Oddi musculature and ductules that are lined by pancreatobiliary-type epithelium (**Fig. 1**). These compartments have not only distinctive histology but also functional properties, each bringing its own chemical milieu, which makes this small region, and the neoplasms that develop within it, highly complex and diagnostically challenging. Recently, with more standardized grossing protocols,[1,2] careful analysis of the tumors that arise in this area has led to more

refined classification and elucidated more specific characteristics of ampullary cancers.[3–8]

PREINVASIVE NEOPLASMS

Adenomas of the Ampullary Duodenum

In order to qualify as an ampullary duodenal adenoma (ADA), greater than 75% of the lesion must involve the duodenal surface. Depending on size and location, patients may have signs of biliary obstruction prompting endoscopy and discovery

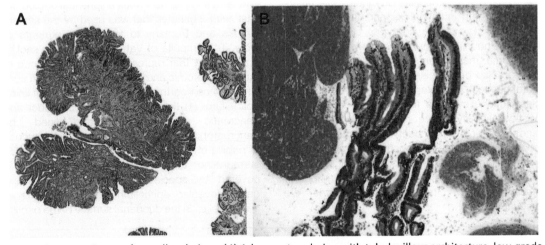

Fig. 2. Biopsy specimens of ampullary lesions. (*A*) Adenomatous lesion with tubulovillous architecture, low-grade dysplasia (lower half of central fragment), and high-grade dysplasia (upper half of central fragment) including basally located cribriform, basophilic glands (hematoxylin-eosin, original magnification ×200). (*B*) Fine-needle aspiration biopsy of ampullary lesion shows adenomatous epithelium with tubulovillous architecture and low-grade dysplasia. Follow-up resection of this patient (see **Fig. 4**A) showed an IAPN with low-grade dysplasia (hematoxylin-eosin, original magnification ×200).

of polypoid tubular, villous, or tubulovillous masses (**Fig. 2**). ADAs are either sporadic or associated with familial adenomatous polyposis (FAP) syndrome. The ampulla is a common extracolonic site of involvement in patients with FAP.[9–11] Intestinal-type ADAs are histologically similar to their colorectal counterparts and, although typically low-grade, they can also show high-grade dysplasia characterized by more significant cytologic atypia and architectural complexity, including greater nuclear enlargement, pseudostratification and irregularity, high nuclear to cytoplasmic ratio, nuclear angulation, prominent nucleoli, increased mitoses and fusion, and/or branching of tubules, with single cell necrosis and luminal necrotic debris (see **Fig. 2**). Reactive mucosal changes may closely mimic ADA, and, depending on severity, the 2 may be impossible to distinguish.[12,13]

Adenomas of the ampullary duodenum are more likely to harbor invasive carcinoma than similarly sized colorectal adenomas. Invasive carcinoma that arises in ADAs is often hidden in the polyp's base and is difficult to detect in superficial biopsies (see **Fig. 2**). The presence of a large, firm, or eroded mucosal nodule that converges with adjacent duodenal mucosa and is associated with duct dilatation should prompt careful examination for an invasive component on limited biopsies. Adenomatous epithelium may extend into ductules of the nearby normal papilla and can thus simulate invasive adenocarcinoma on biopsy. The presence of paradoxic differentiation with cuboidal, eosinophilic, pancreatobiliary-type epithelium; nonlobular architecture and irregularly shaped glands; micropapillary tufting; marked cytologic atypia; and loss of polarity are all suggestive of an invasive carcinoma component. In addition, traditional architectural markers of invasion (tumor budding, desmoplasia, perineural and lymphvascular invasion) are even more helpful but may not be seen on superficial biopsies.[6,7] Another diagnostic differential to consider when evaluating duodenal and ampullary biopsies is mucosal basement membrane colonization (so-called cancerization) by an underlying invasive carcinoma of the ampulla.[14,15] This colonization can simulate high-grade dysplasia or even reactive atypia (**Fig. 3**). Identifying the features described earlier, as well as a 2-cell population, and abrupt transition between benign and atypical epithelium/glands, helps with recognition of this phenomenon. Because invasive carcinoma

is often pancreatobiliary (rather than intestinal), immunohistochemical stains can potentially distinguish between the 2, because pancreatobiliary adenocarcinoma is positive for CK7 and MUC1, whereas intestinal (adenomatous) epithelium expresses intestinal markers CK20, MUC2, and CDX2, plus or minus CK7 (see **Fig. 3**). A low threshold of suspicion for colonization is required to accurately identify these cases. Other potentially useful immunohistochemical markers include p53, MUC5AC, and S100P, which can show either abnormal expression (p53) or positive staining (MUC5AC and S100P) in pancreatobiliary-type carcinoma/colonization and wild-type expression (p53) or negative staining (MUC5AC and S100P) in benign/reactive epithelium, whereas SMAD4 is lost in pancreatobiliary-type carcinoma (if *SMAD4* is mutated) and retained in reactive epithelium (see **Fig. 3**).[5,16,17]

Intra-ampullary Papillary-Tubular Neoplasm

Unlike ADAs, intra-ampullary papillary-tubular neoplasms (IAPNs) are (noninvasive) adenomatous masses (tumoral intraepithelial neoplasms) in which the bulk (at least 75%) of the lesion is located within the ampullary channel.[7,18–20] IAPNs are considered by some to represent the intra-ampullary counterpart of intraductal papillary (mucinous) neoplasms of the pancreas (IPMN) and biliary tract (IPN-B). Large papillary or polypoid tumors can fill and distend the ampullary channel and may minimally (<25%) extend into the distal common bile duct and main pancreatic duct (**Fig. 4**). The mean age of affected patients is 64 years, and tumors show a male predominance.[12,21]

On gross examination of the ampullary duodenum, IAPNs typically cause domelike elevation of intact mucosa, often with a patent papilla orifice from which nodules of friable granular material may protrude into the duodenum. On bivalving of the pancreatic head and ampulla, IAPNs grow as exophytic granular masses.[1,3,7] Ulceration may be evident, but overt mucinous discharge, characteristic of IPMNs of the pancreatic head, is seldom encountered. Microscopically, IAPNs show varying degrees of papillary and/or tubular growth with a (frequently mixed) spectrum of dysplasia. Unlike ADAs, ~50% of IAPNs are of hybrid/mixed phenotype (ie, intestinal, gastric, and/or pancreatobiliary), which is reflected in their immunoprofiles, where they coexpress

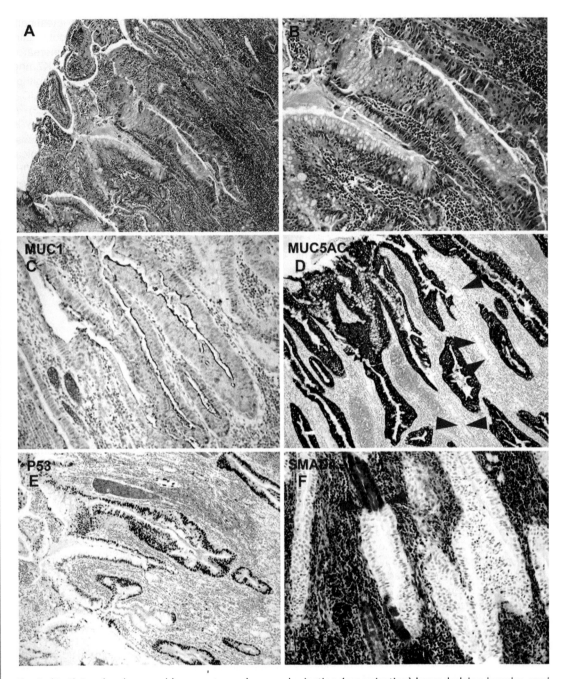

Fig. 3. (*A, B*) Duodenal mucosal basement membrane colonization (cancerization) by underlying invasive carcinoma of ampulla. There is a 2-cell population, with abrupt transition between benign intestinal-type epithelium/glands and atypical, eosinophilic, pancreatobiliary-type epithelium (hematoxylin-eosin, original magnification X 40× [*A*] and [*B*] hematoxylin-eosin, original magnification X 200×). The colonizing pancreatobiliary-type adenocarcinoma is positive for MUC1 (*C*), MUC5AC (*D*), and p53 (*E*), and shows loss of SMAD4 (*F*). These stains highlight the sharp transition between colonized cancer cells and benign intestinal surface epithelium and glands (arrowheads indicate normal glands with opposite immunoprofile to the carcinoma).

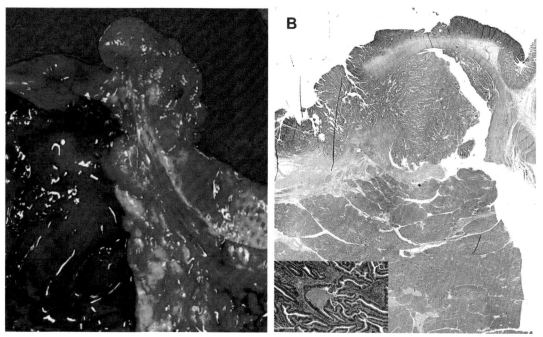

Fig. 4. (*A*) Gross specimen shows growth of IAPN as an exophytic/polypoid lesion that focally extends into the common bile duct. (*B*) Whole-mount slide of IAPN with predominant papillae filling the intra-ampullary channel with occasional luminal debris (*inset*).

the keratins CK7 and CK20 in more than 50% of cases, as well as intestinal (MUC2 and CDX2) and gastropancreatobiliary (MUC1, MUC5AC, and MUC6) markers.[4,7]

Approximately 75% of IAPNs are associated with invasive carcinoma (intestinal, pancreatobiliary, or mixed phenotype).[3,7] The invasive component is usually deeply placed, microscopic (>1.0 cm), and subject to being overlooked (or not sampled on superficial biopsies), hence the importance of extensive or total sampling of these lesions.[7] If completely resected, IAPNs have an excellent prognosis. Recurrence is common, particularly when high grade, and can be seen even years after the initial resection. Hence, long-term follow-up is critical even when noninvasive.[7] Nonetheless, IAPNs with an associated invasive adenocarcinoma component have far better survival (perhaps because of early biliary obstruction) than conventional (invasive) ampullary carcinomas that are unaccompanied by an IAPN (3-year survival of 69% vs 44%).[7]

Key Points
PREINVASIVE NEOPLASMS OF THE AMPULLA

	ADA	IAPN
Location	>75% of lesion involves duodenal surface	>75% of lesion is within ampullary channel
Bile Duct Obstruction	Uncommon (because of size)	Common
Architecture	Tubular, villous, or tubulovillous	Papillary or tubular
Morphology	Intestinal	Intestinal, pancreatobiliary (or gastric), mixed
High-grade Dysplasia	Uncommon	Common
Invasive Carcinoma	Uncommon	Common (75%)

Differential Diagnosis
PREINVASIVE NEOPLASMS
OF THE AMPULLA

ADA and IAPN

Entity	Associations
Reactive changes	Inflammation, Low nuclear to cytoplasmic ratio, Smooth nuclear contours, Increased mitoses but no atypical mitoses
Extension of adenomatous epithelium to ductules	Glands with smooth regular contours, Lack of stromal response, single cell necrosis, or confluent necrosis; No evidence of paradoxic differentiation, gland fusion, or complexity
Invasive carcinoma	Large, firm, eroded mucosal nodule, Convergence with duodenal mucosa, Bile duct obstruction and dilatation, Marked cytologic atypia, loss of polarity, paradoxic differentiation with pancreatobiliary-type epithelium, nonlobular arrangement of glands, irregularly shaped glands, or glands with micropapillary tufting
Surface colonization by underlying invasive carcinoma	May mimic high-grade dysplasia Frequently pancreatobiliary (rather than intestinal) type, 2-cell population, Abrupt transition between benign and carcinomatous epithelium/glands; Pancreatobiliary: + for CK7, MUC1, MUC5AC, S100P, ±SMAD4 loss, abnormal p53 expression Intestinal: + for CK20, MUC2, CDX2, ±CK7, abnormal p53 expression

INVASIVE ADENOCARCINOMAS

Invasive ampullary carcinomas (ACs) are rare and comprise 0.5% of all gastrointestinal cancers and 6% to 9% of all periampullary cancers.[3,19] Although usually sporadic, they can also arise in FAP.[9–11] Based on their gross appearance and location, ACs are divided into site-specific categories that are now incorporated into the College of American Pathologists (CAP) synoptic reporting cancer protocols.[22] Detailed description of the bivalving grossing technique for pancreatoduodenectomy specimens, which ensures identification of even minute ACs, exceeds the limits of this article but is outlined in detail in Adsay and colleagues. "Whipple Made Simple for Surgical Pathologists,".[1]

SITE-SPECIFIC CLASSIFICATION OF INVASIVE ADENOCARCINOMA

Based on location, invasive AC can be divided into 3 main categories, which have been incorporated into the CAP cancer protocols.[22] These categories are (1) intra-ampullary, (2) periampullary-duodenal, and (3) ampullary carcinoma, not otherwise specified (NOS) (mixed).[3,8,13,22,23]

1. Intra-ampullary:
   A. IAPN-associated ACs are associated with a large preinvasive (IAPN) component (75% of which must be within the ampulla).[3,6–8,13] From the duodenal surface, they dilate and may protrude from the ampullary orifice. On bivalving of the pancreatic head, common bile duct, and pancreatic ducts, the bulk of the tumor appears as a tan, friable, noninvasive mass (see **Fig. 4**) (discussed earlier in relation to IAPN) with only a limited (often microscopic) invasive component. This subtype often has a relatively good prognosis if completely resected (median survival >10 years).
   B. Ampullary-ductal AC is the other intra-ampullary tumor, but it is biologically different from IAPN-associated AC and is considered the ampullary counterpart of pancreatic ductal adenocarcinoma (PDAC) or distal common bile duct carcinoma. Unlike IAPN-associated AC, ampullary-ductal AC does not have a significant adenomatous/preinvasive component but instead forms small scirrhous (often circumferential) infiltrating tumors that may extend into and constrict the pancreatic and distal common bile ducts, while preserving (or minimally altering) the papilla of Vater and ampullary-

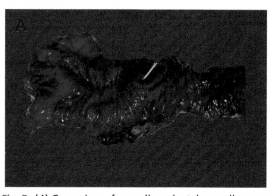
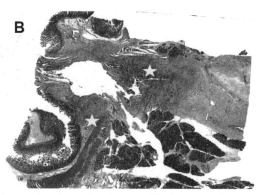

Fig. 5. (*A*) Gross view of ampullary-ductal ampullary carcinoma showing volcanic crater–like lesion on the ampullary orifice. (*B*) Whole-mount slide showing the lesion (indicated by stars) involving the distal segments of main PD and common bile duct.

duodenal mucosa (**Fig. 5**).[3,6,13] Ampullary-ductal AC typically may produce a subtle buttonlike duodenal mucosal elevation, and, if the bivalving grossing technique is not used, it can easily be missed. Some tumors can significantly undermine the duodenal mucosa, leading to ulceration (see **Fig. 5**). Although frequently small (<2.0 cm), ampullary-ductal ACs are frequently high T stage, metastatic to lymph nodes (57%), and have the shortest median survival (38 months) of all (site-specific) AC subtypes (discussed later), but significantly better survival than PDAC.[3,4,6,8,13] Microscopically, ampullary-ductal AC often proves to be of pancreatobiliary phenotype.

2. Periampullary:
   A. Periampullary-duodenal AC arises from the ampullary duodenum and is the largest (>4.0 cm) of the invasive ACs. It forms ulcerovegetative masses that are easily identifiable from the mucosal surface, with the ampullary orifice located eccentrically within the tumor.[3,13] Although large, these typically have a better prognosis than the other site-specific subtypes.[3,4,8,13]

3. Ampullary, NOS:
   A. Ampullary carcinoma, NOS is presumed to arise from the papilla of Vater (the duodenal mucosal edge where the main pancreatic duct and common bile duct merge into the duodenal mucosa; **Fig. 6**) and thus is neither truly intra-ampullary nor periampullary/duodenal but a combination of both because it cannot be confidently placed into any of the categories discussed earlier.[3,6,8,13,22]

Fig. 6. Ampullary carcinoma, NOS. The infiltrating glands form an ill-defined mass that involves the papilla of Vater and extends to the duodenal mucosa (hematoxylin-eosin).

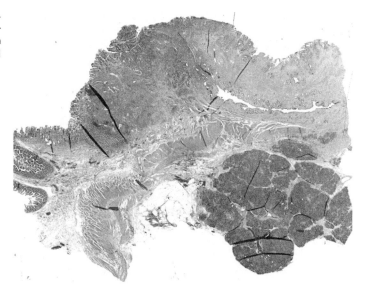

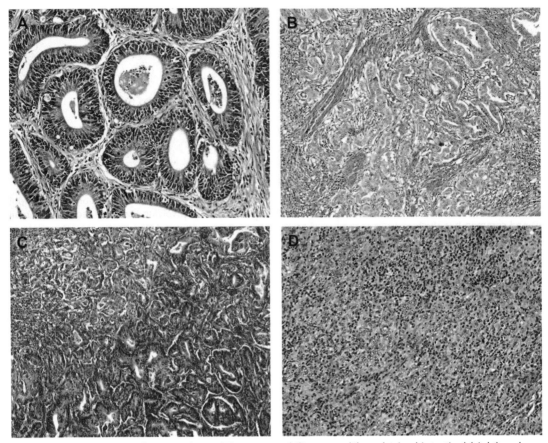

Fig. 7. Invasive carcinoma of intestinal type (*A*), pancreatobiliary type (*B*), and mixed intestinal (*right*) and pancreatobiliary (*left*) phenotype (*C*). (*D*) Medullary carcinoma of ampulla with syncytial growth of tumor cells with numerous lymphocytes interspersed.

HISTOLOGIC CLASSIFICATION OF INVASIVE ADENOCARCINOMA

The ampulla is lined by 3 distinct types of glandular epithelium (intestinal, biliary, and gastric-foveolar), reflecting the transitional nature of this landmark where multiple tributaries converge. As a result, the invasive cancers that develop therein are morphologically disparate. AC is most frequently tubular/glandular, and is divided into 3 main morphologic phenotypes: intestinal, pancreatobiliary, and mixed pancreatobiliary-intestinal (or gastric-foveolar).[4,24,25] Despite their frequent mixed phenotype, an attempt at morphologic classification is always warranted because of the proven correlation between histologic subtype and prognosis (discussed later).[2–4,23]

Intestinal Phenotype

Most invasive ACs are characterized by glandular units that are lined by variably differentiated intestinal-type epithelium with morphologic and immunophenotypic (CK20, MUC2, and CDX2 positive; CK7 and MUC1 negative) kinship to conventional colonic adenocarcinomas (**Fig. 7**A). These types are commonly associated with intestinal-type adenomas.[3,4,7,13] Periampullary-duodenal ACs are often of intestinal phenotype and have an associated intestinal-type adenomatous component from which they are thought to arise. IAPN-associated ACs also frequently have an intestinal component, which may or may not predominate.[7] Intestinal-predominant (or pure) phenotype AC is the largest (mean size 4.5 cm), compared with pure pancreatobiliary-type (2.2 cm) or mixed pancreatobiliary-intestinal (2.7 cm) AC, and has a longer median (although not significant) survival than the pure pancreatobiliary or mixed pancreatobiliary-intestinal AC (80 vs 40 vs 56 months).[4,26–28] All other clinicopathologic characteristics (nodal status, T stage, as well as 3-year and 5-year survival rates) are not significantly different.[4]

Pancreatobiliary Phenotype

Pancreatobiliary ACs are also characterized by variably differentiated glands; clusters or singly dispersed nonstratified cuboidal or low columnar eosinophilic epithelium containing round to oval, irregular, hypochromatic or hyperchromatic nuclei with abundant desmoplastic stroma; as well as morphologic and immunophenotypic kinship (CK7 and MUC1 positive; CK20, MUC2, and CDX2 negative) to pancreatic/biliary carcinomas (**Fig. 7B**).[4] They rarely have an associated adenomatous component. Ampullary-ductal ACs are typically purely of pancreatobiliary phenotype. IAPN-associated ACs can have (pure) pancreatobiliary or (mixed) pancreatobiliary-predominant morphology. Pancreatobiliary-predominant/pure ACs are the smallest (mean size 2.2 cm) of all site-specific subtypes, but have higher T stage, more frequent lymph-vascular and perineural invasion, lymph node metastasis, and comparatively shorter survival (40 months) than intestinal (pure/mixed predominant) AC, but longer survival than PDAC.[3–5,7,8,13,26–28] Although ACs with gastric-type mucin (both histologically and immunophenotypically) have been classified as gastric-type AC, they are more closely related to pancreatobiliary-type AC, and the 2 are often regarded as 1.

Mixed/Hybrid Pancreatobiliary-Intestinal Phenotype

A significant proportion of ACs (>40% in our experience) are of mixed or ambiguous phenotype (**Fig. 7C**).[3,4,6,8] Mixed/hybrid ACs show poor interobserver agreement on morphologic classification and are often immunohistochemically mixed as well, thus making them difficult to definitively categorize.[5,7,24,25,29] These ambiguous cases should be classified as tubular AC with mixed features, but the predominant pattern should be noted in the pathology report. Mixed-phenotype ACs have clinicopathologic characteristics that are between their intestinal and pancreatobiliary counterparts, but their median survival (56 months) is closer to that of pure pancreatobiliary (40 months) than intestinal AC (80 months).[4,27,30–36]

Key Points
CLINICOPATHOLOGIC ASSOCIATIONS OF SITE-SPECIFIC TYPES OF INVASIVE ADENOCARCINOMA OF AMPULLA OF VATER[3,13,19]

	Intra-ampullary (40%)		Periampullary (5%)	Ampullary, NOS (55%)
—	IAPN-Associated (25%)	Ampullary-ductal (15%)	—	—
Preinvasive Component	Large preinvasive (IAPN) component	No/limited preinvasive component	Preinvasive adenomatous component common	± preinvasive component
Duodenal Mucosal Findings	Dilated orifice, protruding polypoid, friable lesion, central AoV	Buttonlike elevation, intact or minimally ulcerated mucosa, central AoV	Large ulcerated, vegetative duodenal mucosal masses, peripheral AoV	Ulcerated ± polypoid ampullary lesion with central AoV
Size of Invasion	Small (1.5 cm)	Small (<2.0 cm)	Large (3.4 cm)	Small (1.8 cm)
Histology	Frequently mixed	Pure/ predominantly pancreatobiliary	Frequently intestinal (pure/ predominant)	Predominantly pancreatobiliary
Lymph Node Metastasis (%)	28	41	50	42
T Stage (T1–2/T3–4 Ratio)	5.8	0.6	2	1.6
5-y Survival (%)	53	29	55	39

Abbreviation: AoV, ampulla of Vater.

<table>
<tr><td colspan="2" align="center">Gross/Site-Specific Classification of Ampullary Carcinoma</td></tr>
</table>

• Intra-ampullary: ampullary-ductal	Typically pancreatobiliary, is the most aggressive despite small size
• Intra-ampullary: intra-ampullary papillary tubular neoplasm	Large noninvasive component; small invasive component; frequent lymph node metastasis; longest survival of the subtypes
• (Peri)ampullary-duodenal (duodenal surface of papilla)	Large size; 50% show lymph node metastasis, but indolent despite large size
• Ampullary, NOS	—
Histologic Classification of Ampullary Carcinoma	
• Intestinal	Better prognosis than pancreatobiliary
• Pancreatobiliary	Worse prognosis than intestinal AC but better than PDAC
• Mixed type (40%)	—
Prognostic correlation of histologic typing is not as strong as previously reported.	

Other Histologic Phenotypes

Nontubular carcinomas may involve the ampulla, but these are far less common. By definition, mucinous adenocarcinoma has greater than 50% mucinous component with a limited intestinal epithelial component that floats within pools of mucin.[19,37] Poorly cohesive cell carcinoma is highly aggressive and composed of single (frequently signet ring) cells that invade the surrounding stroma.[38] Medullary carcinoma accounts for 3% of ACs (**Fig. 7D**) and forms nodular syncytial masses of tumor cells with an associated lymphocytic infiltrate.[13,19] AC may also show squamous or neuroendocrine differentiation or may be undifferentiated with osteoclastlike giant cells, or rhabdoid cells that show SWI/SNF (switch/sucrose non-fermentable) complex deficiency (with resultant loss of nuclear SMARCB1/INI-1).[39–42] Mesenchymal neoplasms have rarely been reported to arise in the ampulla, including ganglioneuroma and rhabdomyosarcoma. Their pathologic features are similar to those that arise in other anatomic locations.[13]

IMMUNOHISTOCHEMICAL PROFILE OF AMPULLARY CARCINOMA

In addition to the site-specific and morphologic classification of ACs, an immunohistochemistry (IHC)-based classification system is also used (discussed earlier) and is endorsed in oncologists' management protocols.[5,24,25,29] Immunohistochemical panels used in IHC classification are based on observations of MUC2, CK20, and CDX2 positivity in intestinal ACs, and MUC1 and CK7 positivity in pancreatobiliary AC.[5,24,25,29] However, multiple studies have shown

that these putative lineage markers fail to definitively classify a significant percentage (up to 40%) of ACs and have no prognostic significance.[5,24,29] These ambiguous cases highlight inherent flaws with these IHC panels. The authors recently found that positivity for MUC5AC, a gastric IHC marker that was overlooked in almost all earlier large-scale AC studies, is an independent poor prognosticator in AC.[5]

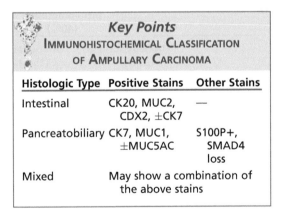

Key Points
IMMUNOHISTOCHEMICAL CLASSIFICATION
OF AMPULLARY CARCINOMA

Histologic Type	Positive Stains	Other Stains
Intestinal	CK20, MUC2, CDX2, ±CK7	—
Pancreatobiliary	CK7, MUC1, ±MUC5AC	S100P+, SMAD4 loss
Mixed	May show a combination of the above stains	

MOLECULAR CHARACTERISTICS OF AMPULLARY CARCINOMA

Recent development in sequencing technologies have provided important advances in the comprehension of the biology of AC, and have highlighted that there is significant genetic overlap, even in seemingly unambiguous cases.[43–46] Sporadic and FAP-associated ampullary adenomas show molecular abnormalities associated with Wnt signaling, including *APC* and *KRAS* mutations,

Fig. 8. This invasive ampullary carcinoma invades duodenum (submucosa, muscularis propria, subserosal adipose tissue, and superficial pancreatic parenchyma, <0.5 cm), and is consistent with stage pT3a carcinoma.

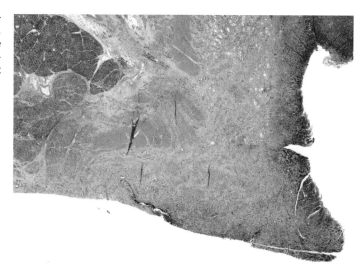

and less frequently mutations in *BRAF* and mismatch repair genes (seen in 15%).[47–50] Like colorectal cancer, intestinal-type ACs show mutation of *APC* in greater than 50% of cases, whereas pancreatobiliary-type ACs show predominant *KRAS*, *TP53*, and *SMAD4* mutations, of similar frequency to PDAC.[17,47,48,50,51] In addition, *ELF3* has been implicated as a novel driver gene in AC[17,50] and, along with *KRAS* and *TP53*, may be mutated in all histologic subtypes, suggesting shared biological mechanisms in development. Mafficini and colleagues[49] showed that *TP53* and *KRAS* status were also independent prognostic predictors of survival regardless of histologic subtype. This finding provides additional support for reconsideration of the histologic and IHC classification, because their genetic landscapes show significant overlap. Molecular profiling also has better prognostic reliability than histologic classification and can better select patients that respond to different chemotherapeutic regimens, regardless of histologic type. *ERBB2* amplification has been shown in up to 23% of ACs and is mutually exclusive with downstream *KRAS/NRAS/BRAF* mutations that are responsible for resistance of therapies targeting *ERBB2*.[43,49]

Key Points
GENOMIC PROFILING OF AMPULLARY CARCINOMA

- Histologic subtypes show differences in prevalence for some genes.

- TP53, KRAS, APC, and ELF3 are often mutated in all histologic subtypes.

- ELF3 is also an important driver gene in ampullary carcinogenesis.

- ERBB2 amplification is seen in up to 23%.

STAGING OF AMPULLARY CARCINOMA

The (2017) eighth edition of the American Joint Committee on Cancer (AJCC) Cancer Staging Manual[52] and updated CAP Cancer Protocol for Carcinoma of the Ampulla of Vater revealed changes to the pathologic T and N classification and have added greater complexity to the staging of an already challenging anatomic site. First, subcategories were introduced for the T stage based on depth of invasion beyond the sphincter of Oddi (T1a) into the duodenal submucosa (T1b), duodenal muscularis propria (T2), superficial (≤0.5 cm) (T3a) or deep pancreas, peripancreatic soft tissue or duodenal serosa (T3b) (**Fig. 8**); or involvement of the celiac axis, superior mesenteric artery, and/or common hepatic artery. In addition, lymph node (pN) staging was subdivided into N1 (1–3 positive nodes) and N2 (±4 positive nodes). This subdivision was done because recent studies have shown that the number of positive lymph nodes independently affects survival in AC.[53,54] A minimum of 12 regional lymph nodes is required for optimal staging. Lymph node metastases are more frequent in pancreatobiliary than intestinal-type AC (55% vs 18%).[27] A recent analysis of the AJCC classification system showed that the 2-tier reclassification of positive lymph nodes was linked to significant differences in survival (including recurrence-free survival) between T3a and T3b tumors (but not between T1b and T2 or between lymphatic/venous invasion/node metastases).[55] These results raise the question of the need for a size-related staging of duodenal involvement, when a 2-tier system (of duodenal involvement present vs absent) may be sufficient.

Key Points
CURRENT
PATHOLOGIC TUMOR-NODE-METASTASIS STAGING OF AMPULLARY CARCINOMA (AMERICAN JOINT COMMITTEE ON CANCER, EIGHTH EDITION)[55]

Definition

Tumor

Tx Primary tumor cannot be assessed

T0 No evidence of primary tumor

Tis Carcinoma in situ

T1 Limited to AoV/Oddi sphincter or invades beyond Oddi sphincter, ±duodenal submucosa

T1a Tumor limited to AoV or sphincter of Oddi

T1b Tumor invades beyond sphincter of Oddi, ± duodenal submucosa

T2 Tumor invades duodenal muscularis propria

T3 Tumor directly invades pancreas (≤0.5 cm) or extends >0.5 cm into pancreas, peripancreatic/periduodenal tissue, or duodenal serosa, but not celiac axis or superior mesenteric artery

T3a Tumor directly invades pancreas (up to 0.5 cm)

T3b Tumor extends >0.5 cm into pancreas, or peripancreatic/periduodenal tissue or duodenal serosa, but not celiac axis or SMA

T4 Tumor involves celiac axis, SMA, and/or common hepatic artery, irrespective of size

Nodes

Nx Regional lymph nodes cannot be assessed

N0 No regional lymph node metastasis

N1 1–3 positive regional lymph nodes

N2 ±4 positive regional lymph nodes

Abbreviation: SMA, superior mesenteric artery.

PROGNOSIS OF AMPULLARY CARCINOMA

Overall, AC has far better rates of survival than pancreatic ductal (PDAC) and distal common bile duct cancers, and has a 5-year survival of ~45%.[3,56,57] Site-specific classification also affects survival, with IAPN-associated ACs showing longer survival than ampullary-ductal AC, which is typically of pancreatobiliary phenotype. Nonetheless, ampullary-ductal AC has a much better prognosis than ordinary pancreatic ductal adenocarcinomas.[3,4,7,57] Pancreatobiliary-type

AC has a worse prognosis than intestinal-type AC.[4,19,23,57] Size of invasive carcinoma is also a key prognostic factor, particularly in IAPN-associated AC.[7,57] Independent prognostic factors in AC include age, number of positive nodes, perineural/lymph-vascular/venous invasion, margin positivity, and tumor budding.[3,4,7,57] Positive margins occur in less than 5% of ampullary carcinomas, compared with at least 35% of pancreatic tumors.[57]

Key Points
PROGNOSTIC FACTORS IN AMPULLARY CARCINOMA

Anatomic/site-specific classification

IAPN-associated ampullary carcinomas show longer survival than ampullary-ductal AC

Ampullary-ductal ampullary carcinoma is more aggressive than all other subtypes

Histologic subtype

Pancreatobiliary-type ampullary carcinoma has a worse prognosis than intestinal-type ampullary carcinoma

Among nontubular carcinomas, poorly cohesive cell carcinoma, high-grade neuroendocrine carcinoma, and undifferentiated carcinoma with SWI/SNF proteins have poor prognosis

T stage

Size of invasive carcinoma is a prognostic factor (larger tumors are more aggressive)

N stage

Number of positive lymph nodes (N2 tumors are more aggressive than N1)

Other factors

Perineural invasion

Lymph-vascular invasion

Venous invasion

Margin positivity

Tumor budding

MUC5AC expression by carcinoma

DISCLOSURE

The authors have nothing to disclose financially.

REFERENCES

1. Adsay NV, Basturk O, Saka B, et al. Whipple made simple for surgical pathologists: orientation, dissection,

and sampling of pancreaticoduodenectomy specimens for a more practical and accurate evaluation of pancreatic, distal common bile duct, and ampullary tumors. Am J Surg Pathol 2014;38(4):480–93.

2. Adsay NV, Basturk O, Altinel D, et al. The number of lymph nodes identified in a simple pancreatoduodenectomy specimen: comparison of conventional vs orange-peeling approach in pathologic assessment. Mod Pathol 2009;22(1):107–12.

3. Adsay V, Ohike N, Tajiri T, et al. Ampullary region carcinomas: definition and site specific classification with delineation of four clinicopathologically and prognostically distinct subsets in an analysis of 249 cases. Am J Surg Pathol 2012;36(11):1592–608.

4. Reid MD, Balci S, Ohike N, et al. Ampullary carcinoma is often of mixed or hybrid histologic type: an analysis of reproducibility and clinical relevance of classification as pancreatobiliary versus intestinal in 232 cases. Mod Pathol 2016;29(12):1575–85.

5. Xue Y, Reid MD, Balci S, et al. Immunohistochemical classification of ampullary carcinomas: critical reappraisal fails to confirm prognostic relevance for recently proposed panels, and highlights MUC5AC as a strong prognosticator. Am J Surg Pathol 2017; 41(7):865–76.

6. Ohike N, Coban I, Kim GE, et al. Tumor budding as a strong prognostic indicator in invasive ampullary adenocarcinomas. Am J Surg Pathol 2010;34(10):1417–24.

7. Ohike N, Kim GE, Tajiri T, et al. Intra-ampullary papillary-tubular neoplasm (IAPN): characterization of tumoral intraepithelial neoplasia occurring within the ampulla: a clinicopathologic analysis of 82 cases. Am J Surg Pathol 2010;34(12):1731–48.

8. Balci S, Basturk O, Saka B, et al. Substaging nodal status in ampullary carcinomas has significant prognostic value: proposed revised staging based on an analysis of 313 well-characterized cases. Ann Surg Oncol 2015;22(13):4392–401.

9. Alexander JR, Andrews JM, Buchi KN, et al. High prevalence of adenomatous polyps of the duodenal papilla in familial adenomatous polyposis. Dig Dis Sci 1989;34(2):167–70.

10. Domizio P, Talbot IC, Spigelman AD, et al. Upper gastrointestinal pathology in familial adenomatous polyposis: results from a prospective study of 102 patients. J Clin Pathol 1990;43(9):738–43.

11. Noda Y, Watanabe H, Iida M, et al. Histologic follow-up of ampullary adenomas in patients with familial adenomatosis coli. Cancer 1992;70(7):1847–56.

12. Thompson LDR, Basturk O, Adsay NV. Pancreas. In: Mills SE, editor. Sternberg's diagnostic surgical pathology. Philadelphia: Lippincott Williams & Wilkins; 2015. p. 1577–662.

13. Adsay NV, Basturk O. Tumors of major and minor ampulla. In: Odze R, Goldblum J, editors. Surgical pathology of the GI tract, liver, biliary tract, and pancreas. Philadelphia: Elsevier; 2015. p. 1120–42.

14. Polydorides AD, Shia J, Tang LH, et al. An immuno-histochemical panel distinguishes colonization by pancreatic ductal adenocarcinoma from adenomas of ampullary and duodenal mucosa. Mod Pathol 2008;21:132A.

15. Xue Y, Obeng RC, Graham R, et al. Morphological features of colonization of ampullary and duodenal mucosa by invasive carcinoma: an interobserver variability study (Abstract). Mod Pathol 2020;33: 1683–4.

16. Schmidt MT, Himmelfarb EA, Shafi H, et al. Use of IMP3, S100P, and pVHL immunopanel to aid in the interpretation of bile duct biopsies with atypical histology or suspicious for malignancy. Appl Immunohistochem Mol Morphol 2012;20(5):478–87.

17. Yachida S, Wood LD, Suzuki M, et al. Genomic Sequencing Identifies ELF3 as a Driver of Ampullary Carcinoma. Cancer Cell 2016;29(2):229–40.

18. Kloppel G, Adsay V, Konukiewitz B, et al. Precancerous lesions of the biliary tree. Best Pract Res Clin Gastroenterol 2013;27(2):285–97.

19. Adsay NV, Reid MD. Ampullary Adenocarcinoma. In: Board WCoTE, editor. WHO classification of tumours: digestive system tumours. 5th edition. Lyon (France): IARC Press; 2019. p. 127–30.

20. Sekine S, Shia J. Ampullary Adenoma. In: Board WCoTE, editor. WHO classification of tumours: digestive system tumours. 5th edition. Lyon (France): IARC Press; 2019. p. 121–3.

21. Klimstra DS, Albores-Saavedra J, Hruban RH, et al. Tumours of the ampullary region, Adenomas and other premalignant neoplastic lesions. In: Bosman FT, Carneiro F, Hruban RH, et al, editors. WHO classification of tumours of the digestive system. Lyon (France): International Agency for Research on Cancer (IARC); 2010. p. 83–6.

22. Kakar S, Shi C, Adsay NV, et al. Protocol for the Examination of Specimens From Patients With Carcinoma of the Ampulla of Vater. Cancer Protocol Templates 2017. 2019. Available at: https://www. cap.org/protocols-and-guidelines/cancer-reporting--tools/cancer-protocol-templates. Accessed November 15, 2019.

23. Adsay NV, Bagci P, Tajiri T, et al. Pathologic staging of pancreatic, ampullary, biliary, and gallbladder cancers: pitfalls and practical limitations of the current AJCC/UICC TNM staging system and opportunities for improvement. Semin Diagn Pathol 2012; 29(3):127–41.

24. Ang DC, Shia J, Tang LH, et al. The utility of immunohistochemistry in subtyping adenocarcinoma of the ampulla of vater. Am J Surg Pathol 2014; 38(10):1371–9.

25. Chang DK, Jamieson NB, Johns AL, et al. Histomolecular phenotypes and outcome in adenocarcinoma of the ampulla of vater. J Clin Oncol 2013; 31(10):1348–56.

26. Bronsert P, Kohler I, Werner M, et al. Intestinal-type of differentiation predicts favourable overall survival: confirmatory clinicopathological analysis of 198 periampullary adenocarcinomas of pancreatic, biliary, ampullary and duodenal origin. BMC Cancer 2013;13:428.

27. Kimura W, Futakawa N, Yamagata S, et al. Different clinicopathologic findings in two histologic types of carcinoma of papilla of Vater. Jpn J Cancer Res 1994;85(2):161–6.

28. Westgaard A, Pomianowska E, Clausen OP, et al. Intestinal-type and pancreatobiliary-type adenocarcinomas: how does ampullary carcinoma differ from other periampullary malignancies? Ann Surg Oncol 2013;20(2):430–9.

29. Costigan D, Sheahan K, Conlon KC, et al. The role of immunohistochemistry in subtyping ampullary adenocarcinoma (Abstract). Mod Pathol 2016; 29(2):167A.

30. Lowe MC, Coban I, Adsay NV, et al. Important prognostic factors in adenocarcinoma of the ampulla of Vater. Am Surg 2009;75(9):754–60, [discussion: 761].

31. Kamisawa T, Honda G, Kurata M, et al. Pancreatobiliary disorders associated with pancreaticobiliary maljunction. Dig Surg 2010;27(2):100–4.

32. Westgaard A, Tafjord S, Farstad IN, et al. Pancreatobiliary versus intestinal histologic type of differentiation is an independent prognostic factor in resected periampullary adenocarcinoma. BMC Cancer 2008; 8:170.

33. Morini S, Perrone G, Borzomati D, et al. Carcinoma of the ampulla of Vater: morphological and immunophenotypical classification predicts overall survival. Pancreas. 2013;42(1):60–6.

34. Kim WS, Choi DW, Choi SH, et al. Clinical significance of pathologic subtype in curatively resected ampulla of vater cancer. J Surg Oncol 2012;105(3): 266–72.

35. Howe JR, Klimstra DS, Moccia RD, et al. Factors predictive of survival in ampullary carcinoma. Ann Surg 1998;228(1):87–94.

36. Fischer HP, Zhou H. Pathogenesis of carcinoma of the papilla of Vater. J Hepatobiliary Pancreat Surg 2004;11(5):301–9.

37. Jang K-T, Balci S, Bagci P, et al. Mucinous Carcinomas of the Ampulla: Clinicopathologic Analysis of 33 Cases (Abstract). Mod Pathol 2014;27(2S):450A.

38. Tuncel D, Basturk O, Bradley KT, et al. Poorly cohesive (signet ring cell) carcinoma of the ampulla of vater. Int J Surg Pathol 2020;28(3):236–44.

39. Fujita T, Konishi M, Gotohda N, et al. Invasive micropapillary carcinoma of the ampulla of Vater with extensive lymph node metastasis: Report of a case. Surg Today 2010;40(12):1197–200.

40. Hoshimoto S, Aiura K, Shito M, et al. Adenosquamous carcinoma of the ampulla of Vater: a case report and literature review. World J Surg Oncol 2015;13:287.

41. Kawamoto Y, Ome Y, Terada K, et al. Undifferentiated carcinoma with osteoclast-like giant cells of the ampullary region: Short term survival after pancreaticoduodenectomy. Int J Surg Case Rep 2016;24:199–202.

42. Agaimy A, Daum O, Markl B, et al. SWI/SNF Complex-deficient Undifferentiated/Rhabdoid Carcinomas of the Gastrointestinal Tract: A Series of 13 Cases Highlighting Mutually Exclusive Loss of SMARCA4 and SMARCA2 and Frequent Co-inactivation of SMARCB1 and SMARCA2. Am J Surg Pathol 2016;40(4):544–53.

43. Hechtman JF, Liu W, Sadowska J, et al. Sequencing of 279 cancer genes in ampullary carcinoma reveals trends relating to histologic subtypes and frequent amplification and overexpression of ERBB2 (HER2). Mod Pathol 2015;28(8):1123–9.

44. Hsu HP, Shan YS, Jin YT, et al. Loss of E-cadherin and beta-catenin is correlated with poor prognosis of ampullary neoplasms. J Surg Oncol 2010; 101(5):356–62.

45. Overman MJ, Zhang J, Kopetz S, et al. Gene expression profiling of ampullary carcinomas classifies ampullary carcinomas into biliary-like and intestinal-like subtypes that are prognostic of outcome. PLoS One 2013;8(6):e65144.

46. Pinto P, Peixoto A, Santos C, et al. Analysis of founder mutations in rare tumors associated with hereditary breast/ovarian cancer reveals a novel association of BRCA2 mutations with ampulla of vater carcinomas. PLoS One 2016;11(8):e0161438.

47. Achille A, Scupoli MT, Magalini AR, et al. APC gene mutations and allelic losses in sporadic ampullary tumours: evidence of genetic difference from tumours associated with familial adenomatous polyposis. Int J Cancer 1996;68(3):305–12.

48. Kawakami M, Kimura Y, Furuhata T, et al. beta-Catenin alteration in cancer of the ampulla of Vater. J Exp Clin Cancer Res 2002;21(1):23–7.

49. Mafficini A, Amato E, Cataldo I, et al. Ampulla of Vater Carcinoma: Sequencing Analysis Identifies TP53 Status as a Novel Independent Prognostic Factor and Potentially Actionable ERBB, PI3K, and WNT Pathways Gene Mutations. Ann Surg 2018;267(1): 149–56.

50. Wong W, Lowery MA, Berger MF, et al. Ampullary cancer: Evaluation of somatic and germline genetic alterations and association with clinical outcomes. Cancer 2019;125(9):1441–8.

51. Moore PS, Orlandini S, Zamboni G, et al. Pancreatic tumours: molecular pathways implicated in ductal cancer are involved in ampullary but not in exocrine nonductal or endocrine tumorigenesis. Br J Cancer 2001;84(2):253–62.

52. Herman JM, Pawlik TM, Merchant NB, et al. Ampulla of Vater. In: Amin MB, editor. AJCC cancer staging

manual. 8th edition. Chicago: Springer; 2017. p. 327–35.

53. Basturk O, Saka B, Balci S, et al. Substaging of Lymph Node Status in Resected Pancreatic Ductal Adenocarcinoma Has Strong Prognostic Correlations: Proposal for a Revised N Classification for TNM Staging. Ann Surg Oncol 2015;22(Suppl 3):S1187–95.

54. Sakata J, Shirai Y, Wakai T, et al. Number of positive lymph nodes independently affects long-term survival after resection in patients with ampullary carcinoma. Eur J Surg Oncol 2007;33(3):346–51.

55. Imamura T, Yamamoto Y, Sugiura T, et al. The Prognostic Relevance of the New 8th Edition of the Union for International Cancer Control Classification of TNM Staging for Ampulla of Vater Carcinoma. Ann Surg Oncol 2019;26(6):1639–48.

56. Gonzalez RS, Bagci P, Basturk O, et al. Intrapancreatic distal common bile duct carcinoma: Analysis, staging considerations, and comparison with pancreatic ductal and ampullary adenocarcinomas. Mod Pathol 2016;29(11):1358–69.

57. Saka B, Tajiri T, Ohike N, et al. Clinicopathologic comparison of ampullary versus pancreatic carcinoma: preinvasive component, size of invasion, stage, resectability and histologic phenotype are the factors for the significantly favorable outcome of ampullary carcinoma (abstract). Mod Pathol 2013;26:429A.

Updates in Appendix Pathology
The Precarious Cutting Edge

Norman J. Carr, FRCPath

KEYWORDS

- Appendix • Appendiceal neoplasia • Goblet cell carcinoid • Goblet cell adenocarcinoma
- Mucinous neoplasia • Pseudomyxoma peritonei

Key points

- It is essential to diagnose appendiceal neoplasia accurately owing to the management options now available, which include radical surgery and intraperitoneal chemotherapy.

- Mucinous neoplasms of the appendix encompass low-grade and high-grade appendiceal mucinous neoplasms and mucinous adenocarcinoma. Nonmucinous adenocarcinoma also occurs.

- Pseudomyxoma peritonei is a characteristic syndrome that usually arises from mucinous appendiceal neoplasia.

- Goblet cell adenocarcinoma, previously known as goblet cell carcinoid, is a distinctive neoplasm that almost always arises in the appendix. Its histologic features are related to prognosis.

ABSTRACT

Mucinous appendiceal tumors include low-grade appendiceal mucinous neoplasm, high-grade appendiceal mucinous neoplasm, and mucinous adenocarcinoma. Nonmucinous adenocarcinomas are less frequent. Recent consensus guidelines and the latest edition of the World Health Organization classification will allow consistent use of agreed nomenclature. Accurate diagnosis is important not only for patient management but also to allow comparison of results between centers and tumor registries. Serrated polyps are the most common benign polyp in the appendix. They need to be distinguished from low-grade appendiceal mucinous neoplasm, which can also mimic other benign conditions. Goblet cell adenocarcinomas are a distinctive type of appendiceal neoplasm.

OVERVIEW

Although appendiceal neoplasms are unusual, they are not rare and they can challenge the diagnostic abilities of the most experienced pathologists.[1–4] Furthermore, the classification and terminology of appendiceal neoplasia has been controversial for decades.[3,5] In 2016, consensus guidelines were published following an international modified Delphi process with the aim of unifying terminology[6] and the 2019 World Health Organization (WHO) classification of appendiceal neoplasia has built on this consensus.[7–9] This article discusses its practical application in diagnosis and differential diagnosis. Pseudomyxoma peritonei, a rare complication of mucinous appendiceal neoplasia, is also covered.

Nonmucinous appendiceal neoplasms are less frequent than mucinous tumors, and their relationship to other types of appendiceal neoplasia is unclear.[10,11] They are discussed briefly along with mucinous adenocarcinomas. Serrated polyps and colonic-type adenomas are considered to be precursors of malignant appendiceal neoplasms and are also discussed.

In addition, this article covers goblet cell tumors separately. The name by which they have been known since 1974, goblet cell carcinoid, has had the unfortunate effect of causing them to be

---

Peritoneal Malignancy Institute, Basingstoke and North Hampshire Hospital, Aldermaston Road, Basingstoke RG24 9NA, UK
E-mail address: norman.carr@hhft.nhs.uk

Surgical Pathology 13 (2020) 469–484
https://doi.org/10.1016/j.path.2020.05.006

confused with neuroendocrine tumors.[12,13] They are not part of the neuroendocrine tumor family; instead they are a type of adenocarcinoma. They have been renamed goblet cell adenocarcinoma in the 2019 WHO classification, a term more appropriate to their nature.[14]

APPENDICEAL MUCINOUS NEOPLASIA

Low-grade appendiceal mucinous neoplasm (LAMN), high-grade appendiceal mucinous neoplasm (HAMN), mucinous appendiceal adenocarcinoma, benign polyps, and pseudomyxoma peritonei are discussed here.

GROSS FEATURES

LAMNs and HAMNs commonly cause the appendix to enlarge because of dilation of the lumen, which becomes filled with mucus (**Fig. 1**).[15–17] The wall is often fibrotic and focally calcified. Diverticulum-like structures can be visible; they generally represent areas of pushing invasion. The term mucocele may be used for a dilated appendix with a fibrous wall filled with mucin, but it is a descriptive term only and it must not be used as a pathologic diagnosis.[6,15] Myxoglobulosis is a rare event in which the intraluminal mucin forms distinct round globules a few millimeters in diameter.[18] Occasionally, the appendix may be grossly normal.

Mucinous adenocarcinomas of the appendix may present as a mucocele, but the appendix is often distorted or surrounded by mucinous tumor. Sometimes, it may be difficult or impossible to identify the appendix because it has been partially or totally destroyed by malignant tumor growth.

Pseudomyxoma peritonei (PMP) is a clinical syndrome caused by the growth of a mucinous neoplasm within the peritoneal cavity.[6] It is characterized by slow but relentless accumulation of intra-abdominal mucin that can lead to marked abdominal distention.[19,20] The omentum is frequently transformed into a firm mass (omental cake). In women, large Krukenberg tumors of the ovary are common (**Fig. 2**). PMP is distinguished from other types of transcoelomic metastasis by the following:

- PMP shows the redistribution phenomenon by flowing with peritoneal fluid to sites of fluid reabsorption.[21] The mucin and the cells it contains accumulate at these sites; for example, the paracolic gutters, diaphragmatic peritoneum, pelvic peritoneum, and omentum. Thus, the tumor is redistributed within the abdominal cavity.
- The appendix is the usual primary site (other possible sites of origin are discussed elsewhere in this article in relation to diagnosis).
- Although the tumor spreads extensively over peritoneal and serosal surfaces, there is usually little or no invasion into the parenchyma of underlying organs.
- Hematogenous and nodal metastases are rare, despite the large peritoneal tumor burden. If they are encountered, it is generally a sign of high-grade disease, although occasionally even low-grade PMP can spread to the thorax.[22,23]

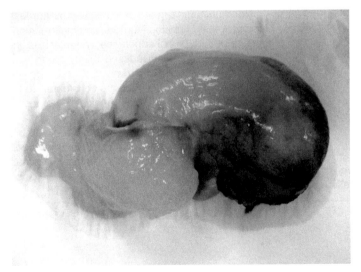

Fig. 1. Mucocele caused by a low-grade appendiceal mucinous neoplasm. There is rupture with extrusion of mucus.

Fig. 2. Ovarian Krukenberg tumor from a patient with pseudomyxoma peritonei of appendiceal origin. The cut surface shows a multilocular mucinous cyst.

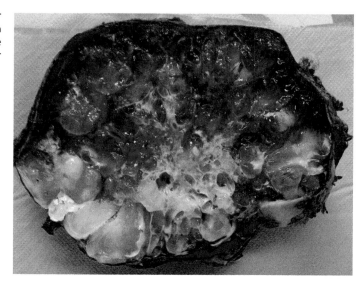

MICROSCOPIC FEATURES

Mucinous appendiceal neoplasms are of 3 main types: LAMN, HAMN, and mucinous adenocarcinoma (**Figs. 3–5, Table 1**).[6] The tumor cells are typically columnar and mucin rich, although they may become cuboidal with less intracytoplasmic mucin.[4,15,24] LAMNs and HAMNs may have attenuated epithelium with squamoid, mucin-poor cells. An essential principle of classification is that LAMN and HAMN are characterized by pushing invasion, whereas infiltrative invasion implies adenocarcinoma (**Box 1**).[7,8]

LAMNs and HAMNs often show widespread ulceration, and such mucosal denudation may mimic an inflammatory process unless the appendix is adequately sampled to show the presence of neoplastic epithelium (**Fig. 6**). As a general rule, it is advisable to entirely process appendiceal mucoceles for histology.[4,25]

Molecular Abnormalities

Mucinous appendiceal neoplasms (LAMNs, HAMNs, and mucinous adenocarcinomas) commonly contain *GNAS* and *KRAS* mutations, whereas *BRAF* and *APC* mutations and microsatellite instability are rare. Mutations of *TP53* and abnormal immunoexpression of p53 are associated with HAMNs or adenocarcinomas.[26–31]

Benign Polyps

There are several benign lesions that occur in the appendix (**Box 2**). In all of them, the muscularis mucosae is generally intact.

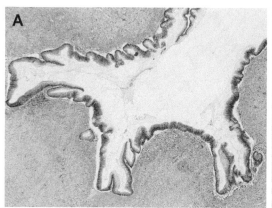
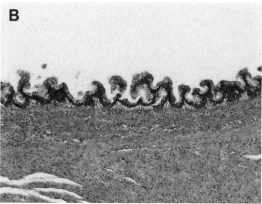

Fig. 3. Low-grade appendiceal mucinous neoplasm. (*A*) Low power shows diverticulum-like pushing invasion (hematoxylin-eosin, original magnification ×4). (*B*) Low-grade columnar epithelium with an undulating pattern of growth (hematoxylin-eosin, original magnification ×20).

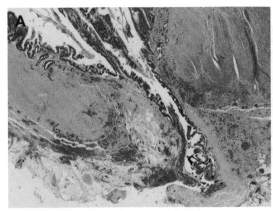
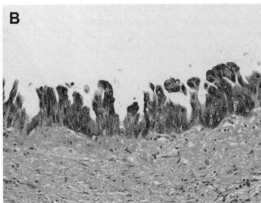

Fig. 4. HAMN. (*A*) Pushing invasion is present (hematoxylin-eosin, original magnification ×4). (*B*) The epithelium shows high-grade features with pseudopapillae (hematoxylin-eosin, original magnification ×40).

The most common is the serrated polyp. They precisely recapitulate the histologic appearances of sessile serrated lesions of the colorectum (**Fig. 7**).[32] However, the term serrated polyp is preferred in the appendix because the molecular pathologic changes are different from those found in colorectal lesions. In particular, *KRAS* mutations are more common and *BRAF* mutations less common in appendiceal serrated polyps.[27] The noncommittal term serrated polyp was recommended by an international panel of experts, reflecting the fact that the serrated pathway in the appendix is probably different from that in the colorectum.[6] The WHO classification allows both sessile serrated lesion and serrated polyp as acceptable terms.[9] Most serrated polyps lack dysplasia, but dysplastic changes are found in some (**Fig. 8**).

Hyperplastic polyps, as defined in **Box 2**, are rare in the appendix (**Fig. 9**). Also rare are conventional colorectal-type adenomas (**Fig. 10**)[33]; they resemble their colorectal counterparts and some

are dysplastic serrated polyps that have lost conspicuous serration.

DIFFERENTIAL DIAGNOSIS

The main differential diagnoses for LAMNs are both nonneoplastic and neoplastic, as summarized in **Table 2**. In the experience of referral centers, overinterpretation of ruptured diverticulosis with reactive mucosal changes as LAMN is one of the most common diagnostic discrepancies (**Fig. 11**).[34–37]

Retention cysts or inflammatory mucoceles are rare. The appendix is mildly dilated and the wall is fibrotic and chronically inflamed. The mucosa is ulcerated or atrophic. Sometimes, it is impossible to exclude LAMN if there is complete mucosal denudation.

DIAGNOSIS

Mucinous appendiceal neoplasms are commonly asymptomatic or are found incidentally in

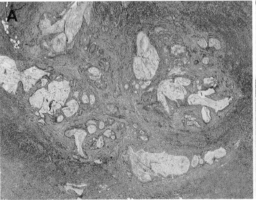
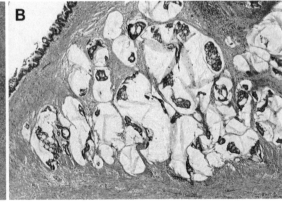

Fig. 5. Mucinous adenocarcinoma, G2. (*A*) Infiltrative glands within a desmoplastic stroma (hematoxylin-eosin, original magnification ×2). (*B*) The small cellular mucin pool pattern of infiltrative invasion (hematoxylin-eosin, original magnification ×10).

Table 1
Key histologic features of mucinous appendiceal neoplasms

	Type of Invasion (see Box 1)	Architectural Pattern	Nuclear Features	Mitotic Activity
LAMN	Pushing	Filiform villi, undulating, flat	Basally oriented, minimal atypia	Rare, not atypical
HAMN	Pushing	Filiform villi, undulating, flat with pseudopapillae	Loss of polarity, marked atypia	Frequent, may be atypical
Mucinous adenocarcinoma	Infiltrative	Variably sized glands and islands	Variable	Frequent, may be atypical

appendices removed for acute appendicitis. There may be nonspecific abdominal pain, palpable mass, or abdominal distension, especially if there is PMP.[17,19,20] Occasionally, PMP presents as mucin in a hernia sac.[38]

PMP arises from appendiceal mucinous neoplasia (LAMN, HAMN, or mucinous adenocarcinoma) in most cases. However, other possible primary neoplasms include mucinous tumors of the urachus, pancreas, colon, biliary tract, and pelvicalyceal system.[4,24,39–42] PMP rarely arises from the ovary; studies have shown that the appendix is the primary site when there are synchronous ovarian and appendiceal mucinous tumors.[43] The principal exception to this rule is mature cystic teratoma of the ovary. Mucinous neoplasms arising in ovarian teratomas can have morphologic appearances and genetic abnormalities identical to those found in appendiceal mucinous neoplasms, and such lesions can produce true PMP.[44,45]

The term HAMN is used for those rare mucinous neoplasms with high-grade dysplasia but no evidence of infiltrative invasion. HAMN is a relatively new entity; in previous case series they have been variably included either with LAMNs or adenocarcinoma.[6] Therefore, their behavior is unclear and requires further study. In our experience, HAMNs limited to the appendix probably have a low risk of progression, but cases in which pseudomyxoma peritonei develop tend to pursue a more aggressive course than LAMNs.

Many appendiceal mucinous neoplasms show mixed features. A lesion with features of LAMN in some areas may show focal high-grade atypia or infiltrative invasion leading to a diagnosis of HAMN or adenocarcinoma, respectively. This principle is the rationale for recommending that any appendix containing a mucinous neoplasm should be entirely processed for histology.

Sometimes, dysplastic serrated polyps resemble traditional serrated adenomas of the colorectum. The significance is unclear, and for reporting purposes it is sufficient to call them serrated polyp with low-grade or high-grade

Box 1
Key histologic features of pushing and infiltrative invasion

1. Pushing invasion:
   - Epithelium extending into appendiceal wall on a broad front
   - Diverticulum-like structures
   - Thinning of appendiceal wall, often circumferential
   - Underlying dense fibrosis, often hyaline
   - The concept of pushing invasion includes dissection of the wall by acellular mucin
2. Infiltrative invasion:
   - Small cellular mucin pool pattern: cytologically malignant cells (strips, clusters, or glands) within pools of extracellular mucin; desmoplasia may not be conspicuous (see **Fig. 5B**)
   - Small, angulated glands within a desmoplastic stroma
   - Tumor budding within a desmoplastic stroma

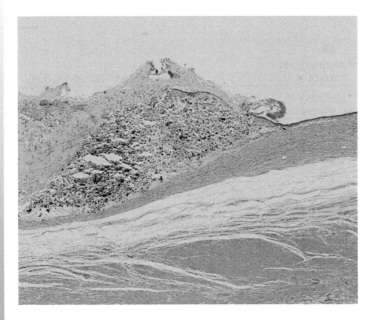

Fig. 6. LAMN with mucosal denudation (left of image). Flattened neoplastic epithelium is visible on the right (hematoxylin-eosin, original magnification ×2).

Box 2
Key histologic features of benign appendiceal polyps

1. Serrated polyp
   - Circumferential growth common
   - Tubular architecture with serrated epithelial profiles
   - Serrations extend into crypt bases
   - Dilatation of crypt bases
   - Expansion of crypt bases by growth parallel to muscularis mucosae
   - No conventional cytologic dysplasia
2. Serrated polyp with dysplasia
   - Architecture commonly features villi, complex branching, and/or crowding of crypts
   - Conventional dysplasia present; may be low grade or high grade
   - Serration may be reduced
3. Hyperplastic polyp
   - Localized, not circumferential
   - Tubular architecture with serrations limited to upper two-thirds
   - Proliferation zone confined to crypt bases
   - Basal parts of crypts morphologically normal
4. Colorectal-type adenomas
   - May be tubular, tubulovillous, or villous
   - Dysplasia may be low grade or high grade
   - Lack serrations (which would imply dysplastic serrated polyp)

Fig. 7. Serrated polyp of appendix. The basal parts of the crypts show serration and dilatation. There is no conventional dysplasia (hematoxylin-eosin, original magnification ×10).

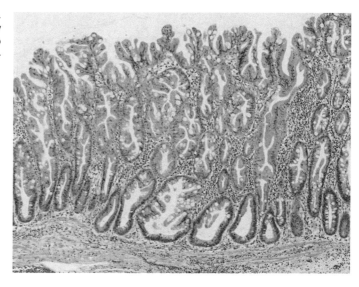

dysplasia, perhaps with a comment on the resemblance to traditional serrated adenoma.[4]

Mucinous adenocarcinomas, by definition, comprise more than 50% extracellular mucin and are the most frequent type of adenocarcinoma in the appendix. Nonmucinous adenocarcinomas also occur and show a range of morphology; they usually resemble colorectal adenocarcinoma, although a few have pale cytoplasm and resemble pancreatobiliary adenocarcinoma.[8] When an invasive component arises in a colorectal-type adenoma of the appendix, it is often nonmucinous.

PROGNOSIS

Prognosis in appendiceal mucinous neoplasia is strongly associated with stage and grade.[7,16,24,25,46–48] Knowledge of the role of biomarkers is limited, but evidence suggests that mutated TP53 and abnormally expressed p53 are associated with reduced survival.[26,28,49,50] In patients with PMP, preoperative tumor marker levels correlate with overall survival and risk of recurrence.[51]

Survival has improved with the introduction of cytoreductive surgery and hyperthermic intraperitoneal chemotherapy (HIPEC) for patients with PMP or peritoneal metastases.[52] Right hemicolectomy is indicated for invasive adenocarcinoma, which allows regional lymph node resection,[53–55] but this should be performed at the same time as HIPEC if the latter treatment is indicated to prevent the possibility of neoplastic cells seeding scar tissue.[56]

Fig. 8. Dysplastic serrated polyp of appendix. The epithelium is atypical. Serrations are reduced (hematoxylin-eosin, original magnification ×20).

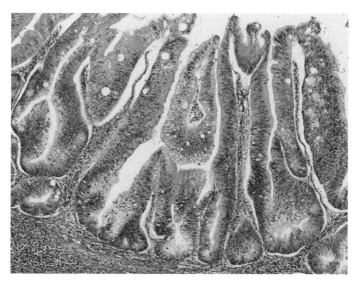

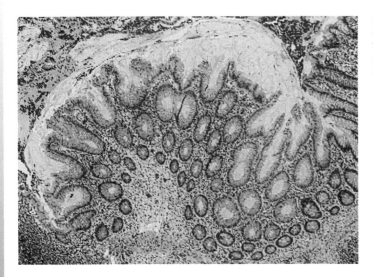

Fig. 9. Hyperplastic polyp of appendix. The lesion is localized, and serrations are confined to the upper portions of the crypts (hematoxylin-eosin, original magnification ×10).

Spread and Staging

In LAMN and HAMN, diverticulum-like herniations or broad-front spread can lead to rupture, with consequent seeding of the peritoneal cavity by neoplastic cells.[4,57] Presumably this is the mechanism by which pseudomyxoma peritonei develops, although occasionally no histologic evidence of rupture is found.[58] Mucinous appendiceal adenocarcinoma can also produce pseudomyxoma peritonei, especially if well differentiated,[52] but alternatively it can behave more like conventional adenocarcinoma, with discrete peritoneal implants (rather than pseudomyxoma) and distant metastases. Nonmucinous adenocarcinomas typically behave this way, but even nonmucinous adenocarcinomas have a high frequency of metastatic disease limited to the peritoneum.[10]

The TNM (tumor, node, metastasis) classification of appendiceal neoplasms (which is different from that of colorectal neoplasms) is summarized in **Table 3**.[47] For LAMNs, there is no pT1 or pT2; instead, lesions confined to the submucosa or muscularis propria are designated pTis(LAMN), reflecting the very low risk of recurrence in such lesions. The regional nodes for the appendix are the ileocolic chain. If only mesoappendiceal nodes are sampled, the designation should be pNx. Involvement of the ovaries is typical of the PMP syndrome and is classified pM1b. The designation of pM1c

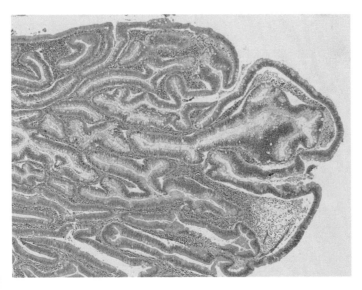

Fig. 10. Appendiceal tubular adenoma with low-grade dysplasia. The lesion is indistinguishable from a colonic adenoma (hematoxylin-eosin, original magnification ×4).

Table 2
Differential diagnosis of low-grade appendiceal mucinous neoplasm

LAMN Vs:	Helpful Distinguishing Features
Reactive mucosal changes	• Commonly associated with ruptured diverticulum-like (see **Fig. 11**) • Mucosal hyperplasia and/or atrophy • Crypt disarray but preservation of lamina propria • Serration and hypermucinosis of epithelium common but mostly confined to superficial parts of mucosa • Intramucosal neuromas common • Muscularis mucosae intact • Extravasation of acellular mucin into periappendiceal tissues common • No filiform villi • No crowding of crypts
Retention cyst (inflammatory mucocele)	• Rare • Appendix <2 cm in diameter • No features of neoplasia • Appendix must be entirely processed before entertaining a diagnosis of retention cyst
Serrated polyp	• Basal parts of crypts show dilatation and serration • Crowding of crypts • No pushing invasion (pushing invasion is diagnostic of LAMN, even in the absence of conventional cytologic dysplasia)
HAMN	• Low-power architecture is indistinguishable from LAMN, but high-power examination reveals high-grade dysplasia • Cribriform architecture may be found in HAMN but is not required for diagnosis
Mucinous adenocarcinoma	• Presence of infiltrative invasion (see **Box 1**)

should be reserved for hematogenous spread (eg, lung or bone metastases) or distant lymphatic spread.

Based on the limited available evidence, HAMNs associated with spread beyond the appendiceal wall are more likely to develop pseudomyxoma peritonei and pursue an aggressive course than LAMNs.[15,25] There is some evidence suggesting that HAMNs confined to the appendix are unlikely to develop pseudomyxoma peritonei, but more data are required.

Grading

Table 4 shows the WHO grading system for mucinous appendiceal neoplasms.[8] Although mucinous adenocarcinomas can be described as well, moderately or poorly differentiated, in the WHO classification system mucinous adenocarcinomas are classified G2 unless signet ring cells are present, when they are classified G3, in keeping with the worse prognosis associated with signet ring morphology.[8,59–61] Lesions showing extensive

sheets of pleomorphic cells can also be classified G3.[3] The grading of nonmucinous adenocarcinomas corresponds to that of colorectal adenocarcinomas.

In patients with PMP, the grade and cellularity are prognostic factors.[15,16,24,25,33,48] Numerous classifications of PMP have been proposed over the years, but a 4-tier system has been shown to be prognostically relevant (**Box 3, Fig 12**).[5,47] The grade of the peritoneal disease and the appendiceal primary is usually the same, but occasionally the grades can be discordant.[6,48]

If only acellular extra-appendiceal mucin is found (ie, mucin without epithelial cells), interpretation depends on the clinical circumstances. Acellular mucin can result not only from ruptured mucinous appendiceal neoplasia but also from other conditions, notably ruptured ovarian cystadenomas. True serosal mucinous deposits can be distinguished from artifactual spillage of intraluminal mucin at the time of specimen dissection by the presence of inflammation, granulation tissue, and neovascularization.

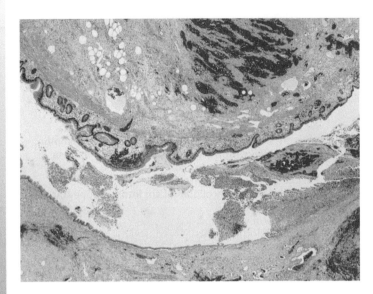

Fig. 11. Ruptured diverticulum of appendix. The mucosa is atrophic and focally attenuated, but lamina propria is preserved (hematoxylin-eosin, original magnification ×2).

GOBLET CELL ADENOCARCINOMA

Goblet cell adenocarcinoma (GCA) has been known by several names, including goblet cell carcinoid, crypt cell carcinoma, and adenocarcinoid. However, the appellation of carcinoid has led to confusion with true neuroendocrine tumors.[12] The 2019 WHO terminology of goblet cell adenocarcinoma recognizes that they are a type of adenocarcinoma.[14] Genetically, GCAs differ from both neuroendocrine tumors and other types of appendiceal adenocarcinoma. For example, mutations in *EGFR*, *KRAS*, or *BRAF* are generally not found.[62,63]

GCAs are rare with a wide age range and have an equal sex distribution.[64–66] They commonly

Table 3
Summary of tumor, node, metastasis classification of appendiceal neoplasms

Primary Tumor		
• LAMNs only	Confined to appendix (not beyond muscularis propria)	pTis
• Adenocarcinomas and HAMNs only	Invades submucosa/muscularis propria	pT1/pT2
• All lesions	Invades subserosa or mesoappendix (includes acellular mucin)	pT3
	Perforates visceral peritoneum, including cells and/or mucin on the serosa	pT4a
	Directly invades other organs or structures	pT4b
Regional Lymph Nodes		
No regional node metastasis		pN0
Metastasis in 1 regional node		pN1a
Metastasis in 2–3 regional nodes		pN1b
Tumor deposits (satellites) without regional nodal metastasis		pN1c
Metastasis in 4 or more regional nodes		pN2
Distant Metastasis		
Intraperitoneal acellular mucin only		pM1a
Intraperitoneal metastasis with mucinous epithelium		pM1b
Nonperitoneal metastasis		pM1c

(*Data from* Overman MJ, Asare EA, Compton CC, et al. Appendix – carcinoma. In: American Joint Committee on Cancer. AJCC Cancer Staging Manual, 8th edition. Chicago: Springer; 2017. p. 237-50.)

Table 4
Summary of World Health Organization grading of mucinous appendiceal neoplasms

LAMN	G1
HAMN	G2
Mucinous adenocarcinoma	G2
Mucinous adenocarcinoma with signet ring cells	G3

present as appendicitis or abdominal pain, although they can be an incidental finding.[67–69] Ovarian metastases can be the presenting feature in women.[70,71] Origin outside the appendix has been described but is exceptionally rare. Most presentations of GCA outside the appendix represent spread from an undetected appendiceal primary.[72]

GROSS FEATURES

GCAs are often grossly inconspicuous or produce ill-defined thickening of the appendiceal wall. Such lesions are rarely suspected until histologic examination. Extensive or high-grade lesions may cause distortion and enlargement of the appendix.

MICROSCOPIC

GCAs are defined by goblet cells forming small clusters that may be solid or have small lumina (**Fig. 13**). The cells have mucin-rich cytoplasm compressing the nuclei against the outer rim.[14,66,67,73] To be classified as a GCA, a lesion must include a component showing these classic features. There are generally smaller numbers of cells with eosinophilic or granular cytoplasm showing neuroendocrine differentiation scattered among the goblet cells. Occasionally, a few Paneth-like cells may also be present.

The tumors are poorly circumscribed and circumferentially infiltrate the appendiceal wall. The appendiceal mucosa generally shows no evidence of epithelial dysplasia. Perineural and lymphatic

vessel invasion may be present. Extracellular mucin may be prominent, and, if it comprises more than 50% of the tumor, the diagnosis of mucinous GCA is appropriate.[6]

The tumor cells generally express CK20, MUC2, and carcinoembryonic antigen (CEA). Many also express CK7.[66,74] Neuroendocrine markers such as synaptophysin and chromogranin A are usually positive, but chromogranin in particular may be confined to the scattered cells that histologically resemble neuroendocrine cells.[66,75] However, the diagnosis of GCA depends on morphologic criteria rather than immunohistochemistry, and occasional cases may be negative for immunohistochemical markers of neuroendocrine differentiation.[13]

DIFFERENTIAL DIAGNOSIS

Certain neuroendocrine neoplasms, particularly the rare tubular neuroendocrine tumor and clear cell neuroendocrine tumor, can resemble GCA.[76–78] However, neuroendocrine neoplasms do not contain intracellular mucin. Signet ring cell carcinoma of the appendix can be difficult to distinguish from GCA, and any appendiceal neoplasm rich in signet ring cells should be scrutinized carefully to identify any diagnostic features of GCA.[79,80] Metastatic carcinomas also enter the differential diagnosis.

PROGNOSIS AND SPREAD

Typical GCAs behave as low-grade malignancies. Transcoelomic spread is common, leading to involvement of peritoneal surfaces and the ovaries.[80] However, some lesions are more aggressive and this behavior is associated with adverse histologic features (**Box 4, Fig. 14**). These features have been incorporated into a variety of grading systems, but a discussion of their relative merits is beyond the scope of this article.[65,67,75,80,81]

Data regarding appropriate management of GCAs are lacking owing to their overall rarity.[65] Various criteria for performing right

Box 3
Classification of pseudomyxoma peritonei

Acellular mucin

Low-grade mucinous carcinoma peritonei (G1)

High-grade mucinous carcinoma peritonei (G2)

High-grade mucinous carcinoma peritonei with signet ring cells (G3)

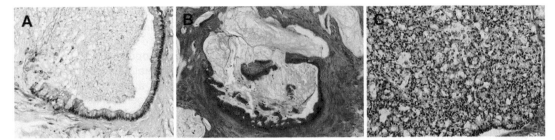

Fig. 12. Pseudomyxoma peritonei of appendiceal origin. (*A*) Low-grade mucinous carcinoma peritonei (G1) (hematoxylin-eosin, original magnification ×20). (*B*) High-grade mucinous carcinoma peritonei (G2) (hematoxylin-eosin, original magnification ×10). (*C*) High-grade mucinous carcinoma peritonei with signet ring cells (G3) (hematoxylin-eosin, original magnification ×10).

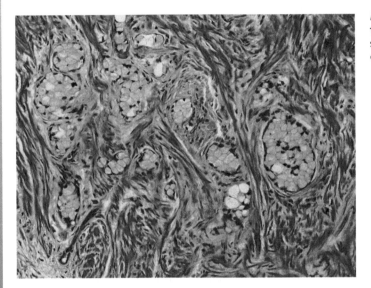

Fig. 13. GCA. This lesion shows the typical clusters of goblet cells with small peripheral nuclei (hematoxylin-eosin, original magnification ×20).

Box 4
Adverse histologic features associated with worse prognosis in goblet cell adenocarcinoma

- Nuclei vesicular and pleomorphic rather than small and dark
- Prominent desmoplasia
- Distortion or destruction of appendiceal wall
- Irregular large clusters or confluent sheets of neoplastic cells
- Discohesive cell growth
- Areas of poorly differentiated gland-forming colorectal-type adenocarcinoma

Fig. 14. GCA with adverse histologic features. Prominent nuclear atypia is visible. There is discohesive growth with individual signet ring–like cells (*arrow*) (hematoxylin-eosin, original magnification ×20).

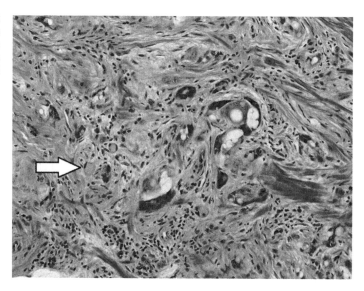

hemicolectomy have been proposed but they are mostly based on small case series.[12,75] Patients with peritoneal involvement may benefit from cytoreductive surgery and HIPEC.[82,83]

SUMMARY

Given the management options now available, accurate diagnosis of the neoplasms discussed in this article is increasingly important. Many are unusual, and histologic diagnosis may not be straightforward. An opinion from a reference center with experience in their diagnosis and treatment may be indicated.

If the principles outlined in this article are followed, reporting practices will be consistent and will allow comparison of results between institutions and cancer registries. However, as with all disease classifications, terminology should be related to prognosis and response to treatment, and may need to change as knowledge accumulates. Thus, the histologic classification of appendiceal neoplasia should be considered a work in progress. Improved understanding of molecular pathways will help with this process, as it has in other organs.

DISCLOSURE

The author has nothing to disclose.

REFERENCES

1. Marmor S, Portschy PR, Tuttle TM, et al. The rise in appendiceal cancer incidence: 2000-2009. J Gastrointest Surg 2015;19:43–750.

2. Smeenk RM, van Velthuysen ML, Verwaal VJ, et al. Appendiceal neoplasms and pseudomyxoma peritonei: a population based study. Eur J Surg Oncol 2008;34:196–201.

3. Valasek MA, Pai RK. An update on the diagnosis, grading and staging of appendiceal mucinous neoplasms. Adv Anat Pathol 2018;25:38–60.

4. Carr NJ, Bibeau F, Bradley RF, et al. The histopathological classification, diagnosis and differential diagnosis of mucinous appendiceal neoplasms, appendiceal adenocarcinomas and pseudomyxoma peritonei. Histopathology 2017;71:847–58.

5. Bradley RF, Carr NJ. Pseudomyxoma peritonei: pathology, a historical overview, and proposal for unified nomenclature and updated grading. AJSP Rev Rep 2019;24:88–93.

6. Carr NJ, Cecil TD, Mohamed F, et al. A consensus for classification and pathologic reporting of pseudomyxoma peritonei and associated appendiceal neoplasia. Am J Surg Pathol 2016;40:14–26.

7. Misdraji J, Carr NJ, Pai RK. Appendiceal mucinous neoplasm. In: WHO classification of tumours editorial board. digestive system tumours. 5th edition. Lyon (France): IARC; 2019. p. 144–6.

8. Misdraji J, Carr NJ, Pai RK. Appendiceal adenocarcinoma. In: WHO classification of tumours editorial board. digestive system tumours. 5th edition. Lyon (France): IARC; 2019. p. 147–8.

9. Misdraji J, Carr NJ, Pai RK. Appendiceal serrated lesions and polyps. In: WHO classification of tumours editorial board. digestive system tumours. 5th edition. Lyon (France): IARC; 2019. p. 141–3.

10. Uemura M, Qiao W, Fournier K, et al. Retrospective study of nonmucinous appendiceal adenocarcinomas: role of systemic chemotherapy and cytoreductive surgery. BMC Cancer 2017;17:331.

11. Kabbani W, Houlihan PS, Luthra R, et al. Mucinous and nonmucinous appendiceal adenocarcinomas: different clinicopathological features but similar genetic alterations. Mod Pathol 2002;15:599–605.

12. Wen KW, Hale G, Shafizadeh N, et al. Appendiceal goblet cell carcinoid: common errors in staging and clinical interpretation with a proposal for an improved terminology. Hum Pathol 2017;65:187–93.

13. van Velthuysen MF, van Eeden S, Carr NJ. The enigma of goblet cell tumors of the appendix. AJSP Rev Rep 2019;24:98–104.

14. Misdraji J, Carr NJ, Pai RK. Appendiceal goblet cell adenocarcinoma. In: WHO classification of tumours editorial board. digestive system tumours. 5th edition. Lyon (France): IARC; 2019. p. 149–51.

15. Misdraji J, Yantiss RK, Graeme-Cook FM, et al. Appendiceal mucinous neoplasms: a clinicopathologic analysis of 107 cases. Am J Surg Pathol 2003;27:1089–103.

16. Pai RK, Beck AH, Norton JA, et al. Appendiceal mucinous neoplasms: Clinicopathologic study of 116 cases with analysis of factors predicting recurrence. Am J Surg Pathol 2009;33:1425–39.

17. Li X, Zhou J, Dong M, et al. Management and prognosis of low-grade appendiceal mucinous neoplasms: a clinicopathologic analysis of 50 cases. Eur J Surg Oncol 2018;44:1640–5.

18. Gonzalez JEG, Hann SE, Trujillo YP. Myxoglobulosis of the appendix. Am J Surg Pathol 1988;12:962–6.

19. Esquivel J, Sugarbaker PH. Clinical presentation of the pseudomyxoma peritonei syndrome. Br J Surg 2000;87:1414–8.

20. Jarvinen P, Lepisto A. Clinical presentation of pseudomyxoma peritonei. Scand J Surg 2010;99:213–6.

21. Sugarbaker PH. Pseudomyxoma peritonei: a cancer whose biology is characterized by a redistribution phenomenon. Ann Surg 1994;219:109–11.

22. Pestieau SR, Esquivel J, Sugarbaker. Pleural extension of mucinous tumor in patients with pseudomyxoma peritonei syndrome. Ann Surg Oncol 2000;7:199–203.

23. Geisinger KR, Levine EA, Shen P, et al. Pleuropulmonary involvement in pseudomyxoma peritonei: morphologic assessment and literature review. Am J Clin Pathol 2007;127:135–43.

24. Carr NJ, Finch J, Ilesley IC, et al. Pathology and prognosis in pseudomyxoma peritonei: a review of 274 cases. J Clin Pathol 2012;65:919–23.

25. Yantiss RK, Shia J, Klimstra DS, et al. Prognostic significance of localized extra-appendiceal mucin deposition in appendiceal mucinous neoplasms. Am J Surg Pathol 2009;33:248–55.

26. Singhi AD, Davison JM, Choudry HA, et al. GNAS is frequently mutated in both low-grade and high-grade disseminated appendiceal mucinous neoplasms but does not affect survival. Hum Pathol 2014;45:1737–43.

27. Pai RK, Hartman DJ, Gonzalo DH, et al. Serrated lesions of the appendix frequently harbor KRAS mutations and not BRAF mutations indicating a distinctly different serrated neoplastic pathway in the appendix. Hum Pathol 2014;45:227–35.

28. Hara K, Saito T, Hayashi T, et al. A mutation spectrum that includes GNAS, KRAS and TP53 may be shared by mucinous neoplasms of the appendix. Pathol Res Pract 2015;211:657–64.

29. Liu X, Mody K, de Abreu FB, et al. Molecular profiling of appendiceal epithelial tumors using massively parallel sequencing to identify somatic mutations. Clin Chem 2014;60:1004–11.

30. Gleeson EM, Feldman R, Mapow BL, et al. Appendix-derived pseudomyxoma peritonei (PMP): molecular profiling toward treatment of a rare malignancy. Am J Clin Oncol 2018;41:777–83.

31. Tsai JH, Yang CY, Yuan RH, et al. Correlation of molecular and morphological features of appendiceal epithelial neoplasms. Histopathology 2019;75:468–77.

32. Rubio CA. Serrated adenomas of the appendix. J Clin Pathol 2004;57:946–9.

33. Carr NJ, McCarthy WF, Sobin LH. Epithelial noncarcinoid tumours and like-like lesions of the appendix. A clinicopathologic study of 184 patients with a multivariate analysis of prognostic factors. Cancer 1995;75:757–68.

34. Hsu M, Young RH, Misdraji J. Ruptured appendiceal diverticula mimicking low-grade appendiceal mucinous neoplasms. Am J Surg Pathol 2009;33:1515–21.

35. Lowes H, Rowaiye B, Carr NJ, et al. Complicated appendiceal diverticulosis versus low-grade appendiceal mucinous neoplasms: a major diagnostic dilemma. Histopathology 2019;75:478–85.

36. Amin A, Carr N. Diagnostic concordance in cases of appendiceal mucinous neoplasia referred to a tertiary referral centre. J Clin Pathol 2019;72:639–41.

37. Valasek MA, Thung I, Gollapalle E, et al. Overinterpretation is common in pathological diagnosis of appendix cancer during patient referral for oncologic care. PLoS One 2017;12:e0179216.

38. Esquivel J, Sugarbaker PH. Pseudomyxoma peritonei in a hernia sac: analysis of 20 patients in whom mucoid fluid was found during a hernia repair. Eur J Surg Oncol 2001;27:54–8.

39. Delhorme JB, Severac F, Averous G, et al. Cytoreductive surgery and hyperthermic intraperitoneal chemotherapy for pseudomyxoma peritonei of appendicular and extra-appendicular origin. Br J Surg 2018;105:668–76.

40. Rao P, Pinheiro N, Franco M, et al. Pseudomyxoma peritonei associated with primary mucinous

borderline tumor of the renal pelvicalyceal system. Arch Pathol Lab Med 2009;133:1472–6.

41. Lee SE, Jang JY, Hoon S, et al. Intraductal papillary mucinous carcinoma with atypical manifestations: report of two cases. World J Gastroenterol 2007; 13:1622–5.

42. Vora C, Tzivanakis A, Dayal, et al. Pseudomyxoma peritonei arising from a low-grade mucinous neoplasm of the urachus. AJSP Rev Rep 2019;24: 117–20.

43. Misdraji J. Appendiceal mucinous neoplasms: controversial issues. Arch Pathol Lab Med 2010; 134:864–70.

44. Choi YJ, Lee SH, Kim MS, et al. Whole-exome sequencing identified the genetic origin of a mucinous neoplasm in a mature cystic teratoma. Pathology 2016;48:372–6.

45. Stewart CJ, Tsukamoto T, Cooke B, et al. Ovarian mucinous tumour arising in mature cystic teratoma and associated pseudomyxoma peritonei: report of two cases and comparison with ovarian involvement by low-grade appendiceal mucinous tumour. Pathology 2006;38:534–8.

46. Fournier K, Rafeeq S, Taggart M, et al. Low-grade appendiceal mucinous neoplasm of uncertain malignant potential (LAMN-UMP): prognostic factors and implications for treatment and follow-up. Ann Surg Oncol 2017;24:187–93.

47. Overman MJ, Asare EA, Compton CC, et al. Appendix – carcinoma. In: American Joint Committee on Cancer. AJCC cancer staging manual. 8th edition. Chicago: Springer; 2017. p. 237–50.

48. Ronnett BM, Zahn CM, Kurman RJ, et al. Disseminated peritoneal adenomucinosis and peritoneal mucinous carcinomatosis. A clinicopathologic analysis of 109 cases with emphasis on distinguishing pathologic features, site of origin, prognosis, and relationship to "pseudomyxoma peritonei. Am J Surg Pathol 1995;19:1390–408.

49. Nummela P, Saarinen L, Thiel A, et al. Genomic profile of pseudomyxoma peritonei analyzed using next-generation sequencing and immunohistochemistry. Int J Cancer 2015;136:E282–9.

50. Taggart MW, Galbincea J, Mansfield PF, et al. High-level microsatellite instability in appendiceal carcinomas. Am J Surg Pathol 2013;37:1192–200.

51. Taflampas P, Dayal S, Chandrakumaran K, et al. Preoperative tumour marker status predicts recurrence and survival after complete cytoreduction and hyperthermic intraperitoneal chemotherapy for appendiceal pseudomyxoma peritonei: analysis of 519 patients. Eur J Surg Oncol 2014;40:515–20.

52. Mehta A, Mittal R, Chandrakumaran K, et al. Peritoneal involvement is more common than nodal involvement in patients with high-grade appendix tumors who are undergoing prophylactic

cytoreductive surgery and hyperthermic intraperitoneal chemotherapy. Dis Colon Rectum 2017;60: 1155–61.

53. Nitecki SS, Wolff BG, Shclinkert R, et al. The natural history of surgically treated primary adenocarcinoma of the appendix. Ann Surg 1994;219:51–7.

54. Cortina R, McCormick J, Kolm P, et al. Management and prognosis of adenocarcinoma of the appendix. Dis Colon Rectum 1995;38:848–52.

55. Conte CC, Petrelli NJ, Stulc J, et al. Adenocarcinoma of the appendix. Surg Gynecol Obstet 1988; 166:451–3.

56. Spiliotis J, Efstathiou E, Halkia E, et al. The influence of tumor cell entrapment phenomenon on the natural history of pseudomyxoma peritonei syndrome. Hepatogastroenterology 2012;59:705–8.

57. Lamps LW, Gray GF, Dilday BR, et al. The coexistence of low-grade mucinous neoplasms of the appendix and appendiceal diverticula: a possible role in the pathogenesis of pseudomyxoma peritonei. Mod Pathol 2000;13:495–501.

58. McDonald JR, O'Dwyer ST, Rout S, et al. Classification of and cytoreductive surgery for low-grade appendiceal mucinous neoplasms. Br J Surg 2012; 99:987–92.

59. Davison JM, Choudry HA, Pingpank JF, et al. Clinicopathologic and molecular analysis of disseminated appendiceal mucinous neoplasms: identification of factors predicting survival and proposed criteria for a three-tiered assessment of tumor grade. Mod Pathol 2014;27:1521–39.

60. Shetty S, Natarajan B, Thomas P, et al. Proposed classification of pseudomyxoma peritonei: influence of signet ring cells on survival. Am Surg 2013;79: 1171–6.

61. Sirintrapun SJ, Blackham AU, Russell G, et al. Significance of signet ring cells in high-grade mucinous adenocarcinoma of the peritoneum from appendiceal origin. Hum Pathol 2014;45:1597–604.

62. Johncilla M, Stachler M, Misdraji J, et al. Mutational landscape of goblet cell carcinoids and adenocarcinoma ex goblet cell carcinoids of the appendix is distinct from typical carcinoids and colorectal adenocarcinomas. Mod Pathol 2018;31:989–96.

63. Dimmler A, Geddert H, Faller G. EGFR, KRAS, BRAF-mutations and microsatellite instability are absent in goblet cell carcinoids of the appendix. Pathol Res Pract 2014;210:274–8.

64. Stancu M, Wu TT, Wallace C, et al. Genetic alterations in goblet cell carcinoids of the vermiform appendix and comparison with gastrointestinal carcinoid tumours. Mod Pathol 2003;16: 1189–98.

65. Taggart MW, Abraham SC, Overman MJ, et al. Goblet cell carcinoid tumor, mixed goblet cell carcinoid-adenocarcinoma, and adenocarcinoma

of the appendix. Arch Pathol Lab Med 2015;139: 782–90.

66. van Eeden S, Offerhaus GJ, Hart AA, et al. Goblet cell carcinoid of the appendix: a specific type of carcinoma. Histopathology 2007;51:763–73.

67. Nonaka D, Papaxoinis G, Lamarca A, et al. A study of appendiceal crypt cell adenocarcinoma (so-called goblet cell carcinoid and its related adenocarcinoma). Hum Pathol 2018;72:18–27.

68. Park K, Blessing K, Kerr K, et al. Goblet cell carcinoid of the appendix. Gut 1990;31:322–4.

69. Berardi RS, Lee SS, Chen HP. Goblet cell carcinoids of the appendix. Surg Gynecol Obstet 1988;167:81–6.

70. Klein EA, Rosen MH. Bilateral Krukenberg tumours due to appendiceal mucinous carcinoid. Int J Gynecol Pathol 1996;15:85–8.

71. Hirschfield LS, Kahn LB, Winkler B, et al. Adenocarcinoid of the appendix presenting as bilateral Krukenberg's tumour of the ovaries. Immunohistochemical and ultrastructural studies and literature review. Arch Pathol Lab Med 1985; 109:930–3.

72. Gui X, Qin L, Gao ZH, et al. Goblet cell carcinoids at extraappendiceal locations of gastrointestinal tract: an underrecognized diagnostic pitfall. J Surg Oncol 2011;103:790–5.

73. Burke AP, Sobin LH, Federspiel BH, et al. Goblet cell carcinoids and related tumors of the vermiform appendix. Am J Clin Pathol 1990;94:27–35.

74. Alsaad KO, Serra S, Schmitt A, et al. Cytokeratins 7 and 20 immunoexpression profile in goblet cell and classical carcinoids of appendix. Endocr Pathol 2007;18:16–22.

75. Tang LH, Shia J, Soslow RA, et al. Pathologic classification and clinical behavior of the spectrum of goblet cell carcinoid tumors of the appendix. Am J Surg Pathol 2008;32:1429–43.

76. Matsukuma KE, Montgomery EA. Tubular carcinoids of the appendix: the CK7/CK20 immunophenotype can be a diagnostic pitfall. J Clin Pathol 2012;65: 666–8.

77. Chetty R, Serra S. Lipid-rich and clear cell neuroendocrine tumors ("carcinoids") of the appendix: potential confusion with goblet cell carcinoid. Am J Surg Pathol 2010;34:401–4.

78. La Rosa S, Finzi G, Puppa G, et al. Lipid-rich variant of appendiceal well-differentiated endocrine tumor (carcinoid). Am J Clin Pathol 2010;133:809–14.

79. Ng D, Falck V, McConnell YJ, et al. Appendiceal goblet cell carcinoid and mucinous neoplasms are closely associated tumors: lessons from their coexistence in primary tumors and concurrence in peritoneal dissemination. J Surg Oncol 2014; 109:548–55.

80. Reid MD, Basturk O, Shaib WL, et al. Adenocarcinoma ex-goblet cell carcinoid (appendiceal-type crypt cell adenocarcinoma) is a morphologically distinct entity with highly aggressive behavior and frequent association with peritoneal/intra-abdominal dissemination: an analysis of 77 cases. Mod Pathol 2016;29:1243–53.

81. Lee LH, McConnell YJ, Tsang E, et al. Simplified 2-tier histologic grading system accurately predicts outcomes in goblet cell carcinoid of the appendix. Hum Pathol 2015;46:1881–9.

82. McConnell YJ, Mack LA, Gui X, et al. Cytoreductive surgery with hyperthermic intraperitoneal chemotherapy: an emerging treatment option for advanced goblet cell tumors of the appendix. Ann Surg Oncol 2014;1:1975–82.

83. Radomski M, Pai RK, Shuai Y, et al. Curative surgical resection as a component of multimodality therapy for peritoneal metastases from goblet cell carcinoids. Ann Surg Oncol 2016;23:4338–43.

HER2 in Colorectal Carcinoma: Are We There yet?

Jonathan A. Nowak, MD, PhD

KEYWORDS

• Colon cancer • Colorectal cancer • HER2 • ERBB2 • Targeted therapy

Key points

- *ERBB2* (HER2) alterations, including amplifications and activating mutations, occur in approximately 5% of colorectal cancers (CRCs), and are often mutually exclusive with other oncogenic drivers in the RAS/RAF/MEK/ERK and PI3K/AKT/mTOR signaling pathways.

- Immunohistochemistry, in situ hybridization, and next-generation sequencing are appropriate modalities for detection of ERBB2 overexpression/amplification.

- *ERBB2* amplification does not have clear prognostic significance, although it may predict lack of response to anti-EGFR therapy in metastatic CRC.

- Evidence from multiple phase 2 clinical trials suggests that *ERBB2* amplification in metastatic CRC predicts response to anti-ERBB2 dual-targeted therapy.

- Treatment with trastuzumab and either pertuzumab or lapatinib is now recommended for *RAS* wild-type, ERBB2-amplified metastatic CRC in National Comprehensive Cancer Network guidelines.

ABSTRACT

HER2 (ERBB2) is a member of the ERBB family of receptor tyrosine kinases and functions to drive signaling in the RAS/RAF/MEK/ERK and PI3K/AKT/mTOR pathways. Overall, approximately 2-3% of CRCs exhibit *ERBB2* amplification. Multiple phase II clinical trials have now shown that *ERBB2* amplification can be predictive of response to anti-ERBB2 targeted therapy. Consequently, recently released guidelines from the National Comprehensive Cancer Network recommend treatment with anti-ERBB2 targeted therapy for *RAS* wild-type, *ERBB2*-amplified metastatic CRC. While circumspection is still needed, *ERBB2* amplification has now emerged as the next standard-of-care biomarker for metastatic CRC, expanding targeted therapy options for these patients.

OVERVIEW

HER2 (hereinafter referred to ERBB2 [protein] or *ERBB2* [gene]) is a member of the ERBB family of receptor tyrosine kinases (RTKs), which also includes EGFR (ERBB1), HER3 (ERBB3), and HER4 (ERBB4). These RTKs drive multiple downstream signaling pathways, most notably the RAS/RAF/MEK/ERK and PI3K/AKT/mTOR pathways, and play essential and diverse roles in both normal biology and oncogenesis[1] (**Fig. 1**). Binding of extracellular ligands, such as epidermal growth factor and neuregulins, to EGFR, HER3, and HER4 induces heterodimerization with other ERBB family members and results in autophosphorylation, thereby providing docking sites for downstream signaling molecules and driving intracellular signaling. Unlike the other members of the ERBB family, ERBB2 is unique in that it does not bind any known ERBB ligands directly, although it readily participates in heterodimer formation and transphosphorylation of its dimerization partner. Notably, overexpression of ERBB2, most commonly driven by *ERBB2* amplification, can result in ERBB2 homodimerization and ligand-independent activation, whereas mutations within *ERBB2* itself can enhance kinase activity via several mechanisms.[2,3] Over the past 3 decades,

Department of Pathology, Brigham and Women's Hospital, Harvard Medical School, 75 Francis Street, Boston, MA 02115, USA
E-mail address: janowak@bwh.harvard.edu

Surgical Pathology 13 (2020) 485–502
https://doi.org/10.1016/j.path.2020.05.007
1875-9181/20/© 2020 Elsevier Inc. All rights reserved.

surgpath.theclinics.com

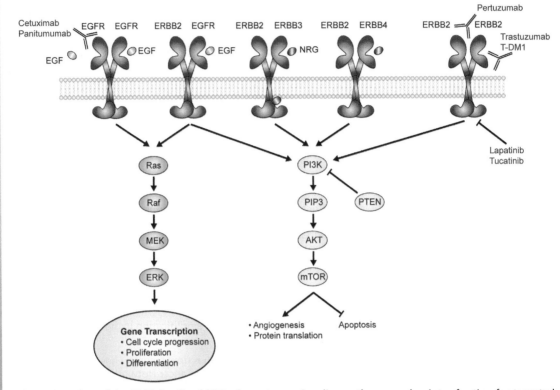

Fig. 1. Overview of the ERBB family of RTKs, downstream signaling pathways and points of action for targeted therapies. Cetuximab and panitumumab are monoclonal antibodies directed against the extracellular domain of EGFR. Trastuzumab is a monoclonal antibody directed against the extracellular domain of ERBB2, whereas T-DM1 is a version of trastuzumab that is conjugated to the cytotoxic agent emtansine (DM1). Pertuzumab is a monoclonal antibody directed against the extracellular domain of ERBB2 that inhibits receptor dimerization. Lapatinib is a small molecule tyrosine kinase inhibitor with activity against both ERBB2 and EGFR. Tucatinib is a small molecule tyrosine kinase inhibitor with high selectivity for ERBB2.

it has become clear that alterations either in ERBB family members themselves or in key components of downstream signaling pathways driven by ERBB family RTKs are some of the most common oncogenic drivers across a broad variety of malignancies.[4]

Across common tumor types, *ERBB2* amplification has been most frequently identified in breast and gastroesophageal cancer, with amplification rates of approximately 15% to 20% in breast cancer and 7% to 38% in gastroesophageal cancer.[5–10] In breast cancer, *ERBB2* amplification characterizes a specific molecular subtype, provides significant prognostic information, and determines eligibility for multiple targeted therapies.[5,11] In gastroesophageal cancer, *ERBB2* amplification also carries prognostic significance and is predictive of response to trastuzumab, a monoclonal antibody directed against ERBB2.[12] In addition, *ERBB2* amplification has also been identified at a lower rate in a variety of other tumor types, such as lung adenocarcinoma, and at a higher frequency in several rare tumor

types, such as salivary duct carcinoma, and studies evaluating the prognostic and predictive utility of *ERBB2* amplification in these tumors are ongoing.[13,14]

THE SPECTRUM OF HER2 ALTERATIONS IN COLORECTAL CANCER

In colorectal adenocarcinoma, recurrent activation of the RAS/RAF/MEK/ERK signaling pathway was one of the first key molecular characteristics to be identified and generally represents an early step in oncogenesis.[15] More recent comprehensive surveys show that approximately 60% to 80% of colorectal adenocarcinomas harbor activating alterations in this pathway and approximately 50% harbor activating alterations in the PI3K pathway.[16] Although activating hotspot mutations in *KRAS*, *BRAF*, and *NRAS* represent the most common mechanisms for RAS/RAF/MEK/ERK pathway activation, activating alterations in ERBB family members themselves are also well-described, although less frequent, events in colorectal adenocarcinoma.

Activating alterations in *ERBB2* in colorectal adenocarcinoma consist of both amplifications and mutations within ERBB2 itself[4,16] (**Fig. 2**). Although both types of alterations may represent targetable vulnerabilities in cancer, *ERBB2* amplification has historically been considered the predominant ERBB2 alteration, and has been the most extensively studied type of alteration, owing to the widespread availability of immunohistochemistry and in situ hybridization methods. Consequently, over the past 2 decades, many studies have evaluated the rate of ERBB2 overexpression in colorectal cancer (**Table 1**). The

reported rates of positivity varied widely in earlier studies, ranging from 1% to more than 40%. The results of these studies may be affected by many variables, most notably antibody clone selection, staining platform, cohort composition, and scoring criteria used to define positivity. Notably, several studies have reported significantly higher rates of positivity when cytoplasmic expression is included in criteria for positivity. However, evaluation of this particular cellular compartment is not considered in the standard scoring methodologies for breast or gastroesophageal cancer, and is of uncertain biologic significance with respect to our current understanding of ERBB2-mediated signaling pathways.[17,18] In addition, artifactual or

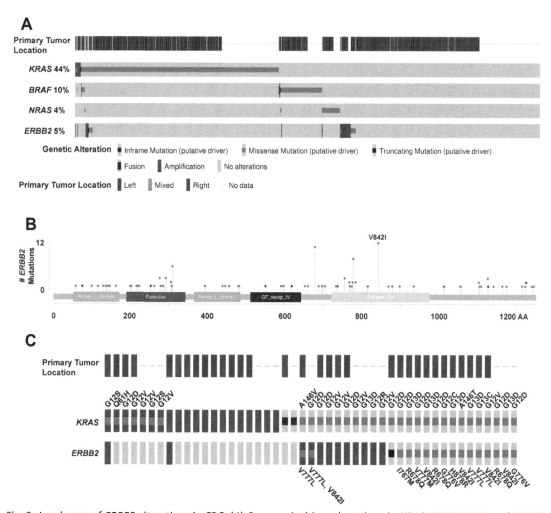

Fig. 2. Landscape of *ERBB2* alterations in CRC. (*A*) Oncogenic driver alterations in *KRAS, BRAF, NRAS,* and *ERBB2* are typically mutually exclusive, although a subset of tumors harbor co-occurring drivers. Amplifications of *ERBB2* are more common than *ERBB2* driver mutations.[16,31] (*B*) The distribution of mutations in *ERBB2* highlights enrichment for known activating, hotspot mutations.[16,31,72] (*C*) The distribution of co-occurring *KRAS* and *ERBB2* drivers alterations in CRC underscores the finding that *KRAS* and *ERBB2* alterations are not completely mutually exclusive.[16,31] All data were accessed and visualized through cBioPortal.[73,74]. (*Data from* Refs.[16,31,72–74]).

Table 1
Rates and prognostic significance of ERBB2 positivity in colorectal cancer

Study, Year	Patients	Stage	Tumor Location	Molecular Subtypes	HER2 Immunohistochemistry Results, % Positive	Prognostic Significance[a]
Sawada et al,[23] 2018	359	I-IV	Colorectal	Trends toward association with KRAS/BRAF wild-type status	4.1 (IHC and reflex FISH)	No association with OS
Park et al,[27] 2018	145	I-III	Rectal, post-neoadjuvant therapy	Significant association with KRAS/BRAF wild-type status	1.4	No association with DFS or cancer-free survival
Ni et al,[20] 2017	4913	–	Colorectal	–	1.4	–
Laurent-Puig et al,[21] 2016	1795	III	Colon	–	2.2	–
Richman et al,[22] 2016	1914 1342	II-III IV	Colorectal	Significant association with KRAS/BRAF wild-type status	1.3 2.2	No association with PFS or OS
Valtorta et al,[19] 2015	1086	–	Colorectal	Significant association with KRAS codon 12/13 wild-type status	4.1	Not assessed
Ingold Heppner et al,[39] 2014	1645	I-IV	Colorectal	Not assessed	1.6	No association with OS
Song et al,[65] 2014	106	pT1-3	Colorectal	Not assessed	7.5 (4B5 clone) 3.8 (SP3 clone)	No association with OS
Conradi et al,[45] 2013	264	II-IV	Rectal	Not assessed	12.4 (biopsies) 26.7 (resections)	ERBB2+ associated with better CSS, no association with OS
Kruszewski et al,[66] 2010	202	I-IV	Colorectal	Not assessed	15.3	No association with OS
Kountoruakis et al,[67] 2006	106	Dukes' B-D	Colorectal	Not assessed	2.8	No association with OS
Schuell et al,[43] 2006	77	Dukes' A-D	Colorectal	Not assessed	3	No association with OS

Essapen et al.[18] 2004	170	Dukes' B-C	Colorectal	Not assessed	~40 (membranous staining)	No association with OS
McKay et al,[24] 2002	249	Dukes' A-D	Colorectal	Not assessed	3.2	No association with OS
Rossi et al,[68] 2002	156	I-III	Colorectal	Not assessed	4 (2^+ or 3^+)	No association with OS
Osako et al,[44] 1998	146	Dukes' A-D	Colorectal	Not assessed	2.1 (membranous staining)	Not assessed for membranous staining

Abbreviations: CSS, cancer-specific survival; DFS, disease-free survival; FISH, fluorescence in situ hybridization; IHC, immunohistochemistry; OS, overall survival.
[a] Prognostic significance noted only for membranous staining.

nonspecific background staining may theoretically be more likely to manifest as cytoplasmic rather than membranous expression, thereby overestimating the number of truly positive cases.

Although these early studies borrowed scoring criteria from other cancer types or developed their own scoring criteria, a validated scoring system designed specifically for CRC was defined and published for use in the HERACLES-A (HER2 Amplification for ColorectaL Cancer Enhanced Stratification) trial of dual-targeted ERBB2 inhibition in 2016.[19] In the first test phase of the study, a scoring system was adapted from existing breast and gastroesophageal scoring systems and designed to capture ERBB2 expression patterns that were observed in unselected archival CRC specimens. ERBB2 expression was compared with silver or fluorescent in situ hybridization (FISH) to directly assess ERBB2 gene copy number status. In the validation phase of the study, this CRC-specific system was applied to KRAS wild-type patients being screened for inclusion within the HERACLES-A trial. In this system, the pattern of ERBB2 expression, intensity of staining, and percent positive cells are jointly considered to classify tumors, similar to existing systems for breast and gastroesophageal cancer (Table 2). Notably, only membranous ERBB2 expression that is circumferential, basolateral, or lateral counts toward positivity (Fig. 3). Intense (3+) expression in ≥50% of cells is categorized as positive, whereas intense (3+) expression in greater than 10% but <50% is still considered positive but requires confirmation by in situ hybridization. Although moderate (2+) expression in ≥50% of cells is categorized as equivocal and requires further evaluation via in situ hybridization, cases that do not meet these criteria are considered negative. While all cases that displayed positive 3+ ERBB2 reactivity in both the testing and validation cohorts were confirmed to be ERBB2 amplified, variable rates of ERBB2 amplification were observed in ERBB2 2+ equivocal cases, although most of these tumors were not ERBB2 amplified. Interestingly, several differences in the typical expression patterns for ERBB2 in colorectal cancer as compared with breast cancer and gastroesophageal cancer were identified (Box 1). Overall, despite greater anatomic relatedness among the esophagus, stomach, and colon, expression of ERBB2 in CRC appears to more closely mirror the pattern seen in breast cancer than in gastroesophageal cancer. Although the reasons for similarity remain speculative, it is noteworthy that CRC and breast cancer both exhibit stronger correlation between ERBB2 amplification by FISH and ERBB2 protein expression than

gastroesophageal cancer, and that both CRC and breast cancer show greater intratumoral homogeneity in ERBB2 amplification.[19]

Application of the HERACLES CRC-specific scoring criteria to both patient cohorts in the initial study demonstrated that approximately 5% of KRAS wild-type tumors were positive for ERBB2 overexpression. More recent larger-scale studies that have used the HERACLES diagnostic criteria have supported an overall rate of 2% to 3% ERBB2 positivity in CRC and have generally identified a significant enrichment for ERBB2 positivity in KRAS wild-type cases.[20–23] These studies have also demonstrated strong correlation between ERBB2 expression levels and ERBB2 amplification by in situ hybridization. Together, the relative agreement of these recent results underscores the value of adopting uniform scoring criteria for assessment of ERBB2 expression.

The HERACLES diagnostic criteria, as initially defined, were designed to function in 2 stages, with initial screening at a local institution followed by repeat analysis and potentially in situ hybridization for a subset of cases at a central laboratory. However, these criteria and reflex testing rules could be readily adapted for full clinical testing at individual laboratory sites by omission of the repeat immunohistochemical (IHC) analysis of ERBB2 required on referral to central pathology. Nevertheless, it should be noted that these criteria were jointly defined by a small number of pathologists working together, and the degree of reproducibility or interobserver correlation for application of these criteria has not yet been established. It is also likely that this system may be modified and refined over time. In particular, the extent to which the system is applicable to both resection, primary biopsy, and metastatic biopsy specimens is undefined. In recognition of the often limited amounts of invasive cancer that are obtained during upper gastrointestinal biopsies, ERBB2 has distinct scoring criteria for resection and biopsy specimens. In this regard, colorectal cancer biopsies may be more similar to upper gastrointestinal biopsies than breast core biopsies, although the higher degree of homogeneity for ERBB2 positivity in colorectal cancer as opposed to gastroesophageal cancer may obviate the need for separate colorectal resection and biopsy scoring systems.[12,19]

A potential point of concern for pathologists is the degree of concordance between ERBB2 positivity in primary versus metastatic lesions. For KRAS and BRAF mutations, the most widely studied CRC oncogenic drivers, a large body of literature supports a discordance rate of approximately 8% to 10% between matched primary and

Table 2
Interpretation criteria for ERBB2 expression in breast, gastric, and colorectal cancer

Tumor Type	Intensity and Pattern	Positive Tumor Cells, %	Score	HER2 Expression Assessment	Reflex Testing for Final Assessment
Breast cancer	No reactivity	–	0	Negative	
Breast cancer	Weak, incomplete membrane staining	Any	1+	Negative	
Breast cancer	Weak, complete membrane staining	<10	1+	Negative	
Breast cancer	Circumferential membrane staining that is, incomplete and/or weak/moderate	>10	2+	Equivocal, need reflex testing	Single-probe ERBB2 ISH or dual-probe ERBB2/CEP17 ISH
Breast cancer	Complete and circumferential, intense membrane staining	≤10	2+	Equivocal, need reflex testing	Single-probe ERBB2 ISH or dual-probe ERBB2/CEP17 ISH
Breast cancer	Uniform intense membrane staining	>30	3+	Positive	
Gastric Cancer Resection	No reactivity or membranous reactivity only	<10	0	Negative	
Gastric Cancer Resection	Faint/barely perceptible membranous reactivity, cells reactive only in part of their membrane	≥1	1+	Negative	
Gastric Cancer Resection	Weak to moderate, complete, basolateral or lateral membranous reactivity	≥10	2+	Equivocal, need reflex testing	
Gastric Cancer Resection	Strong, complete, basolateral or lateral membranous reactivity	≥10	3+	Positive	
Colorectal Cancer	No reactivity	–	0	Negative	
Colorectal Cancer	Faint reactivity (1+), segmental or granular	Any	1+	Negative	
Colorectal Cancer	Moderate reactivity, any pattern	<50	2+	Negative	

(continued on next page)

Table 2
(continued)

Tumor Type	Intensity and Pattern	Positive Tumor Cells, %	Score	HER2 Expression Assessment	Reflex Testing for Final Assessment
Colorectal Cancer	Moderate reactivity, circumferential, basolateral or lateral	≥50	2+	Equivocal, need reflex testing[a]	Single-probe ERBB2 ISH or dual-probe ERBB2/CEP17 ISH
Colorectal Cancer	Intense reactivity, circumferential, basolateral or lateral	<10	3+	Negative	
Colorectal Cancer	Intense reactivity, circumferential, basolateral or lateral	<10 to <50	3+	Positive, need reflex testing[a]	Single-probe ERBB2 ISH or dual-probe ERBB2/CEP17 ISH
Colorectal Cancer	Intense reactivity, circumferential, basolateral or lateral	≥50	3+	Positive	

Abbreviation: ISH, in situ hybridization.

[a] HERACLES diagnostic criteria additionally specify repeat immunohistochemistry at a central laboratory for evaluation of clinical trial eligibility.

Fig. 3. Representative patterns of ERBB2 expression in colorectal adenocarcinoma by IHC. (*A*) Faint reactivity limited to the basal portion of tumor cells (score 1+, negative). (*B*) Faint, circumferential and basolateral reactivity in more than 50% of tumor cells (score 1+, negative) (*C*) Moderate, circumferential and basolateral reactivity in more than 50% of tumor cells (score 2+, equivocal, reflex in situ hybridization required) (*D*) Intense, circumferential reactivity in more than 50% of tumor cells (score 3+, positive). (*E*) An uncommon example of significant intratumoral heterogeneity for ERBB2 expression, with expression patterns ranging from intense circumferential reactivity to complete absence of reactivity in nearly adjacent glands. (*F*) Moderate basolateral expression of ERBB2 in a region of high-grade dysplasia that abuts and partially involves non-neoplastic colonic crypts suggests that ERBB2 overexpression represents an early oncogenic event in colorectal cancer.

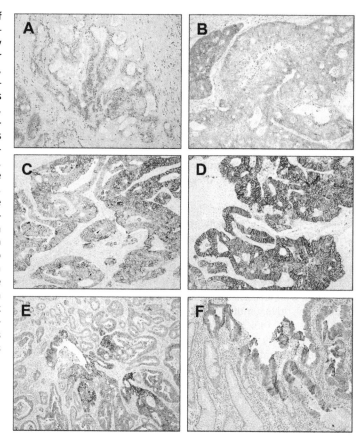

metastatic lesions, suggesting the potential for low but significant discordance with *ERBB2* as well. The limited number of currently available studies have reported varying degrees of concordance. An early study reported a concordance rate of only 52% between primary tumor and lymph node metastasis, although the degree of positivity was not taken into consideration.[24] A more recent study identified a 10% discordance rate between the primary tumor and lymph node metastasis,

and a 27% discordance rate between the primary tumor and liver metastases.[25] Detailed assessment of multiple metastatic sites via a warm autopsy protocol for a small number of patients treated in the HERACLES trials identified significant heterogeneity in ERBB2 expression and amplification between metastatic lesions, supporting the notion that separate metastases may have variable dependence on *ERBB2* amplification as an oncogenic driver irrespective of

---

Box 1
Notable differences in ERBB2 expression among colorectal, breast, and gastroesophageal cancers

- ERBB2 expression in colorectal cancer (CRC) correlates more strongly with *ERBB2* amplification that in gastroesophageal cancer.[19,62]

- ERBB2 expression in CRC is typically uniform across the tumor, unlike gastroesophageal cancer, in which patchy overexpression is often observed.[19,63]

- ERBB2 expression in CRC is often restricted to the basolateral aspects of tumor cells, more closely mirroring gastric instead of breast cancer.[6,19,63,64]

- Most CRC cases with equivocal ERBB2 expression do not exhibit *ERBB2* amplification, although those that are positive for amplification often have more heterogeneous ERBB2 expression than cases with strongly positive ERBB2 expression.[19]

treatment with anti-ERBB2 therapy.[26] An additional point of concern is whether neoadjuvant therapy, common for rectal adenocarcinoma, could influence detection of ERBB2 positivity. Although multiple studies have identified an enrichment for ERBB2 positivity in rectal adenocarcinoma as compared with more proximal locations in the colon, one study specifically focused on post-neoadjuvant rectal adenocarcinoma specimens reported an ERBB2 positivity rate of just 1.4%, lower than overall rates for CRC and hinting at downregulation of expression due to neoadjuvant therapy.[27]

In addition to *ERBB2* amplification and overexpression, a variety of activating mutations in *ERBB2* have now been identified across multiple tumor types, most notably breast and lung cancer.[4,28,29] Such alterations have also been identified in CRC, where they are generally mutually exclusive with *ERBB2* amplification and other oncogenic driver mutations in the RAS/RAF/MEK/ERK and PI3K/AKT/mTOR pathways.[30] In the largest study to date, an overall 4.7% rate of *ERBB2* alteration across 8877 tumors was identified via next-generation sequencing, with amplification in 2.8% of cases, mutations in 1.5% of cases and co-occurring amplifications and mutations in an additional 0.4% of cases.[30] Most *ERBB2* mutations represented known activating alterations, supporting the role of such alterations as true oncogenic drivers. This rate of mutations is similar to that previously identified in CRC by other sequencing studies.[4,31] Although such alterations cannot be detected by IHC or in situ hybridization, they could be detected via next-generation sequencing and may represent targetable alterations that should be borne in mind when considering how ERBB2 can drive CRC oncogenesis. Notably, evaluation of *ERBB2* copy number status using a clinical next-generation sequencing assay has been shown to produce results that are highly concordant with IHC and FISH results for breast and gastroesophageal cancers.[32] A recent study drawing from 1300 CRCs reported perfect concordance with ERBB2 amplification as assessed by next-generation sequencing and ERBB2 positivity by immunohistochemistry as measured by a histo-score ("H-score") criterion, suggesting that this testing methodology is suitable for CRC[33] (**Fig. 4**). Finally, a small number of studies have reported good concordance between cell-free DNA *ERBB2* amplification and tissue-based detection of amplification, although these data are limited and the approach is more generally subject to the limitations of cell-free DNA testing.[34,35]

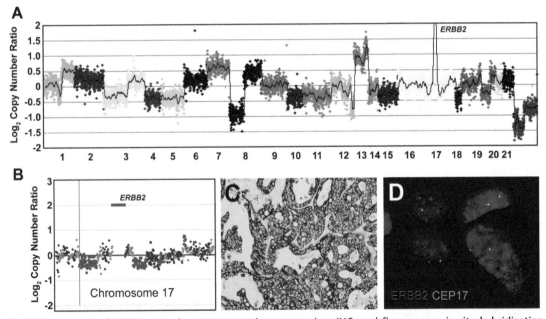

Fig. 4. Assessment of ERBB2 status by next-generation sequencing, IHC, and fluorescence in situ hybridization within a single tumor. (*A*) Global copy number profile highlights an amplification on chromosome 17. (*B*) A focal amplification of *ERBB2*, estimated at 25 copies, is identified on the q arm of chromosome 17. (*C*) IHC for ERBB2 demonstrates intense, circumferential expression in all tumor cells (score 3+, positive). (*D*) Fluorescence in situ hybridization confirms amplification of *ERBB2* as compared with the chromosome 17 centromeric enumeration probe (CEP17).

CLINICOPATHOLOGIC FEATURES OF ERBB2-AMPLIFIED COLORECTAL CANCER

Across studies that have examined rates of ERBB2 positivity in CRC, many studies have identified tumor location as one of the clinicopathologic features most commonly associated with ERBB2 positivity. Overall, the frequency of ERBB2 positivity increases from the right to the left side of the colon, with the highest rates for rectal adenocarcinoma.[36–42] Notably, however, several studies have not supported this association, and the single largest study to date observed an identical rate of 2.8% for ERBB2 amplification in metastatic colonic and rectal cancer when assessed by next-generation sequencing.[21,30,43]

An additional notable association is the relative enrichment of ERBB2 positivity within KRAS and BRAF wild-type tumors (see Fig. 2). Given that both alterations can result in activated RAS/RAF/MEK/ERK signaling, it was initially suspected that ERBB2 amplification would function as a mutually exclusive driver with respect to KRAS, BRAF, and NRAS status. With relatively rare exceptions, activating mutations in KRAS, BRAF, and NRAS are themselves mutually exclusive, suggesting that ERBB2 might behave the same way. However, it is now clear that a subset of CRCs harbor co-occurring ERBB2 amplification and KRAS mutations.[4,30,31] This result has important implications not only for potential prediction of therapeutic response in KRAS-mutant, ERBB2-amplified tumors, but it also has implications for laboratory testing, as identification of a KRAS mutation cannot rule out the possibility of coexisting ERBB2 amplification, nor can identification of ERBB2 positivity by IHC or FISH predict KRAS wild-type status. Finally, ERBB2 amplification is significantly enriched in the mismatch repair proficient/microsatellite stable subset of CRCs, although ERBB2 mutations are enriched with the mismatch repair deficient/microsatellite instability-high subset of CRCs.[30,31]

PROGNOSTIC SIGNIFICANCE OF ERBB2-AMPLIFIED COLORECTAL CANCER

The overall prognostic significance of ERBB2 amplification in CRC is uncertain. Although early studies reported an association with worse prognosis, these studies considered cytoplasmic expression of ERBB2 as a criterion for positivity.[17,44] More recent studies that evaluated only membranous ERBB2 expression have not demonstrated a clear association with prognosis (see Table 1), although a trend toward worse overall survival was identified in one of the largest published studies to date.[39] Notably, a 2013 study focused only on rectal cancer identified ERBB2 positivity as associated with significantly better cancer-specific survival, although not overall survival, suggesting a differential association with prognosis depending on tumor location, or a possible modifying effect due to neoadjuvant therapy.[45] In a study of patients in the PETACC8 trial, a pooled analysis of ERBB2 mutant and amplified tumors revealed an association with shorter time to recurrence and shorter overall survival that was maintained after adjustment for multiple clinicopathologic parameters.[21] However, whether these results translate to purely ERBB2-amplified tumors remains uncertain. Given the relative rarity of ERBB2-amplified tumors, additional large-scale studies will be necessary to determine whether there is a true prognostic significance to ERBB2 amplification status. Nevertheless, even if one exists, it is likely to be smaller in magnitude than other established prognostic factors for CRC, such as mismatch repair status and BRAF mutation status.[46]

ERBB2 STATUS AS A PREDICTOR OF RESISTANCE TO ANTI-EGFR THERAPY

Activating mutations in KRAS, NRAS, and BRAF are known to be associated with resistance to anti-EGFR targeted therapy in colorectal cancer, and testing for such mutations is standard of care for patients with metastatic disease who are being considered for anti-EGFR therapy.[46–48] Given the ability of ERBB2 amplification to also act as an activating alteration in the RAS/RAF/MEK/ERK pathway, it would seem plausible that ERBB2 amplification might similarly serve as a predictor of resistance to anti-EGFR therapy. Studies of patient-derived xenografts supported this notion, with ERBB2-amplified tumors that were wild-type for KRAS, BRAF, NRAS, and PIK3CA mutations exhibiting resistance to the anti-EGFR monoclonal antibody cetuximab.[49] Additional investigation of several CRC patient cohorts with available response data for anti-EGFR therapy revealed a significant enrichment of ERBB2 amplification or overexpression in KRAS wild-type tumors that did not respond to cetuximab, whereas all responding KRAS wild-type tumors were found to be ERBB2 nonamplified or non-overexpressing.[49] In a separate cohort of 233 patients with CRC treated with cetuximab either as monotherapy or in combination with chemotherapy, median progression-free survival (PFS) was 149 days for ERBB2 nonamplified tumors versus 89 days for *ERBB2*-amplified tumors, and overall survival was 515 days for *ERBB2*-nonamplified tumors versus 307 days for *ERBB2*-amplified tumors.[50] Similar results were obtained when analysis was restricted to the *KRAS* wild-type tumor subset. In another cohort of 170 patients with *KRAS* wild-type CRC treated with either etuximab or panitumumab, *ERBB2* amplification was associated with shorter PFS (2.5 vs 6.7 months for *ERBB2*-amplified vs all other *ERBB2* subtypes) and shorter overall survival (4.2 vs 13 months for *ERBB2*-amplified vs all other *ERBB2* subtypes).[51] A more recent study focused on 2 cohorts of *KRAS* and *BRAF* wild-type CRC found that median PFS was significantly shorter in *ERBB2*-amplified patients that received anti-EGFR treatment after first-line therapy in both cohorts (2.9 vs 8.1 months [cohort 1] and 2.8 vs 9.3 months [cohort 2] for amplified and nonamplified tumors, respectively).[52] In contrast to prior studies, overall survival in both cohorts was not significantly different between patients with *ERBB2*-amplified and nonamplified tumors. Notably, none of the 15 *KRAS* codon 12/13 wild-type *ERBB2*-amplified patients included in the HERACLES-A trial who had previously been treated with either cetuximab or panitumumab achieved an objective response.[53] In addition to serving as an intrinsic predictor of lack of response to anti-EGFR therapy, emerging data point to *ERBB2* amplification as a mechanism of acquired resistance to anti-EGFR therapy.[50] Although additional prospective studies will be needed to validate the utility of *ERBB2* amplification as predictive for lack of response to anti-EGFR therapy in *KRAS/NRAS/BRAF* wild-type tumors, it is notable that essentially all existing retrospective studies support such an association.

ERBB2 AMPLIFICATION AS A TARGETABLE ALTERATION IN COLORECTAL CANCER

Building on the initial success of therapies targeting ERBB2 in breast cancer, several early trials evaluated trastuzumab as an anti-ERBB2 therapy in combination with chemotherapy for patients with metastatic CRC with ERBB2-positive IHC[54,55] (**Table 3**). Although these trials did uncover evidence of therapeutic activity for trastuzumab, with partial responses seen in a significant subset of ERBB2-positive patients, these trials closed early due to poor accrual, precluding more definitive evaluation of the efficacy of anti-ERBB2 therapy. An additional phase 1 study combining paclitaxel with trastuzumab and interleukin-12 was completed but did not identify an objective response in any of the treated patients with CRC.[56] However, a critical turning point in the understanding of *ERBB2* as an oncogenic driver in CRC came in 2011, when a study of patient-derived xenograft models found that *ERBB2*-amplified CRC exhibited significant sensitivity to combination lapatinib and pertuzumab or lapatinib and cetuximab, whereas single-agent treatment alone had minimal activity.[49] These results provided a compelling impetus for the HERACLES phase 2 multicenter open-label sequential cohorts trial. HERACLES cohort A was designed to evaluate trastuzumab in combination with lapatinib, whereas HERACLES cohort B was designed to evaluate pertuzumab in combination with the antibody drug conjugate trastuzumab-emtansine (T-DM1). In the HERACLES-A cohort, patients with CRC who were wild-type for *KRAS* exon 12 and 13 mutations were screened for ERBB2 positivity using the HERACLES diagnostic criteria.[53] Of the 33 ERBB2-positive patients who enrolled in HERACLES-A, 23 (70%) patients exhibited disease control, with 10 (30%) objective responses, including 2 complete responses and 8 partial responses, and 13 (39%) patients with stable disease.[40] Notably, this patient population was heavily pretreated, with a median of 5 prior treatment regimens. A favorable overall toxicity profile was observed, with only 18% of patients experiencing grade 3 side effects and no identified drug-related significant adverse events. In the HERACLES-B cohort, *KRAS/BRAF* wild-type patients were also screened for ERBB2 positivity using the HERACLES diagnostic criteria. Although final results have not yet been reported, interim analysis showed that the objective response rate for the first 30 enrolled patients was 10%, whereas 70% of patients showed stable disease.[57] Notably, the median PFS was 4.8 months in HERACLES-B, compared with 4.2 months in HERACLES-A However, patients enrolled in HERACLES-B were less heavily pretreated (median 3 prior regimens) compared with HERACLES-A. Intriguingly, higher *ERBB2* gene copy number in HERACLES-A was associated with longer PFS, and higher ERBB2 expression by IHC was associated with greater objective response rate and longer duration of stable disease in HERACLES-B, suggesting that targeting tumors with the greatest theoretic dependence on *ERBB2* amplification as an oncogenic driver may yield stronger responses.[53]

Based on the positive results from HERACLES-A, multiple additional clinical trials targeting ERBB2 in CRC were initiated. Within the phase 2 basket study MyPathway, patients with treatment-refractory, metastatic CRC with

Table 3
Clinical trials investigating anti-ERBB2 targeted therapy in colorectal cancer

Study	Treatment	Phase	Eligibility Criteria	Line of Treatment	Objective Response Rate	Status
Ramanathan et al,[54] 2004	Trastuzumab + Irinotecan	2	HER2 2+ or 3+ IHC	1st or 2nd	71% (5 of 7)	Terminated early (low accrual)
Clark et al[55]	Trastuzumab + 5-FU, leucovorin, oxaliplatin	2	HER2 2+ or 3+ IHC, progression on 1-2 5-FU and/or irinotecan-containing regimens	2nd or 3rd	24% (5 of 21)	Terminated early (low accrual)
Bekaii-Saab et al,[56] 2009	Trastuzumab + Paclitaxel + IL-12	1	HER2 2+ or 3+ IHC	Any	0% (0 of 6)	Completed
HERACLES-A[53]	Trastuzumab + Lapatinib	2	HERACLES diagnostic criteria, KRAS codon 12/13 wild-type	2nd or greater	30% (8 of 27)	Completed
HERACLES-B[57]	Trastuzumab + Pertuzumab	2	HERACLES diagnostic criteria, KRAS/NRAS wild-type	2nd or greater	10% (3 of 30) 70% stable disease (21 of 30)	Ongoing
HERACLES RESCUE[69]	Trastuzumab-emtansine	2	Progression of disease during or after anti-ERBB2 therapy, including patients in the HERACLES-A cohort	3rd or greater	–	Ongoing
MyPathway[42]	Trastuzumab + Pertuzumab	2	ERBB2 amplification by next-generation sequencing, FISH or CISH	2nd or greater	32% (18 of 57)	Ongoing
MOUNTAINEER[59]	Tucatinib + Trastuzumab	2	RAS wild-type, ERBB2-amplified metastatic CRC as identified by next-generation sequencing, FISH, or immunohistochemistry	2nd or greater	55% (12 of 22)	Ongoing
TRIUMPH[58]	Trastuzumab + Pertuzumab	2	ERBB2 amplified metastatic CRC patients identified either by tissue-based or cell-free DNA testing	2nd or greater	35% (6 of 18) tissue-based cohort 33% (5 of 18) cfDNA-based cohort	Ongoing

(continued on next page)

Table 3
(continued)

Study	Treatment	Phase	Eligibility Criteria	Line of Treatment	Objective Response Rate	Status
SWOG 1613[70]	Trastuzumab + Pertuzumab vs Cetuximab + Irinotecan	2	Anti-EGFR naïve, *KRAS/NRAS/ BRAF* wild-type metastatic CRC patients with *ERBB2* amplification by immunohistochemistry and ISH	2nd or greater	–	Ongoing
MODUL (cohort 3)[71]	Trastuzumab + Pertuzumab	2	ERBB2 positivity	1st	–	Ongoing

Abbreviations: cfDNA, circulating free DNA; ISH, in situ hybridization.

ERBB2 amplification as determined by next-generation sequencing, in situ hybridization, or IHC were treated with trastuzumab and pertuzumab.[42] Across 57 evaluable patients, 18 achieved an objective response (1 complete response and 17 partial responses) and median PFS was 2.9 months. Objective responses were significantly enriched in KRAS wild-type patients, although KRAS status was not evaluated as part of eligibility criteria. The phase 2 TRIUMPH study enrolled patients with previously treated RAS wild-type, ERBB2-amplified metastatic CRC identified either by tissue-based or cell-free DNA testing for dual treatment with trastuzumab plus pertuzumab.[58] Of 18 initial patients evaluable for response, 6 tissue-positive patients (35%) exhibited an objective response, with 1 complete response and 5 partial responses. In the cell-free DNA positive group, 5 patients (33%) exhibited an objective response, including 1 complete response and 5 partial responses. Median progression-free response in both the tissue and cell-free DNA arms was 4 months. Intriguingly, analysis of cell-free DNA at baseline showed that clonal mutations in KRAS, BRAF, PIK3CA, or ERBB2 were present only in patients who exhibited disease progression. The phase 2 MOUNTAINEER study enrolled previously treated RAS wild-type, ERBB2-amplified metastatic CRC as identified by next-generation sequencing, FISH, or IHC for dual treatment with trastuzumab and tucatinib.[59] Of the 22 initial patients evaluable for response, 12 (55%) exhibited an objective response, either complete or partial, whereas 5 (23%) exhibited stable disease. Median PFS was 6.2 months. Across the MyPathway, TRIUMPH, and MOUNTAINEER trials, dual anti-ERBB2 therapy was well tolerated, although grade 3 to 4 treatment-related adverse events were identified in 37% of MyPathway patients. Based on results from HERACLES-A and MyPathway, the National Comprehensive Cancer Network now recommends treatment with trastuzumab and either pertuzumab or lapatinib for RAS wild-type, ERBB2-amplified metastatic CRC.[60] As final results from HERACLES-B, TRIUMPH, and MOUNTAINEER become available, and as initial results from other trials targeting ERBB2 amplification become available, it will be possible to achieve significantly greater clarify about the utility of targeting ERBB2 in CRC.

SUMMARY

ERBB2 has been under investigation in CRC for more than 2 decades. It is now clear that a subset of CRC harbors oncogenic amplifications or mutations in ERBB2. Overall, approximately 2% to 3% of CRCs exhibit ERBB2 amplification. Tumors with amplification are often wild-type for other activating mutations in the RAS/RAF/MEK/ERK pathway, such as those in KRAS, BRAF, and NRAS, although these alterations are not completely mutually exclusive. Thus far, there is little evidence that ERBB2 amplification carries prognostic significance. However, ERBB2 amplification may offer value for predicting resistance to anti-EGFR targeted therapy, similar to activating mutations in KRAS, BRAF, and NRAS. More importantly, ERBB2 amplification appears to predict responsiveness to anti-ERBB2 targeted therapy. Building on the positive findings of the HERACLES-A trial, 7 additional phase 2 trials targeting ERBB2 amplification in CRC are now under way. Interim results from several of these studies appear to support dual-agent targeting of ERBB2 amplification, as in HERACLES-A. Based on results from HERACLES-A and MyPathway, the National Comprehensive Cancer Network now recommends treatment with trastuzumab and either pertuzumab or lapatinib for RAS wild-type, ERBB2-amplified metastatic CRC.[60] However, a note of caution should be taken from the experience of targeting ERBB2 amplification in gastroesophageal cancer, wherein the pivotal phase 3 ToGA trial that helped establish the benefit of adding trastuzumab to first-line chemotherapy was followed by a string of negative trials that did not identify survival benefits for additional therapeutic methods of targeting ERBB2 amplification.[61]

Given that ERBB2 amplification is now a targetable alteration in CRC, pathologists should be well positioned to exploit prior laboratory experience in assessing ERBB2 by IHC and FISH as well as existing IHC interpretation criteria for ERBB2 amplification in CRC. Given that anti-ERBB2 therapy is recommended only for patients with metastatic disease, assessment of ERBB2 amplification via next-generation sequencing is an attraction option, given the relative rarity of amplification and the need for concurrent testing of KRAS, NRAS, and BRAF, and mismatch repair/microsatellite instability status, on such tumors. Encouragingly, the performance of NGS for first-line screening to identify ERBB2 amplification in CRC appears to be excellent.[33] Although additional studies are still needed to more thoroughly evaluate other aspects of testing, such as optimal specimen selection and concordance between ERBB2 amplification in cell-free DNA and tissue, this work will help offer a new therapeutic target to patients with metastatic CRC and leverages drugs already approved for other tumors.

ACKNOWLEDGMENTS

Dr J.A. Nowak thanks Dr Lynette Sholl of Brigham and Women's Hospital for the kind provision of ERBB2 IHC data.

DISCLOSURE

The author has nothing to disclose.

REFERENCES

1. Arteaga CL, Engelman JA. ERBB receptors: from oncogene discovery to basic science to mechanism-based cancer therapeutics. Cancer Cell 2014;25(3):282–303.
2. Tzahar E, Waterman H, Chen X, et al. A hierarchical network of interreceptor interactions determines signal transduction by Neu differentiation factor/neuregulin and epidermal growth factor. Mol Cell Biol 1996;16(10):5276–87.
3. Pahuja KB, Nguyen TT, Jaiswal BS, et al. Actionable activating oncogenic ERBB2/HER2 transmembrane and juxtamembrane domain mutations. Cancer Cell 2018;34(5):792–806.e5.
4. Bailey MH, Tokheim C, Porta-Pardo E, et al. Comprehensive characterization of cancer driver genes and mutations. Cell 2018;174(4):1034–5.
5. Cancer Genome Atlas Network. Comprehensive molecular portraits of human breast tumours. Nature 2012;490(7418):61–70.
6. Bang YJ, Van Cutsem E, Feyereislova A, et al. Trastuzumab in combination with chemotherapy versus chemotherapy alone for treatment of HER2-positive advanced gastric or gastro-oesophageal junction cancer (ToGA): a phase 3, open-label, randomised controlled trial. Lancet 2010;376(9742):687–97.
7. Tanner M, Hollmen M, Junttila TT, et al. Amplification of HER-2 in gastric carcinoma: association with Topoisomerase IIalpha gene amplification, intestinal type, poor prognosis and sensitivity to trastuzumab. Ann Oncol 2005;16(2):273–8.
8. Gravalos C, Jimeno A. HER2 in gastric cancer: a new prognostic factor and a novel therapeutic target. Ann Oncol 2008;19(9):1523–9.
9. Cancer Genome Atlas Research Network, Analysis Working Group, Asan University; BC Cancer Agency, et al. Integrated genomic characterization of oesophageal carcinoma. Nature 2017;541(7636):169–75.
10. Cancer Genome Atlas Research Network. Comprehensive molecular characterization of gastric adenocarcinoma. Nature 2014;513(7517):202–9.
11. Harbeck N, Gnant M. Breast cancer. Lancet 2017; 389(10074):1134–50.
12. Bartley AN, Washington MK, Ventura CB, et al. HER2 Testing and clinical decision making in gastroesophageal adenocarcinoma: guideline from the College of American Pathologists, American Society for Clinical Pathology, and American Society of Clinical Oncology. Arch Pathol Lab Med 2016;140(12): 1345–63.
13. Kim EK, Kim KA, Lee CY, et al. The frequency and clinical impact of HER2 alterations in lung adenocarcinoma. PLoS One 2017;12(2):e0171280.
14. Thorpe LM, Schrock AB, Erlich RL, et al. Significant and durable clinical benefit from trastuzumab in 2 patients with HER2-amplified salivary gland cancer and a review of the literature. Head Neck 2017; 39(3):E40–4.
15. Fearon ER, Vogelstein B. A genetic model for colorectal tumorigenesis. Cell 1990;61(5):759–67.
16. Cancer Genome Atlas Network. Comprehensive molecular characterization of human colon and rectal cancer. Nature 2012;487(7407):330–7.
17. Kapitanovic S, Radosevic S, Kapitanovic M, et al. The expression of p185(HER-2/neu) correlates with the stage of disease and survival in colorectal cancer. Gastroenterology 1997;112(4):1103–13.
18. Essapen S, Thomas H, Green M, et al. The expression and prognostic significance of HER-2 in colorectal cancer and its relationship with clinicopathological parameters. Int J Oncol 2004;24(2):241–8.
19. Valtorta E, Martino C, Sartore-Bianchi A, et al. Assessment of a HER2 scoring system for colorectal cancer: results from a validation study. Mod Pathol 2015;28(11):1481–91.
20. Ni S, Peng J, Huang D, et al. HER2 overexpression and amplification in patients with colorectal cancer: a large-scale retrospective study in Chinese population. J Clin Oncol 2017;35(15_suppl): e15099.
21. Laurent-Puig P, Balogoun R, Cayre A, et al. ERBB2 alterations a new prognostic biomarker in stage III colon cancer from a FOLFOX based adjuvant trial (PETACC8). Ann Oncol 2016;27(suppl_6):vi151.
22. Richman SD, Southward K, Chambers P, et al. HER2 overexpression and amplification as a potential therapeutic target in colorectal cancer: analysis of 3256 patients enrolled in the QUASAR, FOCUS and PICCOLO colorectal cancer trials. J Pathol 2016; 238(4):562–70.
23. Sawada K, Nakamura Y, Yamanaka T, et al. Prognostic and predictive value of HER2 amplification in patients with metastatic colorectal cancer. Clin Colorectal Cancer 2018;17(3):198–205.
24. McKay JA, Loane JF, Ross VG, et al. c-erbB-2 is not a major factor in the development of colorectal cancer. Br J Cancer 2002;86(4):568–73.
25. Shan L, Lv Y, Bai B, et al. Variability in HER2 expression between primary colorectal cancer and corresponding metastases. J Cancer Res Clin Oncol 2018;144(11):2275–81.
26. Siravegna G, Lazzari L, Crisafulli G, et al. Radiologic and genomic evolution of individual metastases

during HER2 blockade in colorectal cancer. Cancer Cell 2018;34(1):148–62.e7.

27. Park JS, Yoon G, Kim HJ, et al. HER2 status in patients with residual rectal cancer after preoperative chemoradiotherapy: the relationship with molecular results and clinicopathologic features. Virchows Arch 2018;473(4):413–23.

28. Greulich H, Kaplan B, Mertins P, et al. Functional analysis of receptor tyrosine kinase mutations in lung cancer identifies oncogenic extracellular domain mutations of ERBB2. Proc Natl Acad Sci U S A 2012;109(36):14476–81.

29. Bose R, Kavuri SM, Searleman AC, et al. Activating HER2 mutations in HER2 gene amplification negative breast cancer. Cancer Discov 2013;3(2):224–37.

30. Ross JS, Fakih M, Ali SM, et al. Targeting HER2 in colorectal cancer: the landscape of amplification and short variant mutations in ERBB2 and ERBB3. Cancer 2018;124(7):1358–73.

31. Yaeger R, Chatila WK, Lipsyc MD, et al. Clinical sequencing defines the genomic landscape of metastatic colorectal cancer. Cancer Cell 2018;33(1): 125–36.e3.

32. Ross DS, Zehir A, Cheng DT, et al. Next-generation assessment of human epidermal growth factor receptor 2 (ERBB2) amplification status: clinical validation in the context of a hybrid capture-based, comprehensive solid tumor genomic profiling assay. J Mol Diagn 2017;19(2):244–54.

33. Cenaj O, Ligon AH, Hornick JL, et al. Detection of ERBB2 amplification by next-generation sequencing predicts HER2 expression in colorectal carcinoma. Am J Clin Pathol 2019;152(1):97–108.

34. Lee J, Franovic A, Shiotsu Y, et al. Detection of ERBB2 (HER2) gene amplification events in cell-free DNA and response to Anti-HER2 agents in a large Asian cancer patient cohort. Front Oncol 2019;9:212.

35. Choi IS, Kato S, Fanta PT, et al. Genomic profiling of blood-derived circulating tumor DNA from patients with colorectal cancer: implications for response and resistance to targeted therapeutics. Mol Cancer Ther 2019;18(10):1852–62.

36. Missiaglia E, Jacobs B, D'Ario G, et al. Distal and proximal colon cancers differ in terms of molecular, pathological, and clinical features. Ann Oncol 2014;25(10):1995–2001.

37. Nam SK, Yun S, Koh J, et al. BRAF, PIK3CA, and HER2 oncogenic alterations according to KRAS mutation status in advanced colorectal cancers with distant metastasis. PLoS One 2016;11(3):e0151865.

38. Marshall J, Lenz H-J, Xiu J, et al. Molecular variances between rectal and left-sided colon cancers. J Clin Oncol 2017;35(4_suppl):522.

39. Ingold Heppner B, Behrens HM, Balschun K, et al. HER2/neu testing in primary colorectal carcinoma. Br J Cancer 2014;111(10):1977–84.

40. Siena S, Sartore-Bianchi A, Trusolino L, et al. Abstract CT005: Final results of the HERACLES trial in HER2-amplified colorectal cancer. Cancer Res 2017;77(13 Supplement):CT005.

41. Sclafani F, Roy A, Cunningham D, et al. HER2 in high-risk rectal cancer patients treated in EXPERT-C, a randomized phase II trial of neoadjuvant capecitabine and oxaliplatin (CAPOX) and chemoradiotherapy (CRT) with or without cetuximab. Ann Oncol 2013;24(12):3123–8.

42. Meric-Bernstam F, Hurwitz H, Raghav KPS, et al. Pertuzumab plus trastuzumab for HER2-amplified metastatic colorectal cancer (MyPathway): an updated report from a multicentre, open-label, phase 2a, multiple basket study. Lancet Oncol 2019; 20(4):518–30.

43. Schuell B, Gruenberger T, Scheithauer W, et al. HER 2/neu protein expression in colorectal cancer. BMC Cancer 2006;6:123.

44. Osako T, Miyahara M, Uchino S, et al. Immunohistochemical study of c-erbB-2 protein in colorectal cancer and the correlation with patient survival. Oncology 1998;55(6):548–55.

45. Conradi LC, Styczen H, Sprenger T, et al. Frequency of HER-2 positivity in rectal cancer and prognosis. Am J Surg Pathol 2013;37(4):522–31.

46. Sepulveda AR, Hamilton SR, Allegra CJ, et al. Molecular biomarkers for the evaluation of colorectal cancer: guideline from the American Society for Clinical Pathology, College of American Pathologists, Association for Molecular Pathology, and American Society of Clinical Oncology. J Mol Diagn 2017;19(2):187–225.

47. Benson AB, Venook AP, Al-Hawary MM, et al. NCCN guidelines insights: colon cancer, version 2.2018. J Natl Compr Canc Netw 2018;16(4):359–69.

48. Messersmith WA. NCCN guidelines updates: management of metastatic colorectal cancer. J Natl Compr Canc Netw 2019;17(5.5):599–601.

49. Bertotti A, Migliardi G, Galimi F, et al. A molecularly annotated platform of patient-derived xenografts ("xenopatients") identifies HER2 as an effective therapeutic target in cetuximab-resistant colorectal cancer. Cancer Discov 2011;1(6):508–23.

50. Yonesaka K, Zejnullahu K, Okamoto I, et al. Activation of ERBB2 signaling causes resistance to the EGFR-directed therapeutic antibody cetuximab. Sci Transl Med 2011;3(99):99ra86.

51. Martin V, Landi L, Molinari F, et al. HER2 gene copy number status may influence clinical efficacy to anti-EGFR monoclonal antibodies in metastatic colorectal cancer patients. Br J Cancer 2013;108(3):668–75.

52. Raghav KPS, Overman MJ, Yu R, et al. HER2 amplification as a negative predictive biomarker for anti-epidermal growth factor receptor antibody therapy in metastatic colorectal cancer. J Clin Oncol 2016; 34(15_suppl):3517.

53. Sartore-Bianchi A, Trusolino L, Martino C, et al. Dual-targeted therapy with trastuzumab and lapatinib in treatment-refractory, KRAS codon 12/13 wild-type, HER2-positive metastatic colorectal cancer (HERACLES): a proof-of-concept, multicentre, open-label, phase 2 trial. Lancet Oncol 2016; 17(6):738–46.

54. Ramanathan RK, Hwang JJ, Zamboni WC, et al. Low overexpression of HER-2/neu in advanced colorectal cancer limits the usefulness of trastuzumab (Herceptin) and irinotecan as therapy. A phase II trial. Cancer Invest 2004;22(6):858–65.

55. Clark JW, Niedzwiecki D, Hollis D, et al. Phase-II trial of 5-fluororuacil (5-FU), leucovorin (LV), oxaliplatin (Ox), and trastuzamab (T) for patients with metastatic. colorectal cancer (CRC) refractory to initial therapy. Onkologie 2003;26(suppl3):13–46.

56. Bekaii-Saab TS, Roda JM, Guenterberg KD, et al. A phase I trial of paclitaxel and trastuzumab in combination with interleukin-12 in patients with HER2/neu-expressing malignancies. Mol Cancer Ther 2009;8(11):2983–91.

57. Sartore-Bianchi A, Martino C, Lonardi S, et al. LBA35Phase II study of pertuzumab and trastuzumab-emtansine (T-DM1) in patients with HER2-positive metastatic colorectal cancer: The HERACLES-B (HER2 Amplification for Colo-rectaL cancer Enhanced Stratification, cohort B) trial. Ann Oncol 2019;30(Supplement_5):v869–70.

58. Nakamura Y, Okamoto W, Kato T, et al. 526PD - TRIUMPH: Primary efficacy of a phase II trial of trastuzumab (T) and pertuzumab (P) in patients (pts) with metastatic colorectal cancer (mCRC) with HER2 (ERBB2) amplification (amp) in tumour tissue or circulating tumour DNA (ctDNA): A GOZILA substudy. Ann Oncol 2019;30:v199–200.

59. Strickler JH, Zemla T, Ou F-S, et al. 527PDTrastuzumab and tucatinib for the treatment of HER2 amplified metastatic colorectal cancer (mCRC): Initial results from the MOUNTAINEER trial. Ann Oncol 2019;30(Supplement_5):v200.

60. Network NCC. Colon cancer (version 1.2020. 2020. Available at: https://www.nccn.org/professionals/physician_gls/pdf/colon.pdf. Accessed February 14, 2020.

61. Zhao D, Klempner SJ, Chao J. Progress and challenges in HER2-positive gastroesophageal adenocarcinoma. J Hematol Oncol 2019;12(1):50.

62. Ross JS, McKenna BJ. The HER-2/neu oncogene in tumors of the gastrointestinal tract. Cancer Invest 2001;19(5):554–68.

63. Hofmann M, Stoss O, Shi D, et al. Assessment of a HER2 scoring system for gastric cancer: results from a validation study. Histopathology 2008;52(7): 797–805.

64. Gomez-Martin C, Plaza JC, Pazo-Cid R, et al. Level of HER2 gene amplification predicts response and overall survival in HER2-positive advanced gastric cancer treated with trastuzumab. J Clin Oncol 2013;31(35):4445–52.

65. Song Z, Deng Y, Zhuang K, et al. Immunohistochemical results of HER2/neu protein expression assessed by rabbit monoclonal antibodies SP3 and 4B5 in colorectal carcinomas. Int J Clin Exp Pathol 2014;7(7):4454–60.

66. Kruszewski WJ, Rzepko R, Ciesielski M, et al. Expression of HER2 in colorectal cancer does not correlate with prognosis. Dis Markers 2010;29(5): 207–12.

67. Kountourakis P, Pavlakis K, Psyrri A, et al. Clinicopathologic significance of EGFR and Her-2/neu in colorectal adenocarcinomas. Cancer J 2006;12(3): 229–36.

68. Rossi HA, Liu Q, Banner B, et al. The prognostic value of invariant chain (Ii) and Her-2/neu expression in curatively resected colorectal cancer. Cancer J 2002;8(3):268–75.

69. Siena S, Bardelli A, Sartore-Bianchi A, et al. HER2 amplification as a 'molecular bait' for trastuzumab-emtansine (T-DM1) precision chemotherapy to overcome anti-HER2 resistance in HER2 positive metastatic colorectal cancer: The HERACLES-RESCUE trial. J Clin Oncol 2016;34(4_suppl):TPS774.

70. Raghav KPS, McDonough SL, Tan BR, et al. A randomized phase II study of trastuzumab and pertuzumab (TP) compared to cetuximab and irinotecan (CETIRI) in advanced/metastatic colorectal cancer (mCRC) with HER2 amplification: S1613. J Clin Oncol 2018;36(15_suppl):TPS3620.

71. Schmoll HJ, Arnold D, de Gramont A, et al. MODUL-a multicenter randomized clinical trial of biomarker-driven maintenance therapy following first-line standard induction treatment of metastatic colorectal cancer: an adaptable signal-seeking approach. J Cancer Res Clin Oncol 2018;144(6):1197–204.

72. Giannakis M, Mu XJ, Shukla SA, et al. Genomic correlates of immune-cell infiltrates in colorectal carcinoma. Cell Rep 2016;15(4):857–65.

73. Cerami E, Gao J, Dogrusoz U, et al. The cBio cancer genomics portal: an open platform for exploring multidimensional cancer genomics data. Cancer Discov 2012;2(5):401–4.

74. Gao J, Aksoy BA, Dogrusoz U, et al. Integrative analysis of complex cancer genomics and clinical profiles using the cBioPortal. Sci Signal 2013; 6(269):pl1.

Histology of Colorectal Carcinoma
Proven and Purported Prognostic Factors

Melanie Johncilla, MD, Rhonda K. Yantiss, MD*

KEYWORDS

• Prognostic features • Colorectal carcinoma • Pathology • Histology

---

Key points

- Histologic grade, subtype, lymphovascular invasion, and perineural invasion are important prognostic indicators for patients with colorectal carcinoma.
- Tumor budding may be even more prognostically relevant than conventional grading schema.
- A host immune response composed of tumor-infiltrating lymphocytes and/or a Crohn-like lymphoid reaction is prognostically relevant, even among mismatch repair–proficient tumors.

ABSTRACT

Although tumor stage has a profound influence on prognosis, several histologic features are also important. These parameters predict biological behavior and can be used by clinicians to determine whether patients are at high risk for disease progression and, thus, are candidates for adjuvant therapy, particularly when they have localized (ie, stage II) disease. This article summarizes the evidence supporting the prognostic values of various histologic parameters evaluated by pathologists who assign pathologic stage to colorectal cancers. Criteria to be discussed include histologic subtype, tumor grade, lymphatic and perineural invasion, tumor budding, and host immune responses.

OVERVIEW

Despite advances in the molecular characterization of colorectal carcinoma, tumor stage assessment remains the gold standard for determining prognosis. Tumor grade, lymphatic vessel invasion, and perineural invasion are also well-established histologic markers of aggressive biological behavior, and other recently described features seem to be predictive of outcome. This article discusses the prognostic importance of histologic features encountered in colorectal carcinoma specimens (**Box 1**).

THE PROGNOSTIC SIGNIFICANCE OF HISTOLOGIC SUBTYPE

Most colorectal carcinomas are adenocarcinomas with intestinal differentiation; mucinous, serrated, and signet ring cell differentiation are less common. The World Health Organization also describes several less common variants that account for less than 10% of colorectal cancers, including adenosquamous, neuroendocrine, squamous cell, and undifferentiated carcinomas.[1] These variants are high-grade neoplasms at risk for aggressive behavior compared with adenocarcinomas. Typical features of colorectal cancer variants are summarized in **Table 1**.

INTESTINAL-TYPE ADENOCARCINOMA

Intestinal-type adenocarcinomas are typically composed of large angulated or fused glands lined by cells with ovoid nuclei, coarse chromatin, and

Department of Pathology and Laboratory Medicine, Weill Cornell Medicine, 525 East 68th Street, New York, NY 10065, USA
* Corresponding author.
E-mail address: rhy2001@med.cornell.edu

Surgical Pathology 13 (2020) 503–520
https://doi.org/10.1016/j.path.2020.05.008

Table 1
Morphologic variants of colorectal carcinoma

Histologic Subtype	Salient Histologic Features
Intestinal-type adenocarcinoma	Gland formation recapitulating colonic mucosa
Mucinous adenocarcinoma	Pools of mucin-containing strips and clusters of tumor cells Pools of mucin-containing signet ring cells
Serrated adenocarcinoma	Serrated glands and cells with clear to eosinophilic cytoplasm
Signet ring cell carcinoma	Infiltrative clusters or single cells with eccentric nuclei
Cribriform carcinoma	Cribriform growth with comedo-type necrosis
Micropapillary carcinoma	Small clusters of neoplastic cells without fibrovascular cores Tumor cells show reverse polarity
Medullary carcinoma	Syncytial nests of medium to large cells with vesicular nuclei and prominent nucleoli Intraepithelial and peritumoral lymphocyte-predominant inflammation
Adenosquamous carcinoma	Malignant glands and squamous components
Carcinoma with sarcomatoid components	Malignant spindle cell tumor with at least focal keratin positivity
Squamous cell carcinoma	Squamous nests with or without keratinization
(Neuro)endocrine carcinoma	Small or large cell carcinoma with high mitotic rate, Ki-67 proliferation index, and immunoexpression of endocrine markers
Undifferentiated carcinoma	High-grade carcinoma without morphologic or immunohistochemical evidence of specific differentiation

numerous mitotic figures. They often contain luminal necrotic debris and are surrounded by desmoplastic stroma (**Fig. 1**). Broders[2] first recognized that extent of glandular differentiation correlated with improved outcome of colorectal carcinoma. His observations ultimately led to implementation of a 4-tiered grading system: carcinomas with greater than 95% glandular elements were classified as well differentiated, whereas those with 50% to 95%, 5% to 49%, and less than 5% gland formation were moderately, poorly, and undifferentiated carcinomas, respectively. More recently proposed schemes classify tumors as low-grade and high-grade based on extent (at least 50%) of glandular differentiation, thereby improving reproducibility and maintaining strong correlations with outcome.[3,4] The World Health Organization recommends that grade be assigned based on the least differentiated areas but notes that the advancing tumor edge should be avoided when determining histologic grade.[1] Most data suggest that this stipulation likely underestimates biological risk. Carcinomas that contain solid elements occupying at least 1 high-power field (400× magnification) are associated with a 69% disease-related 5-year survival compared with 99% 5-year survival rates among patients with cancers containing less than 10 solid tumor cell clusters per low-power field (40× magnification).[5] For this reason, some investigators have proposed a 3-tiered grading system assessing solid cell clusters (<5, 5–9, and ≥10) per intermediate-power field (200× magnification) regardless of their location within the mass. These grade assignments are associated with 5-year disease-free survival rates of 96%, 85%, and

Fig. 1. Intestinal-type adenocarcinomas feature infiltrative glands lined by cells with large, hyperchromatic nuclei and numerous mitotic figures. Low-grade carcinomas are mostly composed of gland-forming elements (*A*), whereas high-grade tumors contain infiltrative cords or single cells with a minor glandular component (*B*).

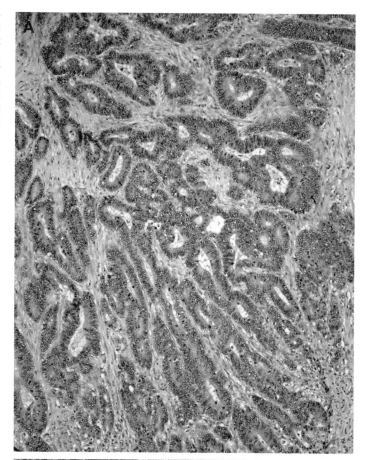

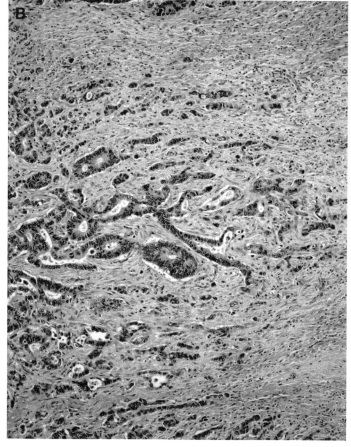

59%, respectively among stage II and III carcinomas.[6] It is also worth mentioning that distinction of tumor grade from tumor budding and poorly differentiated cell clusters is arguably arbitrary in many cases. Tumor buds and poorly differentiated cell clusters are definitionally high grade because they do not form glands. Of note, grading criteria are applicable only to intestinal-type adenocarcinomas; there are no established schema for other variants.

Low-grade tubuloglandular adenocarcinomas are well-differentiated adenocarcinomas consisting of tubular glands lined by remarkably bland epithelial cells unaccompanied by a desmoplastic reaction (**Fig. 2**). Low-grade tubuloglandular carcinomas have distinct molecular features with frequent *IDH1* mutations.[7]

MUCINOUS ADENOCARCINOMA

Mucinous adenocarcinomas account for approximately 10% of colorectal carcinomas.[1,8] Although they are arbitrarily defined by the presence of extracellular mucin accounting for at least 50% of the tumor volume, recent data suggest that extent of mucinous differentiation is not predictive of outcome.[9] Mucinous adenocarcinomas show expansile, pushing growth with strips, clusters, or singly arranged tumor cells floating in mucin pools (**Fig. 3**).

Mucinous adenocarcinomas have historically been classified as high-grade neoplasms owing to their reportedly aggressive behavior.[10,11] Not all of these mucinous tumors are biologically aggressive.[12] Approximately 50% are mismatch repair deficient, in which case they have a better prognosis than morphologically similar stage-matched, mismatch repair–proficient tumors.[8,9,13,14] However, high-grade cytologic features and signet ring cell differentiation are associated with a worse prognosis among mismatch repair–deficient tumors, suggesting that both molecular and morphologic features inform prognosis of mucinous carcinomas.[15,16]

SERRATED ADENOCARCINOMA

Serrated adenocarcinomas account for approximately 8% of all colorectal carcinomas.[17] They are largely composed of neoplastic epithelial cells with clear or eosinophilic cytoplasm, vesicular nuclei, prominent nucleoli, and preserved nuclear polarity (**Fig. 4**).[18] Areas of mucinous differentiation and tumor budding at the advancing tumor edge are frequently identified but serrated carcinomas generally lack abundant luminal necrotic debris typical of intestinal-type carcinomas.[19]

Behavior is related to underlying molecular abnormalities. Approximately 20% show *BRAF* mutations, CpG island hypermethylation, and mismatch repair deficiency, in which case they are associated with a favorable prognosis. The remainder show various combinations of mismatch repair proficiency, *BRAF* or *KRAS* mutations, and extensive or little DNA hypermethylation.[17,20–22] Tumors that are *BRAF* mutated with mismatch repair proficiency are associated with an especially aggressive clinical course.[18,23,24]

SIGNET RING CELL CARCINOMA

Signet ring cell carcinomas account for less than 1% of colorectal carcinomas and are more prevalent among patients less than 40 years of age, particularly those with inflammatory bowel disease.[25,26] These tumors are defined by dyshesive, medium to large cells with abundant mucinous cytoplasm and eccentric, hyperchromatic nuclei that account for at least 50% of the tumor volume.[1] Three patterns of signet ring cell carcinoma have been described: single infiltrating signet ring cells reminiscent of diffuse-type gastric carcinoma, signet ring cells floating in mucin pools, and sheetlike growth of tumor cell nests unaccompanied by a desmoplastic stromal response (**Fig. 5**). The last features nests of mucin-containing cells with peripherally compressed nuclei reminiscent of goblet cell carcinoma of the appendix. Signet ring cell carcinomas with sheetlike growth and those accompanied by extracellular mucin are often associated with mucinous carcinomas.[27]

Approximately one-third of signet ring cell carcinomas are mismatch repair deficient, although mismatch repair status does not seem to influence biological behavior. Signet ring cells are associated with poor prognosis among both mismatch repair–proficient and mismatch repair–deficient carcinomas, even when present as a minor (eg, 10%) component.[15,28,29] For this reason, signet ring cell differentiation warrants designation as high-grade carcinoma, regardless of mismatch repair status.

CRIBRIFORM COMEDO-TYPE CARCINOMA

Cribriform comedo-type carcinomas are composed of expansile sheets and aggregates of tightly packed glands with round lumina and little intervening stroma.[30] They often show a peripheral rim of tumor cells with cribriform growth surrounding necrotic material reminiscent of ductal carcinoma in situ of the breast (**Fig. 6**). This distinctive histologic variant is associated with a worse prognosis than low-

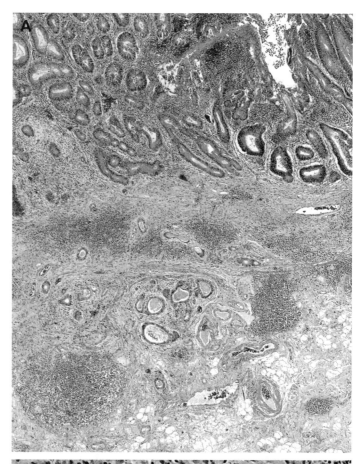

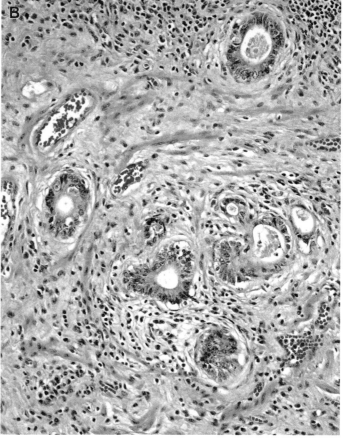

Fig. 2. Low-grade tubuloglandular adenocarcinoma invades the submucosa without destroying the muscularis mucosae (*A*) or eliciting a stromal reaction (*B*).

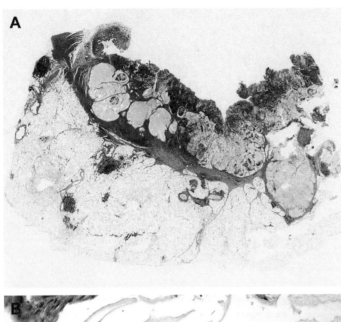

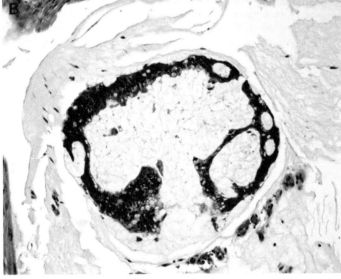

Fig. *3.* Mucinous adenocarcinomas are composed of large mucin pools (*A*) containing strips of neoplastic cells with low-grade (*B*) or high-grade

grade intestinal-type adenocarcinoma despite the presence of extensive glandular differentiation.[31] Cribriform growth of carcinomas in polypectomy specimens is significantly associated with regional lymph node metastases.[32] Many tumors with cribriform areas and comedo-type necrosis also feature other high-grade morphologic patterns, such as mucinous, micropapillary, and serrated differentiation.[33]

MICROPAPILLARY ADENOCARCINOMA

Pure micropapillary carcinomas of the colorectum account for less than 1% of all colorectal carcinomas, but approximately 10% of all colorectal cancers contain areas of micropapillary growth.[33] Micropapillary carcinomas feature lacunar spaces that contain tumor cells and no supportive stroma (**Fig. 7**). Tumor cells show reverse polarity with their apical surfaces oriented toward the periphery of the cluster. They contain eosinophilic cytoplasm and show high-grade nuclear features with frequent lymphovascular invasion. They characteristically show apical MUC1 immunopositivity. This glycoprotein normally inhibits stromal interactions and likely contributes to the morphologic appearance of this tumor type.[34] Micropapillary differentiation is an adverse prognostic factor, even when it accounts for less than 10% of the tumor volume.[33,35–39]

Fig. 3. (continued). (*C*) cytologic features. Adenocarcinomas that contain distended or ruptured glands should be classified as intestinal-type adenocarcinomas rather than mucinous neoplasms (*D*).

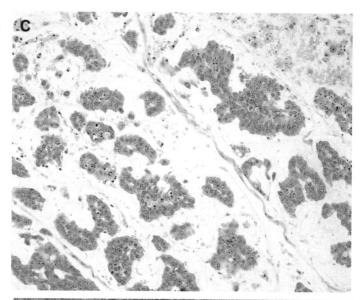

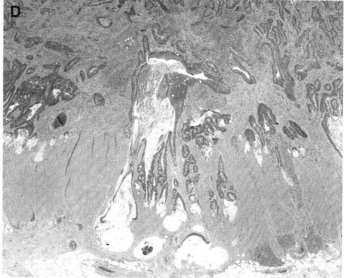

MEDULLARY CARCINOMA

Medullary carcinomas are solid tumors that show minimal gland formation. They contain syncytial nests of polygonal tumor cells with eosinophilic cytoplasm and large vesicular nuclei with prominent nucleoli (**Fig. 8**). Intratumoral and/or peritumoral lymphocytes are frequently present and may be associated with Crohn-type lymphoid aggregates at the advancing tumor edge. Criteria distinguishing medullary carcinoma from poorly differentiated intestinal-type adenocarcinoma with solid growth are not well established.[40–42] As a result, there is a high degree of interobserver variability with respect to classification of solid colorectal carcinomas, even among subspecialty-trained gastrointestinal pathologists.[43] Most medullary carcinomas are mismatch repair deficient and, thus, are associated with better outcomes than stage-matched mismatch repair–proficient adenocarcinomas with solid growth patterns.[42,44]

***

VASCULAR INVASION

LYMPHOVASCULAR AND SMALL VEIN INVASION

Lymphatic channels are present in all layers of the colonic wall, including the deep crypt region of the normal mucosa. Colorectal carcinomas induce lymphangiogenesis, resulting in increased

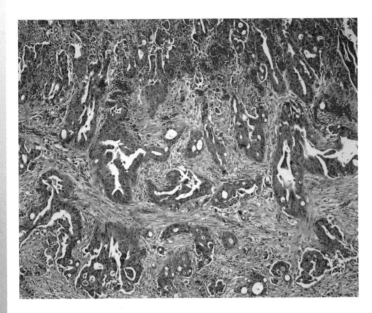

Fig. 4. Serrated adenocarcinomas contain angulated, serrated glands lined by cells with abundant eosinophilic cytoplasm. They often show marked desmoplasia and tumor budding with luminal neutrophils.

microvessel density in and around the tumor.[45] Microvessel density is positively correlated with depth of tumor invasion, lymphatic vessel invasion, regional lymph node metastases, and liver metastases.[46] Both lymphovascular and venous invasion are poor prognostic factors among colorectal carcinomas.[47,48] The diagnosis of small vessel invasion requires identification of single or clustered tumor cell emboli within endothelium-lined spaces. Lymphovascular invasion within the tumor can be obscured by its destructive nature and may be better appreciated at the advancing edge of the tumor or in the adjacent mucosa. Ancillary stains for D240 or other endothelial markers can facilitate detection of vascular invasion.

LARGE VESSEL (VENOUS) INVASION

Large vein invasion is independently associated with a poor prognosis.[49] It may be limited to the vicinity of the tumor in up to one-third of colorectal cancers, in which case its detection can be enhanced by elastin stains.[50,51] Extramural venous invasion is an independent prognostic indicator of recurrence and overall survival in patients with colorectal carcinoma.[51,52] Vascular invasion can result in destruction of the vein wall, appearing as rounded or serpiginous nodules adjacent to large-caliber arteries (**Fig. 9**).

PERINEURAL INVASION

Perineural invasion is detected in approximately 10% of colorectal carcinomas, particularly those with other high-risk features. It is a poor prognostic indicator that is independently associated with regional lymph node metastases and decreased survival, as well as a more than 2.5-fold increased risk of local disease recurrence.[53–55] The presence of extramural perineural invasion is also associated with worse overall survival among patients with neoadjuvantly treated rectal adenocarcinomas.[56]

TUMOR BUDDING AND POORLY DIFFERENTIATED CLUSTERS

Tumor budding is defined by the presence of single infiltrating cells or groups of up to 4 neoplastic cells at the invasive front of the tumor (**Fig. 10A**). Tumor cells may be elongated or spindled and merge imperceptibly with the tumor stroma, a finding that has been termed epithelial-mesenchymal transformation. Tumor budding results from loss of intercellular junctions and is accompanied by expression of CD133, LGR5, and other stem cell markers.[57,58] It is more common among mismatch repair–proficient tumors than mismatch repair–deficient neoplasms and portends increased mortality risk among both types of tumors.[59–62] It is also associated with a high risk of lymph node metastases when detected in polypectomy specimens.[63]

Some investigators recommend that colorectal carcinomas be evaluated for tumor budding by screening at least 10 high-power fields at the invasive front of the tumor and counting the number of cells or clusters per 0.785 mm² in the area of maximal budding.[64] Scores are assigned for low-

Fig. 5. Some investigators classify mucinous tumors with signet ring cells as signet ring cell carcinoma, whereas others consider them to represent high-grade mucinous adenocarcinomas (*A*). Signet ring cells show infiltrative growth (*B*) and may be accompanied by mucin

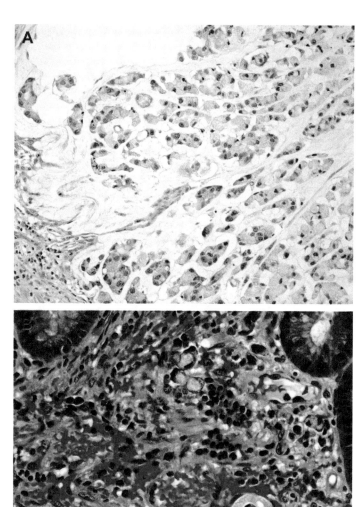

grade (0–4 buds), intermediate-grade (5–9 buds), and high-grade (≥10 buds) tumor budding.[60] Although cytokeratin immunohistochemistry may facilitate evaluation when tumors contain a striking peritumoral lymphocytic infiltrate or a desmoplastic stromal response that obscures small cell clusters, ancillary stains are not clearly superior to routine histologic evaluation when predicting biological behavior.[65]

Poorly differentiated clusters, defined as nests of 5 or more neoplastic cells at the invasive tumor front, are associated with a poor prognosis among mismatch repair–proficient and mismatch repair–deficient carcinomas (**Fig. 10**B).[59,66] Some data suggest that the presence of poorly differentiated clusters is the best predictor of recurrence-free survival among patients with colorectal cancer and can be evaluated with a high degree of interobserver agreement.[67] For this reason, some investigators have proposed that, when present, poorly differentiated clusters should be graded with a 3-tiered system similar to that proposed for assessing tumor budding. The authors have found that poorly differentiated clusters are usually detected in carcinomas that also contain tumor buds, suggesting that the distinction between tumor budding and larger cell clusters is essentially an academic exercise.

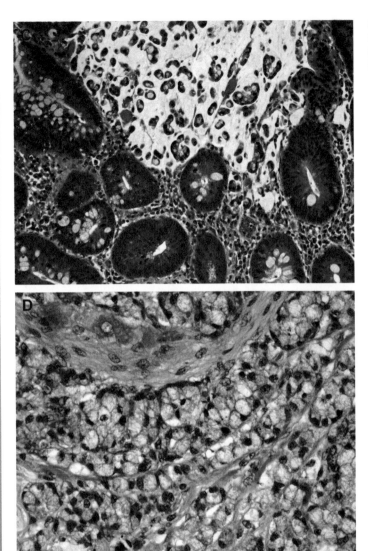

Fig. 5. *(continued).* *(C).* Those associated with mucinous carcinomas often show sheetlike growth of tumor cell nests *(D).*

HOST IMMUNE RESPONSE TO TUMOR

There are 2 patterns of host immune response to colorectal carcinoma: tumor-infiltrating lymphocytes and a Crohn-like lymphoid response at the advancing tumor edge. Both of these histologic findings are more common among mismatch repair–deficient tumors, although the relationship between their detection and outcome is independent of mismatch repair status.[68,69]

TUMOR-INFILTRATING LYMPHOCYTES

Tumor-infiltrating lymphocytes interdigitate between tumor cells and presumably reflect a response to neoantigens elaborated by cancer cells (**Fig. 11A**). They are considered to be increased when at least 2 are detected per high-power field (400× magnification).[70,71] The extent of tumor-infiltrating lymphocytes is generally graded as absent, mild (1–2), or marked (>2) based on the number of tumor-infiltrating lymphocytes present per high-power field (400× magnification).[70]

CROHN-LIKE LYMPHOID REACTION

The Crohn-like lymphoid response features lymphoid aggregates with or without germinal centers located at least 1 mm from the advancing

Fig. 6. Cribriform comedo-type carcinoma resembles ductal carcinoma in situ. Comedo-type necrosis is surrounded by a rim of tumor cells with cribriform architecture.

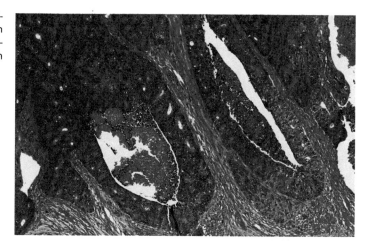

Fig. 7. Micropapillary carcinomas contain clustered tumor cells located within lacunar spaces. They show high-grade cytologic features and lack fibrovascular cores.

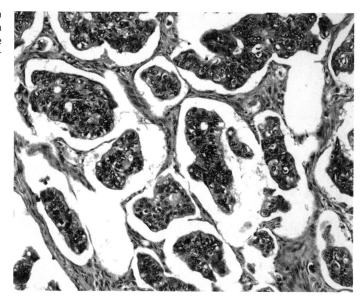

Fig. 8. Medullary carcinomas are composed of syncytia of medium-sized cells with large, vesicular nuclei and numerous intraepithelial lymphocytes.

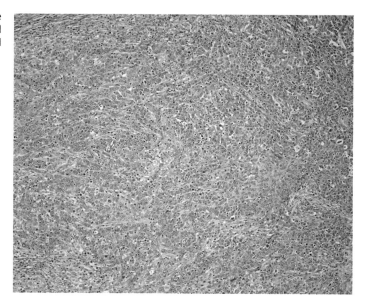

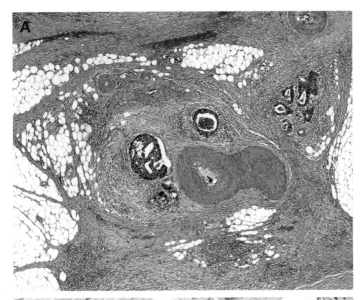

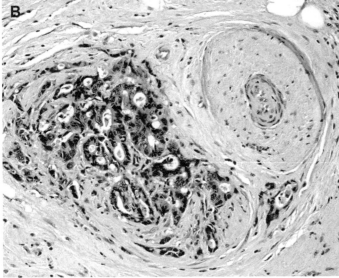

Fig. 9. The presence of a naked artery in the pericolic fat is a clue to the presence of extramural venous invasion (*A*). Extravenous extension should be staged as venous invasion rather than a tumor deposit (*B*).

edge of the tumor (**Fig. 11B**). Although minimal criteria for a Crohn-like lymphoid reaction have not been established, most investigators require 3 to 4 lymphoid aggregates in 1 low-power field (40× magnification) at the advancing edge of tumor.[68,70] A marked Crohn-like lymphoid reaction at the tumor periphery is associated with a decreased incidence of regional lymph node metastases and significantly improved 10-year survival.[72]

NEOADJUVANTLY TREATED RECTAL CARCINOMAS

Locally advanced cancers of the mid to lower rectum are routinely treated with neoadjuvant

therapy to improve resectability and postsurgical quality of life.[73] Treated tumors usually show regression with decreased amounts of viable carcinoma accompanied by mural fibrosis, dystrophic calcifications, and mucin pools. The extent of these changes in the primary tumor and/or metastatic deposits in regional lymph nodes is predictive of prognosis.[74] Tumors with a marked therapeutic response are associated with improved disease-free survival.[75] A variety of regression scoring systems have been proposed, most of which assign the lowest grade to the best treatment response and highest grade to the poorest response. The system accepted by the College of American Pathologists recommends a 4-tier system (complete response, near-

Fig. 10. Tumor buds composed of single cells and small groups are present at the invasive front of the tumor (*A*). Poorly differentiated tumor cell clusters are often present in combination with tumor budding (*B*).

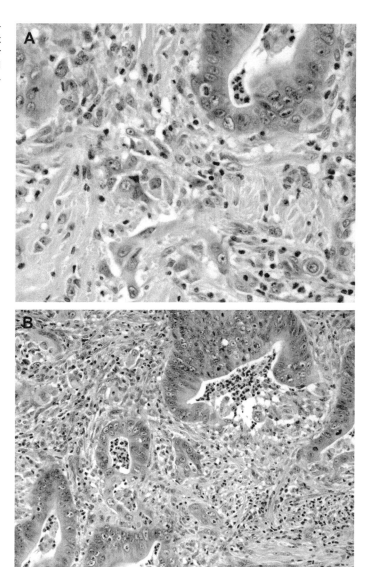

complete response, partial response, or poor response), which is reasonably reproducible with good interobserver agreement.[76] Tumor regression grading should be performed on the primary tumor; a therapeutic response in lymph node deposits is not taken into consideration when grading tumor regression nor does it contribute to overall N stage.[77]

TUMOR BORDER CONFIGURATION AND STROMAL RESPONSE

Colorectal carcinomas are classified as expansile or infiltrative based on the low-power appearance of the advancing tumor front.[78] Tumors with expansile growth have smooth, pushing borders, whereas infiltrative tumors lack sharp demarcation from the adjacent nonneoplastic tissue. An infiltrative growth pattern is associated with decreased survival.[79] The nature of the stromal reaction at the invasive front may be biologically important. Tumors associated with myxoid desmoplastic stroma are associated with poor prognosis and an increased risk of liver metastasis (**Fig. 12**).[67,80] It is possible that the nature of the stromal reaction and its relationship to prognosis is influenced by other features associated with epithelial-mesenchymal transition, such as tumor budding

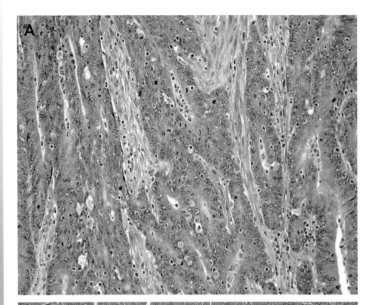

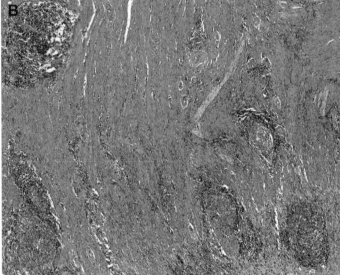

Fig. 11. Numerous intraepithelial lymphocytes are present in this low-grade adenocarcinoma (*A*). A mucinous adenocarcinoma is associated with a rim of rounded lymphoid aggregates (*B*).

and poorly differentiated clusters. The independent predictive value of these features are not well established and, thus, their inclusion in surgical pathology reports is not required at this time.

SUMMARY

Several prognostically important pathologic features should be commented on in colorectal carcinoma surgical pathology reports. Specific cancer types are high-grade neoplasms at risk for biologically aggressive behavior. High-grade features and lymphovascular, venous, and perineural invasion are all associated with decreased overall survival. Colorectal carcinomas that show small nests of tumor cells at the advancing front are more aggressive than those that lack this finding, whereas a host immune response is associated with a better prognosis. For these reasons, information regarding tumor stage and these parameters should be provided in surgical pathology reports for colorectal carcinoma cases.

Fig. 12. Emerging evidence suggests that an exuberant desmoplastic stromal reaction is associated with poor prognosis. However, most tumors with abundant desmoplastic stroma show other high-risk features that predict aggressive behavior.

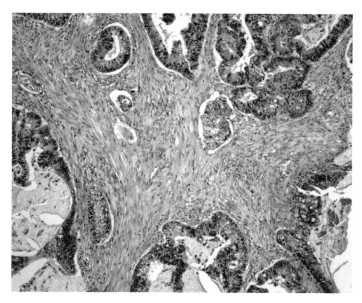

REFERENCES

1. Nagtegaal ID, Arends MJ, Salto-Tellez. Colorectal adenocarcinoma. In: Editorial Board, editor. WHO classification of tumours of the digestive system. WHO classification of tumours. 5th edition. Lyon (France): International Agency for Research on Cancer; 2019. p. 177–87.

2. Broders AC. Grading of carcinoma. Minn Med 1925; 8:726–30.

3. Alexander D, Jhala N, Chatla C, et al. High-grade tumor differentiation is an indicator of poor prognosis in African Americans with colonic adenocarcinomas. Cancer 2005;103(10):2163–70.

4. Harris GJ, Senagore AJ, Lavery IC, et al. Factors affecting survival after palliative resection of colorectal carcinoma. Colorectal Dis 2002;4(1):31–5.

5. Wachtel MS, Haynes AL 3rd, Griswold JA. Signet ring, high grade, and undifferentiated colorectal adenocarcinomas differ. J Surg Res 2010;163(2): 250–6.

6. Chang DT, Pai RK, Rybicki LA, et al. Clinicopathologic and molecular features of sporadic early-onset colorectal adenocarcinoma: an adenocarcinoma with frequent signet ring cell differentiation, rectal and sigmoid involvement, and adverse morphologic features. Mod Pathol 2012;25(8): 1128–39.

7. Hartman DJ, Binion D, Regueiro M, et al. Isocitrate dehydrogenase-1 is mutated in inflammatory bowel disease-associated intestinal adenocarcinoma with low-grade tubuloglandular histology but not in sporadic intestinal adenocarcinoma. Am J Surg Pathol 2014;38(8):1147–56.

8. Andrici J, Farzin M, Sioson L, et al. Mismatch repair deficiency as a prognostic factor in mucinous colorectal cancer. Mod Pathol 2016;29(3):266–74.

9. Gonzalez RS, Cates JMM, Washington K. Associations among histological characteristics and patient outcomes in colorectal carcinoma with a mucinous component. Histopathology 2019;74(3):406–14.

10. Consorti F, Lorenzotti A, Midiri G, et al. Prognostic significance of mucinous carcinoma of colon and rectum: a prospective case-control study. J Surg Oncol 2000;73(2):70–4.

11. Xie L, Villeneuve PJ, Shaw A. Survival of patients diagnosed with either colorectal mucinous or nonmucinous adenocarcinoma: a population-based study in Canada. Int J Oncol 2009;34(4):1109–15.

12. Liddell C, Droy-Dupre L, Metairie S, et al. Mapping clinicopathological entities within colorectal mucinous adenocarcinomas: a hierarchical clustering approach. Mod Pathol 2017;30(8): 1177–89.

13. Leopoldo S, Lorena B, Cinzia A, et al. Two subtypes of mucinous adenocarcinoma of the colorectum: clinicopathological and genetic features. Ann Surg Oncol 2008;15(5):1429–39.

14. Bosman FT, Carneiro F, Hruban RH, et al. WHO classification of the digestive system. 4th edition. Lyon (France): IARC; 2010.

15. Johncilla M, Chen Z, Sweeney J, et al. Tumor grade is prognostically relevant among mismatch repair deficient colorectal carcinomas. Am J Surg Pathol 2018;42(12):1686–92.

16. Hissong E, Crowe EP, Yantiss RK, et al. Assessing colorectal cancer mismatch repair status in the modern era: a survey of current practices and re-

evaluation of the role of microsatellite instability testing. Mod Pathol 2018;31(11):1756–66.

17. Tuppurainen K, Makinen JM, Junttila O, et al. Morphology and microsatellite instability in sporadic serrated and non-serrated colorectal cancer. J Pathol 2005;207(3):285–94.

18. Makinen MJ. Colorectal serrated adenocarcinoma. Histopathology 2007;50(1):131–50.

19. Hirano D, Oka S, Tanaka S, et al. Clinicopathologic and endoscopic features of early-stage colorectal serrated adenocarcinoma. BMC Gastroenterol 2017;17(1):158.

20. Garcia-Solano J, Perez-Guillermo M, Conesa-Zamora P, et al. Clinicopathologic study of 85 colorectal serrated adenocarcinomas: further insights into the full recognition of a new subset of colorectal carcinoma. Hum Pathol 2010;41(10):1359–68.

21. Shida Y, Fujimori T, Tanaka H, et al. Clinicopathological features of serrated adenocarcinoma defined by Makinen in dukes' B colorectal carcinoma. Pathobiology 2012;79(4):169–74.

22. Laiho P, Kokko A, Vanharanta S, et al. Serrated carcinomas form a subclass of colorectal cancer with distinct molecular basis. Oncogene 2007;26(2):312–20.

23. Hirano D, Urabe Y, Tanaka S, et al. Early-stage serrated adenocarcinomas are divided into several molecularly distinct subtypes. PLoS One 2019;14(2):e0211477.

24. Pai RK, Bettington M, Srivastava A, et al. An update on the morphology and molecular pathology of serrated colorectal polyps and associated carcinomas. Mod Pathol 2019;32(10):1390–415.

25. Yantiss RK, Goodarzi M, Zhou XK, et al. Clinical, pathologic, and molecular features of early-onset colorectal carcinoma. Am J Surg Pathol 2009;33(4):572–82.

26. Wang R, Wang MJ, Ping J. Clinicopathological Features and Survival Outcomes of Colorectal Cancer in Young Versus Elderly: A Population-Based Cohort Study of SEER 9 Registries Data (1988-2011). Medicine (Baltimore) 2015;94(35):e1402.

27. Alexander J, Watanabe T, Wu TT, et al. Histopathological identification of colon cancer with microsatellite instability. Am J Pathol 2001;158(2):527–35.

28. Song IH, Hong SM, Yu E, et al. Signet ring cell component predicts aggressive behaviour in colorectal mucinous adenocarcinoma. Pathology 2019;51(4):384–91.

29. Kakar S, Smyrk TC. Signet ring cell carcinoma of the colorectum: correlations between microsatellite instability, clinicopathologic features and survival. Mod Pathol 2005;18(2):244–9.

30. Hamilton SR, Bosman FT, Boffetta P, et al. Tumors of the colon and rectum. In: Bosman FT, Carneiro F, Hruban RH, et al, editors. WHO classification of tumours of the digestive system. 4th edition. Lyon (France): IARC; 2010. p. 134–46.

31. Lino-Silva LS, Salcedo-Hernandez RA, Herrera-Gomez A, et al. Colonic cribriform carcinoma, a morphologic pattern associated with low survival. Int J Surg Pathol 2015;23(1):13–9.

32. Brown IS, Bettington ML, Bettington A, et al. Adverse histological features in malignant colorectal polyps: a contemporary series of 239 cases. J Clin Pathol 2016;69(4):292–9.

33. Gonzalez RS, Huh WJ, Cates JM, et al. Micropapillary colorectal carcinoma: clinical, pathological and molecular properties, including evidence of epithelial-mesenchymal transition. Histopathology 2017;70(2):223–31.

34. Ohtsuki Y, Kuroda N, Umeoka T, et al. KL-6 is another useful marker in assessing a micropapillary pattern in carcinomas of the breast and urinary bladder, but not the colon. Med Mol Morphol 2009;42(2):123–7.

35. Xu F, Xu J, Lou Z, et al. Micropapillary component in colorectal carcinoma is associated with lymph node metastasis in T1 and T2 Stages and decreased survival time in TNM stages I and II. Am J Surg Pathol 2009;33(9):1287–92.

36. Lino-Silva LS, Salcedo-Hernandez RA, Caro-Sanchez CH. Colonic micropapillary carcinoma, a recently recognized subtype associated with histological adverse factors: clinicopathological analysis of 15 cases. Colorectal Dis 2012;14(9):e567–72.

37. Haupt B, Ro JY, Schwartz MR, et al. Colorectal adenocarcinoma with micropapillary pattern and its association with lymph node metastasis. Mod Pathol 2007;20(7):729–33.

38. Kim MJ, Hong SM, Jang SJ, et al. Invasive colorectal micropapillary carcinoma: an aggressive variant of adenocarcinoma. Hum Pathol 2006;37(7):809–15.

39. Kitagawa H, Yoshimitsu M, Kaneko M, et al. Invasive micropapillary carcinoma component is an independent prognosticator of poorer survival in Stage III colorectal cancer patients. Jpn J Clin Oncol 2017;47(12):1129–34.

40. Jessurun J, Romero-Guadarrama M, Manivel JC. Medullary adenocarcinoma of the colon: clinicopathologic study of 11 cases. Hum Pathol 1999;30(7):843–8.

41. Pyo JS, Sohn JH, Kang G. Medullary carcinoma in the colorectum: a systematic review and meta-analysis. Hum Pathol 2016;53:91–6.

42. Ruschoff J, Dietmaier W, Luttges J, et al. Poorly differentiated colonic adenocarcinoma, medullary type: clinical, phenotypic, and molecular characteristics. Am J Pathol 1997;150(5):1815–25.

43. Lee LH, Yantiss RK, Sadot E, et al. Diagnosing colorectal medullary carcinoma: interobserver variability and clinicopathological implications. Hum Pathol 2017;62:74–82.

44. Lanza G, Gafa R, Matteuzzi M, et al. Medullary-type poorly differentiated adenocarcinoma of the large bowel: a distinct clinicopathologic entity characterized by microsatellite instability and improved survival. J Clin Oncol 1999;17(8):2429–38.

45. Schoppmann SF. Lymphangiogenesis, inflammation and metastasis. Anticancer Res 2005;25(6C): 4503–11.

46. Saad RS, Kordunsky L, Liu YL, et al. Lymphatic microvessel density as prognostic marker in colorectal cancer. Mod Pathol 2006;19(10):1317–23.

47. Yamamoto S, Watanabe M, Hasegawa H, et al. The risk of lymph node metastasis in T1 colorectal carcinoma. Hepatogastroenterology 2004;51(58): 998–1000.

48. Compton CC, Greene FL. The staging of colorectal cancer: 2004 and beyond. CA Cancer J Clin 2004; 54(6):295–308.

49. Puppa G, Caneva A, Colombari R. Venous invasion detection in colorectal cancer: which approach, which technique? J Clin Pathol 2009;62(2):102–3.

50. Sternberg A, Amar M, Alfici R, et al. Conclusions from a study of venous invasion in stage IV colorectal adenocarcinoma. J Clin Pathol 2002;55(1): 17–21.

51. Messenger DE, Driman DK, Kirsch R. Developments in the assessment of venous invasion in colorectal cancer: implications for future practice and patient outcome. Hum Pathol 2012;43(7):965–73.

52. Sohn B, Lim JS, Kim H, et al. MRI-detected extramural vascular invasion is an independent prognostic factor for synchronous metastasis in patients with rectal cancer. Eur Radiol 2015;25(5): 1347–55.

53. Huh JW, Kim HR, Kim YJ. Lymphovascular or perineural invasion may predict lymph node metastasis in patients with T1 and T2 colorectal cancer. J Gastrointest Surg 2010;14(7):1074–80.

54. Knijn N, Mogk SC, Teerenstra S, et al. Perineural Invasion is a Strong Prognostic Factor in Colorectal Cancer: A Systematic Review. Am J Surg Pathol 2016;40(1):103–12.

55. Peng J, Sheng W, Huang D, et al. Perineural invasion in pT3N0 rectal cancer: the incidence and its prognostic effect. Cancer 2011;117(7):1415–21.

56. Lino-Silva LS, Salcedo-Hernandez RA, Espana-Ferrufino A, et al. Extramural perineural invasion in pT3 and pT4 rectal adenocarcinoma as prognostic factor after preoperative chemoradiotherapy. Hum Pathol 2017;65:107–12.

57. Ricci-Vitiani L, Lombardi DG, Pilozzi E, et al. Identification and expansion of human colon-cancer-initiating cells. Nature 2007;445(7123):111–5.

58. Vermeulen L, Todaro M, de Sousa Mello F, et al. Single-cell cloning of colon cancer stem cells reveals a multi-lineage differentiation capacity. Proc Natl Acad Sci U S A 2008;105(36):13427–32.

59. Ryan E, Khaw YL, Creavin B, et al. Tumor budding and PDC grade are stage independent predictors of clinical outcome in mismatch repair deficient colorectal cancer. Am J Surg Pathol 2018;42(1):60–8.

60. Lugli A, Karamitopoulou E, Zlobec I. Tumour budding: a promising parameter in colorectal cancer. Br J Cancer 2012;106(11):1713–7.

61. Berg KB, Schaeffer DF. Tumor budding as a standardized parameter in gastrointestinal carcinomas: more than just the colon. Mod Pathol 2018;31(6): 862–72.

62. Wang LM, Kevans D, Mulcahy H, et al. Tumor budding is a strong and reproducible prognostic marker in T3N0 colorectal cancer. Am J Surg Pathol 2009;33(1):134–41.

63. Bosch SL, Teerenstra S, de Wilt JH, et al. Predicting lymph node metastasis in pT1 colorectal cancer: a systematic review of risk factors providing rationale for therapy decisions. Endoscopy 2013;45(10): 827–34.

64. Lugli A, Kirsch R, Ajioka Y, et al. Recommendations for reporting tumor budding in colorectal cancer based on the International Tumor Budding Consensus Conference (ITBCC) 2016. Mod Pathol 2017;30(9):1299–311.

65. Koelzer VH, Assarzadegan N, Dawson H, et al. Cytokeratin-based assessment of tumour budding in colorectal cancer: analysis in stage II patients and prospective diagnostic experience. J Pathol Clin Res 2017;3(3):171–8.

66. Reggiani Bonetti L, Barresi V, Bettelli S, et al. Poorly differentiated clusters (PDC) in colorectal cancer: what is and ought to be known. Diagn Pathol 2016; 11:31.

67. Konishi T, Shimada Y, Lee LH, et al. Poorly differentiated clusters predict colon cancer recurrence: an in-depth comparative analysis of invasive-front prognostic markers. Am J Surg Pathol 2018;42(6): 705–14.

68. Rozek LS, Schmit SL, Greenson JK, et al. Tumor-Infiltrating Lymphocytes, Crohn's-Like Lymphoid Reaction, and Survival From Colorectal Cancer. J Natl Cancer Inst 2016;108(8). https://doi.org/10.1093/jnci/djw027.

69. Ogino S, Nosho K, Irahara N, et al. Lymphocytic reaction to colorectal cancer is associated with longer survival, independent of lymph node count, microsatellite instability, and CpG island methylator phenotype. Clin Cancer Res 2009;15(20):6412–20.

70. Greenson JK, Bonner JD, Ben-Yzhak O, et al. Phenotype of microsatellite unstable colorectal carcinomas: Well-differentiated and focally mucinous tumors and the absence of dirty necrosis correlate with microsatellite instability. Am J Surg Pathol 2003;27(5):563–70.

71. Sinicrope F, Foster NR, Sargent DJ, et al. Model-based prediction of defective DNA mismatch repair

using clinicopathological variables in sporadic colon cancer patients. Cancer 2010;116(7):1691–8.

72. Graham DM, Appelman HD. Crohn's-like lymphoid reaction and colorectal carcinoma: a potential histologic prognosticator. Mod Pathol 1990;3(3): 332–5.

73. Kapiteijn E, Marijnen CA, Nagtegaal ID, et al. Preoperative radiotherapy combined with total mesorectal excision for resectable rectal cancer. N Engl J Med 2001;345(9):638–46.

74. Kuo LJ, Liu MC, Jian JJ, et al. Is final TNM staging a predictor for survival in locally advanced rectal cancer after preoperative chemoradiation therapy? Ann Surg Oncol 2007;14(10):2766–72.

75. Ruo L, Tickoo S, Klimstra DS, et al. Long-term prognostic significance of extent of rectal cancer response to preoperative radiation and chemotherapy. Ann Surg 2002;236(1):75–81.

76. Pai RK, Pai RK. Pathologic assessment of gastrointestinal tract and pancreatic carcinoma after neoadjuvant therapy. Mod Pathol 2018;31(1):4–23.

77. Jessup JM, Goldberg RM, Asare EA, et al. Colon and rectum. In: Amin M, Edge S, Greeme FL, et al, editors. AJCC cancer staging manual. 8th edition. New York: Springer; 2017. p. 251–74.

78. Prall F, Weirich V, Ostwald C. Phenotypes of invasion in sporadic colorectal carcinomas related to aberrations of the adenomatous polyposis coli (APC) gene. Histopathology 2007;50(3):318–30.

79. Halvorsen TB, Seim E. Association between invasiveness, inflammatory reaction, desmoplasia and survival in colorectal cancer. J Clin Pathol 1989;42(2):162–6.

80. Ueno H, Kanemitsu Y, Sekine S, et al. Desmoplastic pattern at the tumor front defines poor-prognosis subtypes of colorectal cancer. Am J Surg Pathol 2017;41(11):1506–12.

Diagnoses and Difficulties in Mesenteric Pathology

Nooshin K. Dashti, MD, MPH[a], Chanjuan Shi, MD, PhD[b],*

KEYWORDS

- Mesenteric vascular disease • Sclerosing mesenteritis • Desmoid-type fibromatosis
- Gastrointestinal stromal tumor

Key points

- Diagnosis of mesenteric vascular diseases can be challenging. Pathologic examination of a resection specimen sometimes is required.
- Mesenteric inflammatory disease can mimic a neoplastic process. Care must be taken in interpreting the pathologic findings.
- Mesenteric neoplasms can be difficult to diagnose. Their diagnosis is based on familiarity with their existence and their clinical, radiologic, and histologic features.
- Secondary involvement of the mesentery/omentum, including lymphomatosis, carcinomatosis, and sarcomatosis, always should be excluded.

ABSTRACT

Mesenteric diseases are broadly separated into 2 groups: non-neoplastic and neoplastic. Common non-neoplastic mesenteric diseases include those involving the mesenteric vasculature and those of inflammatory processes. Mesenteric inflammatory processes can mimic a neoplastic process. Neoplastic diseases of the mesentery are rare. Generally, the morphology, behavior and diagnostic criteria for mesenteric tumors are similar to their soft tissue or organ-specific counterparts. Their recognition can be challenging because they sometimes are overlooked in differential diagnoses.

Mesenteric diseases are uncommon and can be challenging to diagnose, particularly if pathology samples are routed to subspecialty gastrointestinal pathologists not well versed in mesenteric specimens. This article focuses on key non-neoplastic and neoplastic diseases of the mesentery.

SELECTED NON-NEOPLASTIC DISEASES OF THE MESENTERY

MESENTERIC VEIN THROMBOSIS

Introduction

Mesenteric vein thrombosis (MVT) is a rare cause of acute mesenteric ischemia and can be seen in patients with hypercoagulation, surgery, inflammatory bowel disease (IBD), and malignancy.[1] Presentation commonly includes abdominal pain, nausea, vomiting, and melena. Contrast-enhanced CT scan demonstrates a filling defect in mesenteric veins. In cases of bowel ischemia, there is bowel wall thickening, pneumatosis intestinalis, or persistent enhancement of the bowel wall.[1] The jejunum and ileum are the sites affected most commonly.

Gross Features

Grossly, there is profound bowel wall edema, submucosal hemorrhage, or bowel infarct.

[a] Department of Pathology, Microbiology and Immunology, Vanderbilt University Medical Center, 1161 21st Avenue South, Medical Center North, Nashville, TN 37232, USA; [b] Department of Pathology, Duke University School of Medicine, Room 3119, Duke South, 40 Duke Medicine Circle, DUMC 3712, Durham, NC 27710, USA
* Corresponding author.
E-mail address: Chanjuan.Shi@Duke.edu

Surgical Pathology 13 (2020) 521–556
https://doi.org/10.1016/j.path.2020.06.001
1875-9181/20/© 2020 Elsevier Inc. All rights reserved.

Microscopic Features

Microscopically transmural necrosis and mural hemorrhage are seen in severely affected segments (**Fig. 1A**). Other areas may show mucosal ischemia and congestion (**Fig. 1B**). Examination of mesenteric tissue reveals venous thrombosis (**Fig. 1C**). The mesenteric arteries are spared.

Diagnosis and Differential Diagnosis

CT scan is diagnostic in approximately 60% to 70% cases.[1] In other cases, the diagnosis is confirmed only after microscopic examination of the resection specimens. The differential diagnosis includes idiopathic myointimal hyperplasia of mesenteric veins (IMHMV), enterocolic lymphocytic phlebitis (ELP), systemic vasculitis, and other mesenteric vascular diseases.

Key Features

- There is acute mesenteric ischemia

- Affected bowel displays ischemic necrosis and hemorrhage

- Mesenteric venous thrombosis is seen

CHRONIC ATHEROSCLEROTIC MESENTERIC ARTERIAL DISEASE

Introduction

Chronic atherosclerotic mesenteric arterial disease is the main cause of chronic mesenteric ischemia, which typically occurs in patients with severe atherosclerosis involving at least 2 of the following: celiac axis, superior mesenteric artery, and inferior mesenteric artery.[2] Risk factors include smoking, hypertension, diabetes, and hypercholesterolemia. The classic symptoms are postprandial pain, weight loss, and concurrent vascular comorbidities.[2] Computed tomography (CT) angiography is the diagnostic test of choice, which shows atherosclerotic stenosis of the mesenteric vessels.

Gross Findings

There is diffuse atherosclerosis in the mesenteric vessels. Bowel strictures may be seen. Mucosal findings include erosions and ulceration.[3] Inflammatory-type polyps may develop in some patients (**Fig. 2A**).

Microscopic Findings

Microscopically, the affected bowel shows chronic ischemic changes, including villous atrophy, erosion, fibrosis, architectural distortion, and other chronicity (**Fig. 2B, C**). The mesenteric arteries have severe atherosclerosis with almost complete obliteration of the lumen (**Fig. 3**).

Diagnosis and Differential Diagnosis

Chronic artherosclerotic mesenteric arterial disease is diagnosed based on clinical history and radiographic findings. The differential diagnosis includes Crohn's disease and other mesenteric vascular abnormalities/vasculitides.

Key Features

- There are Chronic ischemic changes in affected bowel

- Mesenteric arteries show severe atherosclerosis

INTESTINAL BEHÇET DISEASE

Introduction

Behçet disease is a rare form of vasculitis characterized by recurrent oral ulcers, genital ulcers, and uveitis. Intestinal involvement is seen in 3% to 25% of the patients, with the areas affected most commonly the terminal ileum and ileocecal regions.[4,5] The most common symptom for intestinal Behçet disease is abdominal pain due to ulceration that may penetrate. CT scan shows concentric bowel wall thickening or a polypoid mass with marked contrast enhancement.[6] Mesenteric infiltration around the involved bowel also is present in cases with complications.

Gross Features

Grossly, there may be single or multiple ulcers. Perforation, fistula formation, or hemorrhage sometimes is associated with ulcers.

Microscopic Features

Diffuse vascular dilatation with perivascular lymphocytic infiltration is seen in the mucosa and submucosa (**Fig. 4A, B**). Like Crohn's disease, there may be chronic nonspecific inflammation with normal intervening mucosa and multiple ulcers that can be deeply penetrating (**Fig. 4C**). The vasculitis usually involves small veins and venules, with destruction of the media and fibrous thickening of the intima and adventitia accompanied by intense inflammation around the vasa vasorum (**Fig. 4D**).

Fig. 1. Mesenteric venous thrombosis. (*A*) Transmural necrosis and hemorrhage (hematoxylin-eosin, original magnification ×20). (*B*) Mild mucosal ischemia with congestion (hematoxylin-eosin, original magnification ×100). (*C*) thrombosis in a mesenteric vein (hematoxylin-eosin, original magnification ×40).

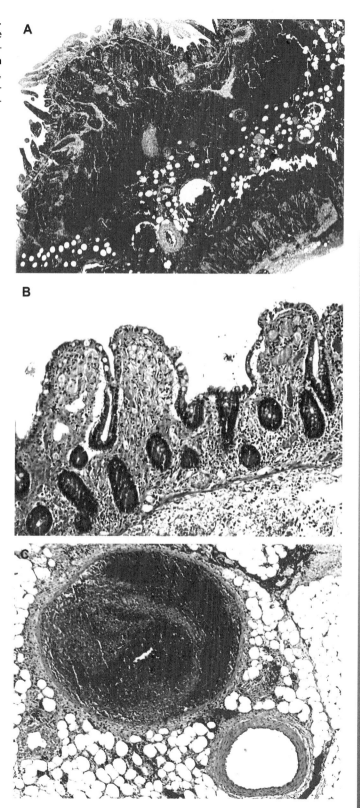

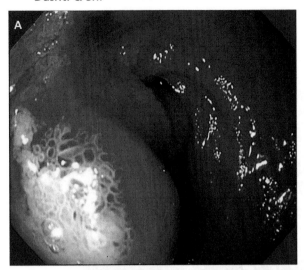

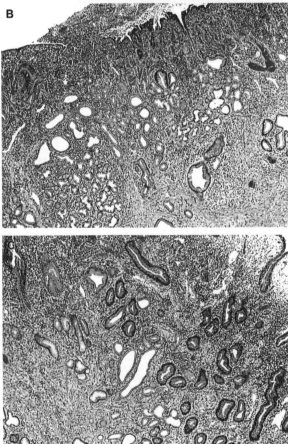

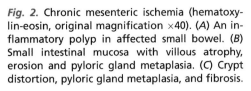

Fig. 2. Chronic mesenteric ischemia (hematoxylin-eosin, original magnification ×40). (*A*) An inflammatory polyp in affected small bowel. (*B*) Small intestinal mucosa with villous atrophy, erosion and pyloric gland metaplasia. (*C*) Crypt distortion, pyloric gland metaplasia, and fibrosis.

Diagnosis and Differential Diagnosis

The diagnostic criteria are not well established. Generally, the diagnosis is confirmed when a patient has Behçet disease and intestinal lesions. The primary differential diagnosis is Crohn's disease. Surgical resection is indicated when patients have no response to medical treatments or have intestinal complications. The recurrence rate, however, is high.

Fig. 3. Mesenteric artery with severe atherosclerosis. (*A*) A mesenteric vessel showing severe atherosclerosis, which is an artery (hematoxylin eosin stain, original magnification ×40), as confirmed by (*B*) Movat stain (original magnification ×40).

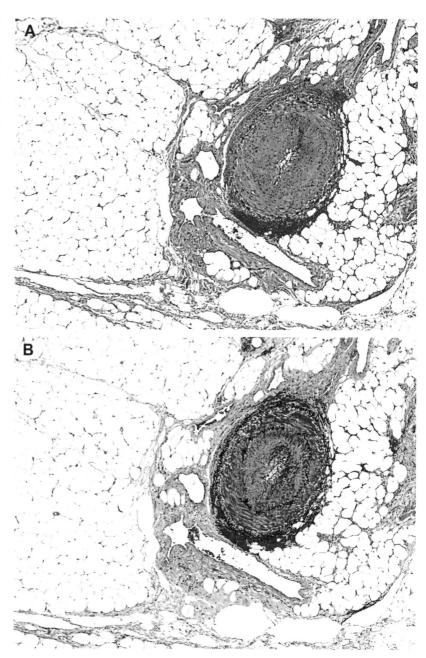

Key Features

- Systemic vasculitis is always present

- Mucosa shows diffuse vascular dilatation and perivascular lymphocytic infiltration

- There is one or multiple ulcers that can be deep

- Vasculitis in venules and small veins is present

ENTEROCOLIC LYMPHOCYTIC PHLEBITIS

Introduction

ELP is a rare condition caused by phlebitis of the bowel wall and mesentery, which results in intestinal congestive injury.[7] No reported patients have a history of systemic vasculitis. It typically affects the small intestine and right colon. Its common clinical presentations include acute abdominal pain, nausea, vomiting, diarrhea, and rectal bleeding.[7] CT scan typically shows bowel wall thickening/edema and increased density of

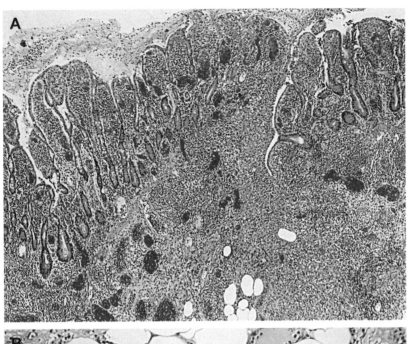

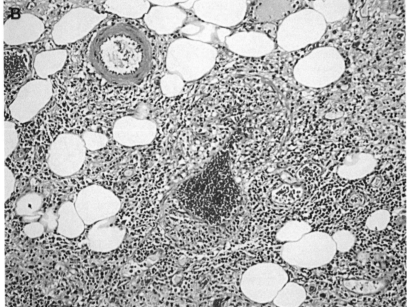

Fig. 4. Intestinal Behçet disease. (A) Small intestinal mucosa with congestion and ulcers (hematoxylin-eosin, original magnification×40). (B) Submucosa with venulitis (hematoxylin-eosin, original magnification×100).

mesenteric fat. Mesenteric angiography shows absence of draining veins from the involved segments.

Gross Features

Grossly, most cases have intestinal infarct. Other findings include stenosis, thickening of bowel wall, tumorlike mass, or ulcer.[7]

Microscopic Features

Mucosal changes include villous expansion by dilation of capillaries (Fig. 5A), thickened capillary walls, and mucosal ischemia. There is submucosal congestion or vascular ectasia (Fig. 5B). Crypt distortion (see Fig. 5A) and ulcer (Fig. 5C) can be present, mimicking Crohn's disease.

Veins of all sizes in the intestinal wall and mesenteric fat are affected by lymphocytic inflammation,

Fig. 4. *(continued).* *(C)* A deep ulcer extending to the submucosa (hematoxylin-eosin, original magnification×40). *(D)* Vasculitis with neutrophilic and lymphocytic infiltrates (hematoxylineosin, original magnification×200).

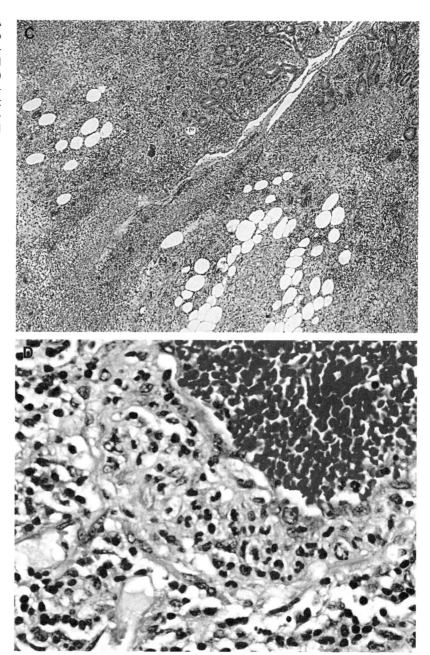

whereas arteries are spared (**Fig. 6**). Other types of pathology include necrotizing phlebitis with neutrophilic infiltration and fibrin deposition, granulomatous phlebitis with epithelioid histiocytes and multinucleated giant cells, and myointimal hyperplasia with near-complete occlusion of vessel lumen (**Fig. 7**). In addition, ELP frequently is associated with fresh and/or organized venous thrombosis.

Diagnosis and Differential Diagnosis

The mucosal findings are nonspecific. The definite diagnosis typically is made after examination of a resection specimen. The differential diagnosis includes Crohn's disease, mesenteric vasculitis (ie, Behçet disease), IMHMV, and MVT. Surgical resection of the affected bowel is curative with only rare recurrences.

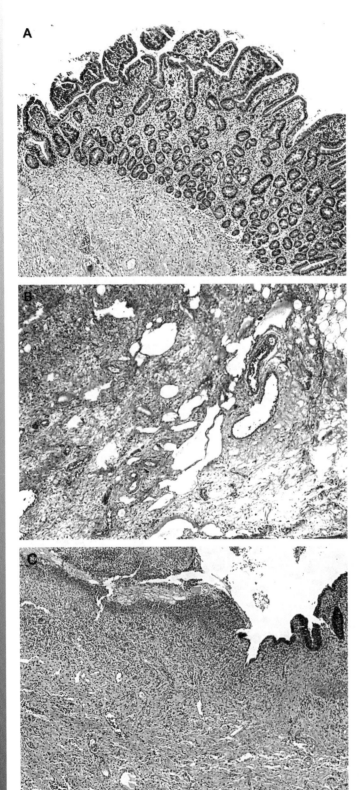

Fig. 5. ELP (Hematoxylin-eosin, original magnification ×40). (*A*) Villous blunting with capillary dilation and mild crypt distortion. (*B*) Submucosal vascular ectasia. (*C*) Ulceration with adjacent reactive mucosa.

Fig.   6. Lymphocytic inflammation of the mesenteric vein. (*A*) Phlebitis with an adjacent normal artery (hematoxylin-eosin, original magnification ×10). (*B*) A high-power field showing infiltration by lymphocytes, plasma cells, and rare eosinophils (hematoxylin-eosin, original magnification ×200).

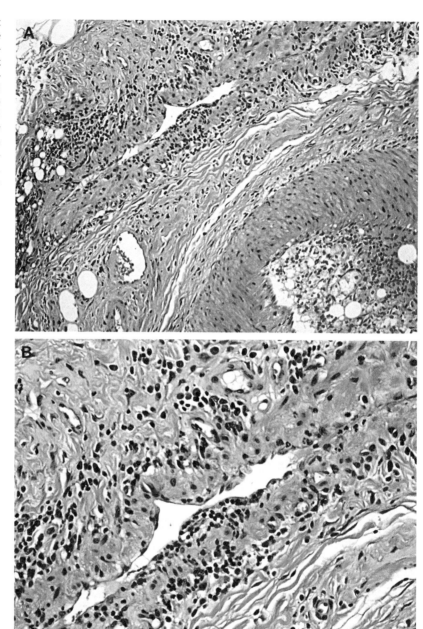

Key Features

- There is no systemic vasculitis

- Intestinal ischemia with dilated capillaries is present

- There is mesenteric venulitis/phlebitis with sparing of arteries

IDIOPATHIC MYOINTIMAL HYPERPLASIA OF MESENTERIC VEINS

Introduction

IMHMV is a rare disease caused by noninflammatory obliteration of medium-sized to large-sized veins in the mesentery and bowel wall, resulting in chronic ischemic changes in involved bowel.[8] The rectosigmoid colon is the site most commonly involved. Most patients are middle-aged,

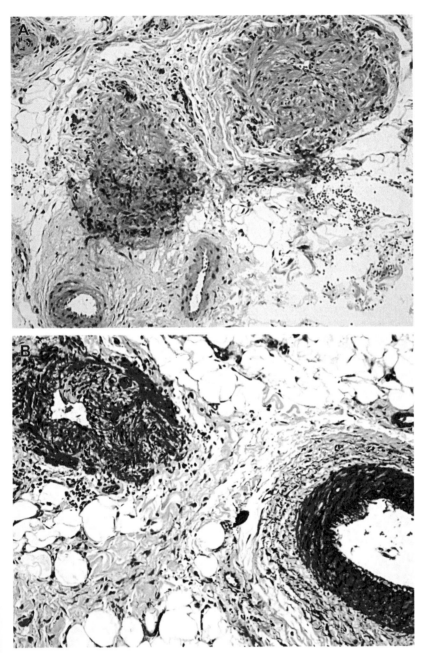

Fig. 7. Additional findings in ELP. (*A*) Marked myointimal hyperplasia in addition to mild inflammation (hematoxylin eosin, original magnification ×100). (*B*) Elastin stain confirming affected vein (elastin stain, original magnification ×100).

previously healthy men presenting with recurrent, progressively severe abdominal pain, weight loss, and bloody diarrhea.[8] In CT cross-sectional imaging, there is segmental colonic thickening/edema (**Fig. 8**).

Gross Features

Gross examination shows segmental involvement of the colon with features of ischemia, including erythema, edema, and friability (**Fig. 9**A). Ulcers and strictures frequently are resent (**Fig. 9**B). In

addition, the mesenteric fat shows abnormal large-caliber veins.

Microscopic Features

Mucosal changes are featured by congestive ischemic changes, including withered microcrypts, hemorrhage, and fibrin deposits in the lamina propria (**Fig. 10**A). Among the glands, there are numerous dilated thick-walled capillaries containing fibrin thrombi (**Fig. 10**B). There is no significant architectural distortion or

Fig. 8. CT showing segmental thickening and edema of the distal colorectum.

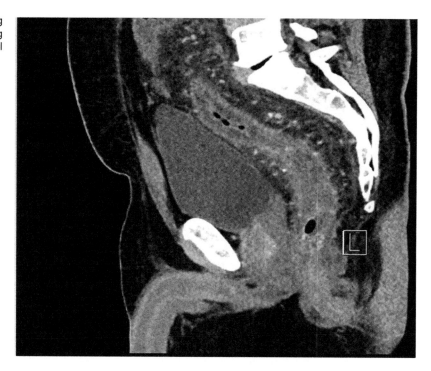

prominent lamina propria lymphoplasmacytic inflammation. The mesenteric veins have a thickened wall due to prominent intimal smooth muscle hyperplasia (**Fig. 11**), which mimics arteries. There is no inflammation associated with abnormal mesenteric veins. The mesenteric arteries are uninvolved.

Diagnosis and Differential Diagnosis

The findings in mucosal biopsy only indicate an ischemic etiology. Definite diagnosis is possible only after examination of mesenteric veins in the resection specimens. The rectosigmoid location, segmental involvement, and mucosal ischemic change, however, are highly suggestive of IMHMV. The primary differential diagnosis includes IBD, ELP, and MVT. Surgical resection of the affected bowel usually is curative.

Key Features

- There is noninflammatory obliteration of medium-sized to large-sized veins in the mesentery and bowel wall

- Affected bowel shows congestive ischemic changes, dilated capillaries, and fibrin thrombi

SCLEROSING MESENTERITIS

Introduction

Sclerosing mesenteritis is a rare disease with fat necrosis and inflammation/fibrosis of the mesentery. Patients with sclerosing mesenteritis often present with abdominal pain, nausea/vomiting, weight loss, and fever.[9] Sclerosing mesenteritis may lead to bowel obstruction and mesenteric ischemia. Reported risk factors include prior abdominal surgery/trauma, autoimmune disease and a history of malignancy.[9] On multidetector CT, it can present as misty mesentery, with increased attenuation of the mesenteric fat, a masslike area of homogenously or heterogeneously increased fat attenuation that does not displace the surrounding mesenteric vascular structures (**Fig. 12**), or as a mass infiltrating the adjacent structures.[10]

Gross Features

Grossly, there is diffuse thickening of the mesentery, an isolated nodular mass at the mesenteric root, or multiple discrete mesenteric nodules.

Microscopic Features

Microscopic findings show variable components of fat necrosis, chronic inflammation, and fibrosis (**Fig. 13**). Several terms have been used to describe sclerosing mesenteritis, including mesenteric lipodystrophy with prominent fat necrosis, mesenteric panniculitis with prominent

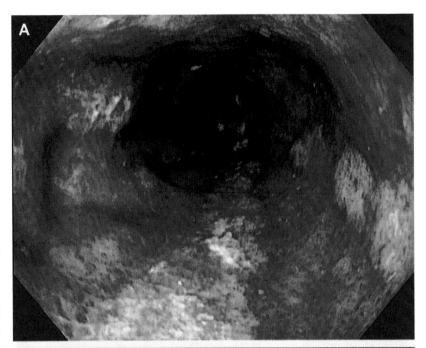

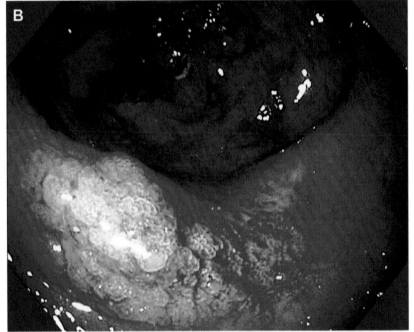

Fig. 9. IMHMV. (*A*) Colonic mucosa showing erythema, edema, and friability. (*B*) Colonic ulcer and stricture.

chronic inflammation, and retractile mesenteritis with extensive fibrosis.

Diagnosis and Differential Diagnosis

Mesenteric biopsy usually is required to confirm the diagnosis. The primary differential diagnosis includes mesenteric malignancies, for example, mesenteric involvement by midgut neuroendocrine tumor (NET).

Key Features

- It presents as a mesenteric mass or masses, mimicking mesenteric malignancies

- There are variable components of fat necrosis and inflammation/fibrosis of the mesentery

Fig. 10. IMHMV. (*A*) Colonic mucosa with ischemic change (hematoxylin-eosin, original magnification ×100). (*B*) A high-power field showing dilated thick-walled capillaries with fibrin thrombi (hematoxylin-eosin, original magnification ×200).

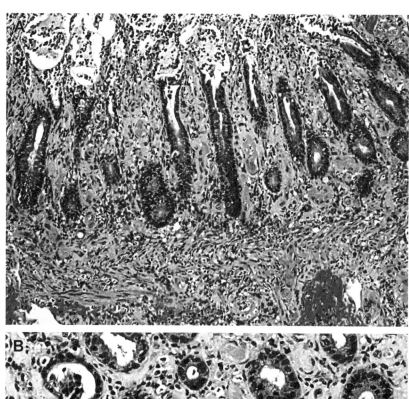

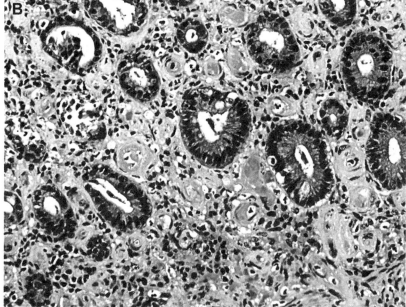

SELECTED PRIMARY NEOPLASMS OF THE MESENTERY

WELL-DIFFERENTIATED LIPOSARCOMA AND DEDIFFERENTIATED LIPOSARCOMA

Introduction

Liposarcomas are the most common soft tissue sarcomas in the adult population, accounting for 15% to 20% of all sarcomas. The World Health Organization[11] recognizes 4 subtypes of liposarcoma: atypical lipomatous tumor (ALT)/well-differentiated liposarcoma (WDL), dedifferentiated liposarcoma (DL), myxoid/round cell liposarcoma, and pleomorphic liposarcoma. ALT is the accepted designation in superficial and intramuscular locations in the extremity and WDL in deep soft tissue (inguinal, paratesticular,

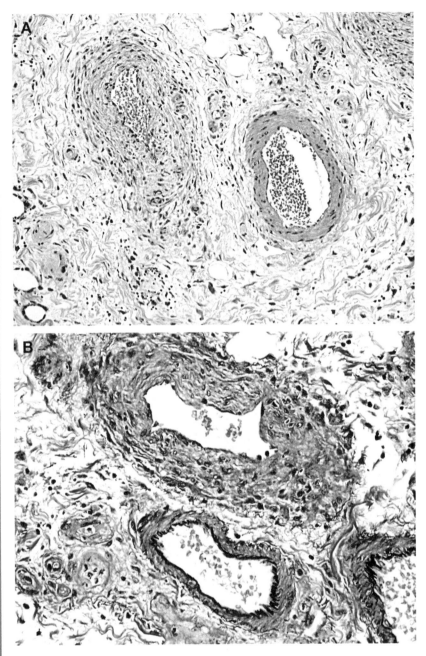

Fig. 11. Vascular changes associated with IMHMV. (*A*) Mesenteric veins with thickened walls and prominent intimal smooth muscle hyperplasia (hematoxylin-eosin, original magnification ×100). (*B*) Elastin stain confirming the vein with adjacent normal arteries (elastin, original magnification ×200).

retroperitoneal, and mediastinal). In contrast to common retroperitoneal liposarcomas, primary liposarcomas of the mesentery are rare. Primary liposarcomas of the mesentery usually arise from the root of the mesentery.

Gross Features

Grossly, the tumor is a multilobulated large mass with a solid, yellow cut surface, demonstrating fibrous bands. Areas of hemorrhage, calcification, and degenerative cystic changes may be present. These intra-abdominal liposarcomas can achieve very large size before becoming symptomatic. Depending on the extent of involvement of the bowel loops, they may have ill-defined borders, rendering resection with adequate margins difficult.

Fig. 12. Sclerosing mesenteritis presenting as a mesenteric mass at CT.

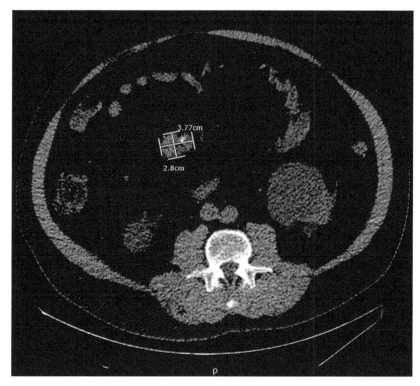

Microscopic Features

Histologically, WDL can be divided into the following subtypes: lipoma-like, sclerosing, and inflammatory. Most liposarcomas show a combination of lipoma-like and sclerosing subtypes. Sections show proliferation of mature-appearing adipocytes intersected with bands of fibrous zones (**Fig. 14**A). These fibrotic zones of collagen contain atypical stromal cells with spindled to multipolar, hyperchromatic nuclei (**Fig. 14**B, C). Traditionally, identifying lipoblasts has been emphasized for the diagnosis of liposarcoma (**Fig. 14**D). Atypical hyperchromatic stromal cells are equally diagnostic. These cells are best found in the fibrous bands and around the vessels. Similarly, they can be identified in the mature adipocytic component.

Diagnosis and Differential Diagnosis

Imaging studies identify a large intra-abdominal mass with a significant component of fat. Identifying classic atypical hyperchromatic stromal cells is essential for diagnosis. Biopsy material may be limited. Both WDL and DL harbor giant marker and ring chromosomes containing amplified sequences of 12q13-15. This amplicon is the site of *MDM2*, *CDK4* and *GLI* genes.[12–14] Fluorescence in situ hybridization (FISH) studies are a highly reliable method for identifying *MDM2* gene amplification, even in small biopsy material.[15,16]

ALT/WDL occurs in the age range of 50 years to 70 years and has a high rate of local recurrence. The metastatic rate is low and it has a 5% to 15% risk of progression to DL. DL has a similar age range, with high local recurrence rate and high risk of metastasis. Morphologically, DL shows transition from WDL to high-grade sarcoma. Traditionally DL shows juxtaposition of a WDL component to a nonlipogenic high-grade sarcoma (**Fig. 15**). Currently, low-grade dedifferentiation[17–19] and lipogenic high-grade differentiation[20] are acceptable concepts in the pathology of liposarcomas. Generous sampling of a WDL to evaluate for possible dedifferentiation is essential.

Large areas of fat necrosis, in particular, due to bowel perforation/inflammation and prior instrumentation, may be mass-forming and need to be distinguished from liposarcoma. Morphologically, fat necrosis is characterized by damaged fat, presenting as fat dropout and finely granular and vacuolated macrophages. The vacuoles are evenly distributed and the nuclei have smooth borders (**Fig. 16**). In difficult cases, FISH testing for *MDM2* amplification is a valuable tool.

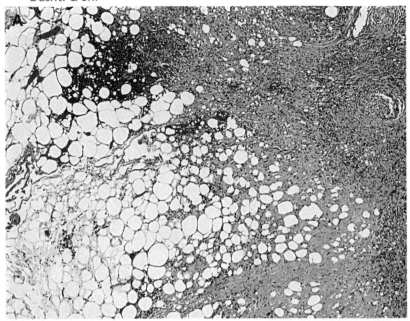

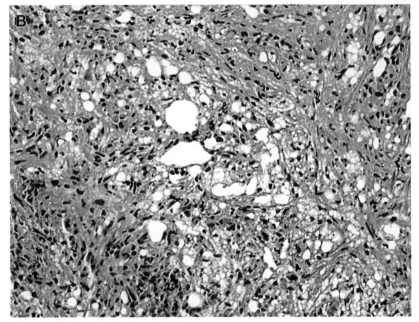

Fig. 13. Sclerosing mesenteritis. (*A*) A section showing fat necrosis, chronic inflammation, and fibrosis (hematoxylin-eosin, origination magnification ×40). (*B*) Prominent fat necrosis with macrophages (hematoxylin-eosin, origination magnification ×100).

Key Features

- Primary liposarcomas of the mesentery are rare.

- Morphologically, they are similar to liposarcomas of other locations.

- FISH for *MDM2* amplification is highly sensitive and specific for diagnosis of both WDL and DL.

- Ample sampling to evaluate for dedifferentiation is prudent.

EXTRAGASTROINTESTINAL STROMAL TUMOR

Gastrointestinal stromal tumors (GISTs) arise from interstitial cells of Cajal or their precursor[21] and are among the most common mesenchymal tumors of the gastrointestinal tract. Stomach is the most common location, followed by jejunum, ileum, duodenum, and colorectum.[22] A small percentage of GISTs are not connected to the gastrointestinal tract and involve omentum, mesentery, retroperitoneum, and pelvic cavity (extragastrointestinal stromal tumors [EGISTs]).[23,24] GISTs usually

Fig. 13. (continued). (*C*) Prominent chronic inflammation (hematoxynlineosin, original magnification ×100). (*D*) Prominent fibrosis (hematoxylineosin, original magnification ×100).

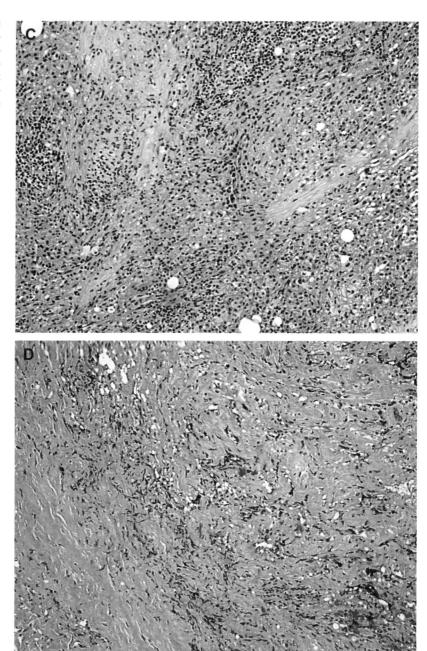

spread through liver metastasis and tumor nodules in the peritoneal cavity. Lymph node metastasis is uncommon (except for the succinate dehydrogenase [SDH]-deficient type).

Gross Features

Grossly, GISTS and EGISTS often are well-circumscribed masses with solid, fleshy, tan cut surfaces. Areas of hemorrhage and degeneration may be present.

Microscopic Features

GISTs can have a predominantly epithelioid or spindle cell morphology. Approximately 10% show a combination of both patterns (**Fig. 17**). The epithelioid morphology has a nested, sheetlike architecture composed of relatively uniform cells with minimal atypia. The spindle cell morphology is composed of uniform spindle cells arranged in fascicles. GISTs can be variably cellular with hyalinized stroma, hyalinized vessels, and calcification.

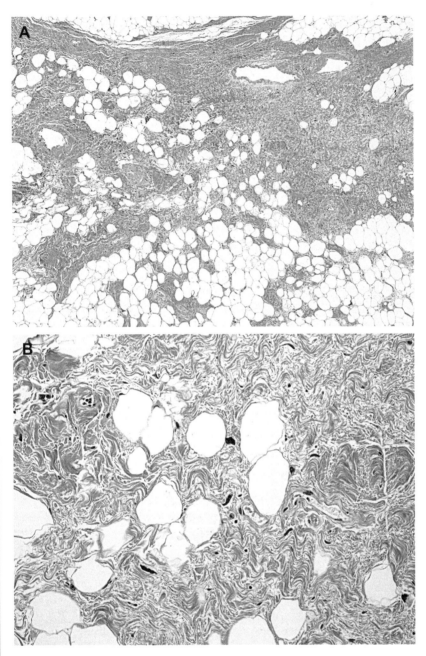

Fig. 14. WDL. (hematoxylin eosin, original magnification ×100) (*A*) Mature-appearing adipocytes intersected with bands of fibrous zones. (*B*, *C*)

Diagnosis and Differential Diagnosis

A panel of immunostains is helpful in diagnosing GISTs and distinguishing them from histologic mimics, such as leiomyoma and schwannoma. GISTs show diffuse and strong expression of KIT (CD117). DOG1 is a sensitive and specific immunomarker, which is positive in a majority of GISTs, including the ones that are negative for KIT. CD34 also is positive in 70% of GISTs. GISTs frequently are tested for mutations of multiple genes at the same time by sequencing. The testing panel includes *KIT*, *PDGFRA*, *BRAF*, *RAS*, *SDHA*, *SDHB*, *SDHC*, *SDHD*, and *NF1*. *KIT* and *PDGFRA* mutations have treatment implications.[25] The Food and Drug Administration has approved small molecule tyrosine kinase

Fig. 14. (continued). These fibrotic zones of collagen contain atypical stromal cells with spindled to multipolar, hyperchromatic nuclei (hematoxylin eosin, original magnification ×200 [for B]; hematoxylin eosin, original magnification ×400 [for C]). (*D*) Lipoblasts with hyperchromatic indented nuclei and lipid-rich vacuoles (photo taken from a case of pleomorphic liposarcoma for comparison) (hematoxylin eosin, original magnification ×400).

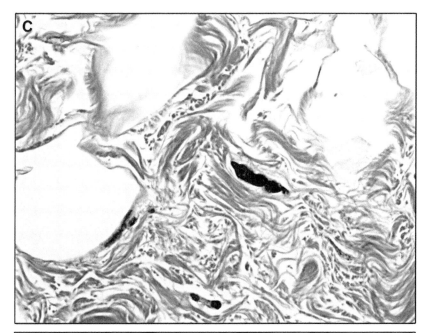

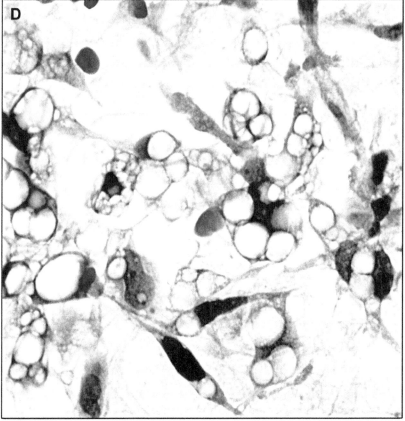

inhibitors, namely imatinib mesylate (Gleevec, Novartis Pharmaceuticals, Basel, Switzerland) and sunitinib malate (Sutent, Pfizer Pharmaceuticals, New York, New York) for treatment of GISTs. In contrast to carcinoma, schwannoma, and smooth muscle tumors, GISTs do not

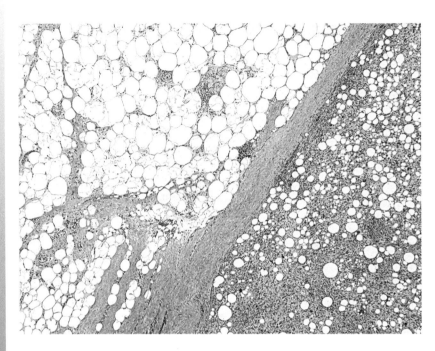

Fig. 15. DL with juxtaposition of WDL component (*left*) to a high-grade sarcoma (*right*) (hematoxylin eosin, original magnification ×100).

exhibit diffuse expression of S100, SOX10, or desmin; focal expression of these markers can be seen (**Fig. 18, Table 1**).

Key Features

- EGISTs are similar to GISTs of other locations.

- Mutation analysis for *KIT* and *PDGFRA* is performed by sequencing and yields important therapeutic information.

DESMOID-TYPE FIBROMATOSIS, INTRA-ABDOMINAL

Introduction

Intra-abdominal desmoid-type fibromatosis includes pelvic and mesenteric desmoid-type fibromatosis and is the most common primary tumor of the mesentery. Most cases are sporadic but some are associated with Gardner syndrome/familial adenomatous polyposis (FAP).[26–28] Due to available space, most of the tumors have a large size and the patients may have compression/obstructive symptoms.

Gross Features

Grossly, desmoid-type fibromatosis is densely fibrotic with tan-white cut surface and infiltrative borders.

Microscopic Features

The morphologic features of intra-abdominal desmoid-type fibromatosis are similar to other types of fibromatosis. The tumor is composed of bland, uniform spindle cells arranged in long sweeping fascicles (**Fig. 19**A). Collapsed vessels with perivascular edema may be present (**Fig. 19**B, C). If the tumor interface is present, infiltration into surrounding soft tissue, keloid-like collagen, and lymphoid aggregates are appreciated.

Diagnosis and Differential Diagnosis

Morphology of desmoid-type fibromatosis is quite distinctive, but at times diagnosis can be difficult. This is true, especially in small biopsies and in cases of recurrence, residual disease, and scar formation. Cases of Gardner syndrome are characterized by germline mutations in *APC*, leading to nuclear accumulation of beta-catenin.[26–28] Most sporadic cases harbor mutations of *CTNNB1*, similarly leading to nuclear accumulation of beta-catenin.[29] Mutational analysis is highly sensitive and specific for desmoid-type

Fig. 16. Fat necrosis with fat dropout and finely granular and vacuolated macrophages. The vacuoles are evenly distributed, and the nuclei have smooth borders. (hematoxylin eosin, original magnification ×400).

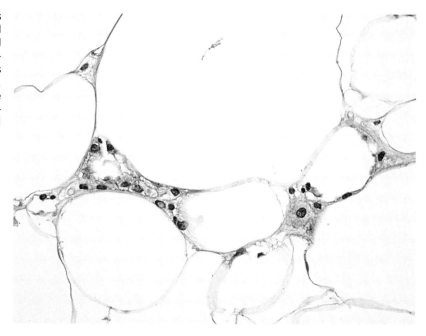

fibromatosis. Immunophenotypically, desmoid-type fibromatosis shows variable expression of smooth muscle actin (SMA) and to a lesser extent desmin. Sclerosing mesenteritis, inflammatory myofibroblastic tumor, idiopathic retroperitoneal fibrosis, and reactive changes due to perforation and procedures enter the differential diagnosis. None of these entities harbor *CTNNB1* mutations.

Key Features

- Some are associated with Gardner/FAP.

- They can achieve large size.

- Beta-catenin mutational analysis is diagnostic.

- They have propensity for local recurrence.

DESMOPLASTIC SMALL ROUND CELL TUMOR

Introduction

Desmoplastic small round cell tumor (DSRCT) is a rare type of small blue round cell tumor that occurs predominantly in young men and has an aggressive course.[30] The tumor usually involves the intra-abdominal or pelvic cavity with extensive spread and large mass, even though it has been identified in other non–peritoneum-covered locations as well.[31–33] The cell of origin and line of differentiation are not clear.

Gross Features

Grossly, DSRCT presents as a large, multilobulated mass with tan to white-gray cut surface.

Microscopic Features

Morphologically, DSRCT is composed of sharply demarcated islands, nests, trabeculae, and cords of primitive cells in a desmoplastic stroma (**Fig. 20A, B**). Nests may show central necrosis. The small round to oval neoplastic cells have an undifferentiated appearance with dense chromatin, scant cytoplasm, and inconspicuous nuclei. Mitotic activity is frequent and apoptotic bodies are easy to find (**Fig. 20C, D**).

Diagnosis and Differential Diagnosis

DSRCT has a distinct epithelial, mesenchymal, and neural polyphenotypic profile with expression of desmin (peculiar dotlike pattern), keratin, epithelial membrane antigen (EMA), and vimentin.[30] The tumor is positive for WT-1 immunostain aimed at the carboxy terminus of WT-1. DSRCT harbors a unique translocation, t(11;22)

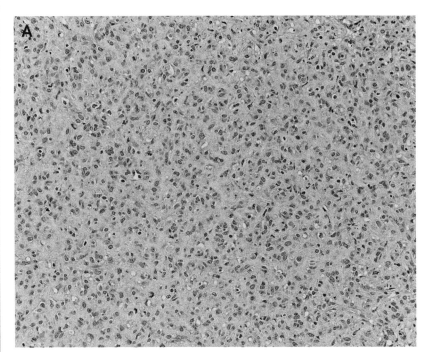

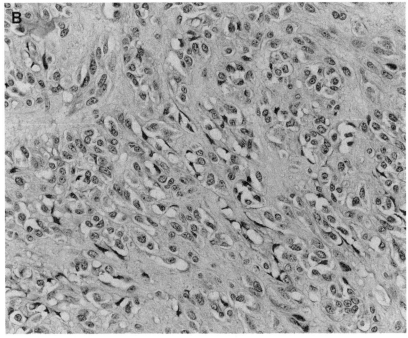

Fig. 17. GISTs. GISTs can have a predominantly epithelioid and ([*A*] hematoxylin-eosin, original magnification ×200 and [*B*] hematoxylin-eosin, original magnification ×400) or spindle cell morphology

Fig. 17. (continued). ([C] hematoxylin-eosin, original magnification ×200 and [D] hematoxylin-eosin, original magnification ×400). Approximately 10% show a combination of epithelioid and spindle cell morphology.

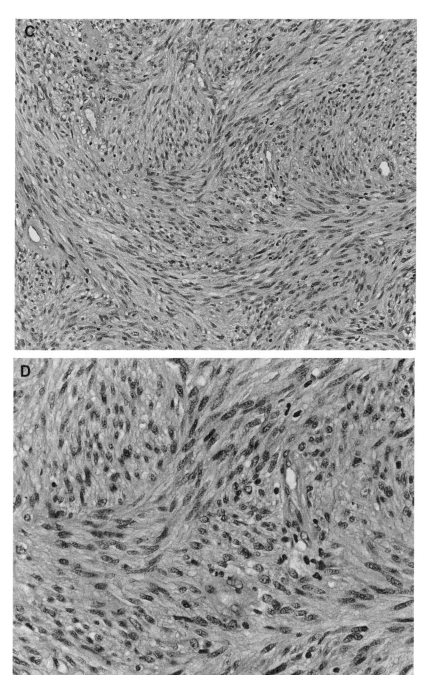

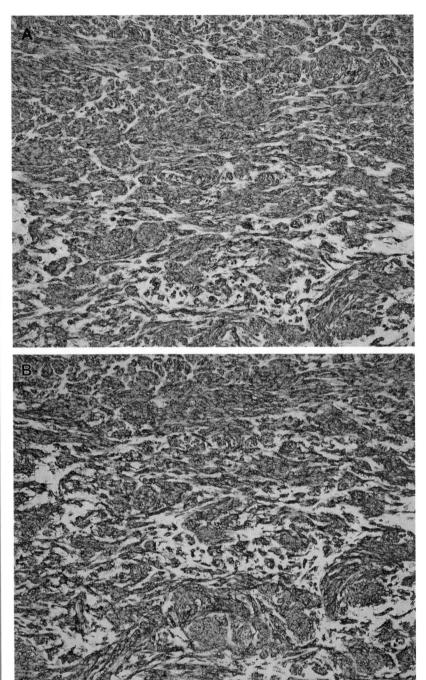

Fig. 18. GIST immunostains. (*A*) KIT (CD117), diffuse membranous and cytoplasmic staining (original magnification ×200). (*B*) Diffuse and intense DOG1 expression (original magnification ×200).

Fig. 18. (continued). (*C*) CD34 expression is seen in approximately 70% of GISTs (original magnification ×200). (*D*) S100 is negative, distinguishing GIST from schwannoma (original magnification ×200).

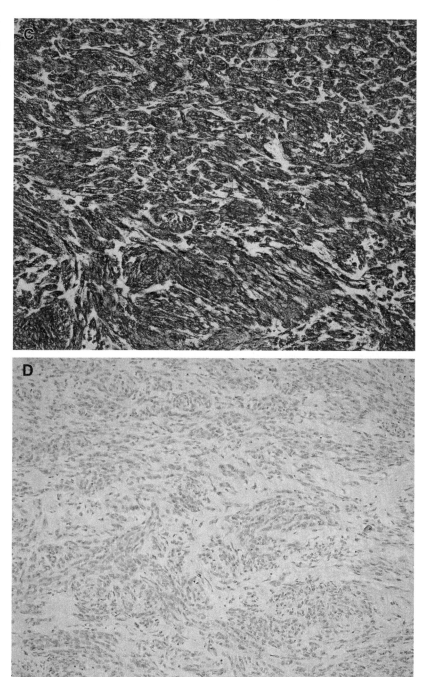

Table 1
Differential diagnosis for gastrointestinal stromal tumor

GIST	Positive for KIT (CD117), DOG1, and CD34 Negative for keratin, S100, SOX10 Pitfall: may have SMA and focal S100 and focal desmin expression
Schwannoma	Negative for KIT (CD117), DOG1, and CD34 Positive for S100, SOX10 Pitfall: may have focal desmin, keratin, and CD34 expression
Leiomyoma and leiomyosarcoma	Negative for KIT (CD117), DOG1, and CD34 Positive for SMA, desmin, and caldesmon Negative for S100, SOX10 Pitfall: can show keratin expression
Carcinoma	Negative for KIT (CD117), DOG1, and CD34 Strong expression of keratin

(p13;q12), involving *EWSR1* and *WT1* genes.[34] FISH or reverse transcriptase–polymerase chain reaction can identify the rearrangement. Similar to other small round cell tumors, DSRCT has to be distinguished from Ewing sarcoma, alveolar and sclerosing rhabdomyosarcoma, neuroblastoma, Wilms tumor, malignant rhabdoid extrarenal tumor, and lymphoma. Due to its specific intra-abdominal and pelvic cavity location and expression of keratin, mesothelioma and small cell carcinoma also enter the differential diagnosis list (**Table 2**).

Key Features

- Predominantly occurs in young men
- Intra-abdominal and pelvic cavity
- Wide differential diagnosis list
- Polyphenotypic profile
- Harbors genetic alteration of t(11;22) (p13;q12), involving *EWSR1* and *WT1*

INFLAMMATORY MYOFIBROBLASTIC TUMOR

Introduction

Inflammatory myofibroblastic tumors (IMTs) have been reported in virtually every body site. Mesentery and omentum are the most common extrapulmonary sites.[35,36] They have potential for local aggressive behavior and metastasis.

Gross Features

The mass usually is lobulated with fleshy tan-white cut surface.

Microscopic Features

IMTs can have variable morphology, ranging from bland spindled to stellate myofibroblastic cells loosely embedded in a myxoid stroma, admixed with inflammatory cells, to more cellular tumors with more compact fascicular architecture (**Fig. 21**).

Diagnosis and Differential Diagnosis

IMTs express SMA and desmin. Approximately half of IMTs harbor mutations of *ALK*. The association between *ALK* status and ALK immunostain is not perfect, and negative immunostain does not exclude the diagnosis.[36–40]

New genetic abnormalities other than *ALK* involvement are identified in IMTs, including *ROS1*, *NTRK1*, and rarely *RET*.[41,42]

GIST, inflammatory leiomyosarcoma, IgG4 disease, and reactive processes due to procedure/perforation enter the differential diagnosis. An important tumor to distinguish is epithelioid inflammatory myofibroblastic sarcoma.[43] This tumor shows epithelioid morphology, marked pleomorphism, aggressive behavior, and nuclear membrane or perinuclear ALK expression. All 11 cases reported in the original study[43] were intra-abdominal.

Key Features

- Distinct neoplasm; should not be confused with pseudotumors and reparative lesions
- Clonal *ALK* mutations can be seen in up to 50% of cases.
- *ALK* mutation status has treatment implications.
- New actionable genes are identified, including *ROS1*, *NTRK1*, and rarely *RET*.

Fig. 19. Desmoid-type fibromatosis. (*A*) Long sweeping fascicles of bland spindle cells. Thin-walled collapsed vessels ([*B*] and [*C*]); (*C*) shows more collagenous background than (*B*). A, C: hematoxylin eosin, original magnification ×100; B. hematoxylin eosin, original magnification ×200.

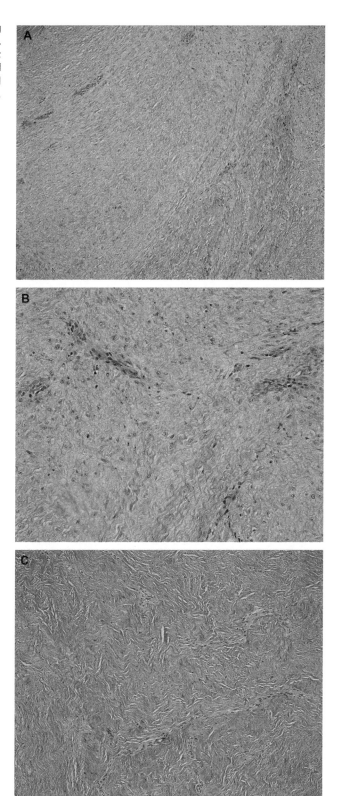

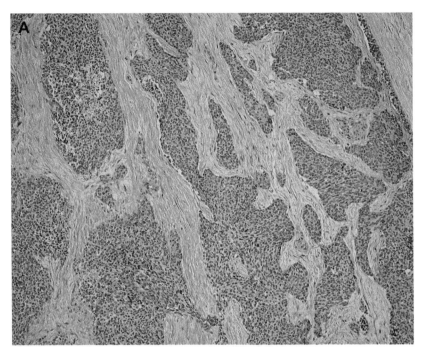

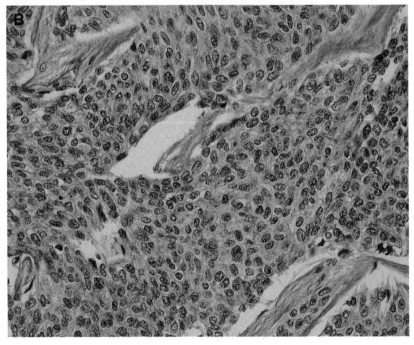

Fig. 20. Desmoplastic round cell tumor. (*A*, *B*) The small round to oval neoplastic cells have an undifferentiated appearance with dense chromatin, scant cytoplasm, and inconspicuous nuclei in a desmoplastic background.

Fig. 20. (*continued*). (*C, D*) Mitotic activity is frequent and apoptotic bodies are easy to find. Tumor necrosis is present. A. hematoxylin eosin, original magnification ×100 B. hematoxylin eosin, original magnification ×400 C. hematoxylin eosin, original magnification ×40 D. hematoxylin eosin, original magnification ×400.

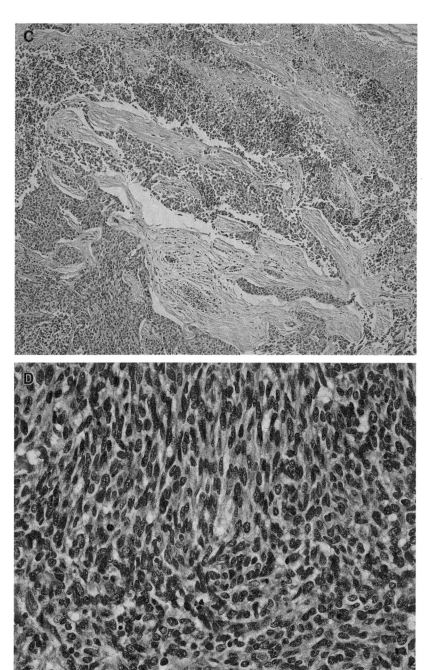

Table 2
Differential diagnosis for desmoplastic small round cell tumor

DSRCT	Positive for pankeratin, EMA, desmin, vimentin, neuron specific enolase, and CD57 Up to one-third positive for CD99 Negative for myogenin, MyoD1, synaptophysin, chromogranin, CK20, and CK5/6 *EWSR1-WT1* fusion
Ewing sarcoma	Positive for CD99 *EWSR1-FLI1* and *EWSR1-ERG* are the most common fusions Pitfall: may express epithelial markers
Alveolar rhabdomyosarcoma	Positive for desmin, myogenin, MyoD1 *FOXO1-PAX3, FOXO1-PAX7* fusions
Sclerosing rhabdomyosarcoma	Positive for desmin, myogenin, MyoD1
Neuroblastoma	*MYCN* amplification Lacks abnormalities in *EWSR1*
Wilms tumor	WT-1
Extrarenal malignant rhabdoid tumor	Loss of INI-1
Lymphoma	Positive for lymphocytic markers depending on subtype: CD45, CD43, TdT, CD3, CD20 Pitfall: can have CD99 positivity
Mesothelioma	Ck 5/6, WT-1, calretinin
Small cell carcinoma	CK, synaptophysin, chromogranin

SECONDARY MESENTERIC INVOLVEMENT BY MIDGUT NEUROENDOCRINE TUMOR

Introduction

Although primary midgut NET often is small, it frequently is associated with a large mesenteric tumor mass with dense fibrosis,[44,45] resulting in small bowel obstruction or ischemia. At CT, the mesenteric mass often displays as an enhancing soft tissue mass with linear bands radiating in the mesenteric fat (**Fig. 22**A), caused by the intense fibrotic proliferation and desmoplastic reaction in the mesenteric fat.

Gross Features

Grossly, there is a large fibrotic mesenteric mass with retraction of adjacent small bowel loops. Examination of the small bowel reveals 1 or more small primary tumors.

Microscopic Features

Microscopically, mesenteric mass has an irregular contour with dense fibrosis at periphery (**Fig. 22**B). Venous invasion may be present (**Fig. 23**A). In advanced disease, there is complete obliteration of mesenteric veins with only entrapped mesenteric arteries visible (**Fig. 23**B). In addition, there

are entrapped large nerves (see **Fig. 23**B) and lymphoplasmacytic inflammation (**Fig. 23**C).

Diagnosis and Differential Diagnosis

In most instances, diagnosis is straightforward and is based on clinical history, classic radiographic findings with presence of primary tumor and liver metastases, and positive ^{111}In-octreotide scintigraphy or [68]G positron emission tomography. Radiographically the primary differential diagnosis is sclerosing mesenteritis.[46] In patients with no distant metastases, complete resection of primary tumor and mesenteric mass is curative.

Key Features

- A large mesenteric mass is frequently associated with midgut NET

- Mesenteric mass is associated with dense fibrosis, inflammation, and entrapped mesenteric arteries, and nerves

DISCLOSURE

None.

Fig. 21. IMTs. IMTs can have variable morphology ranging from bland spindled to stellate myofibroblastic cells loosely embedded in a myxoid stroma, admixed with inflammatory cells (*A–C*) to more cellular tumors (*D*). A, B and D: hematoxylin eosin, original magnification ×200. C: hematoxylin eosin, original magnification ×400.

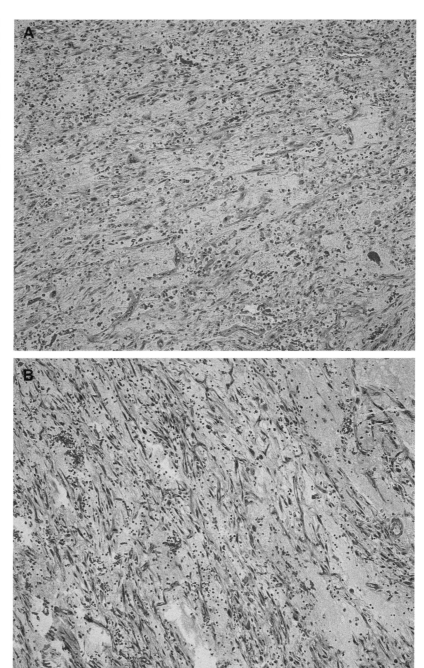

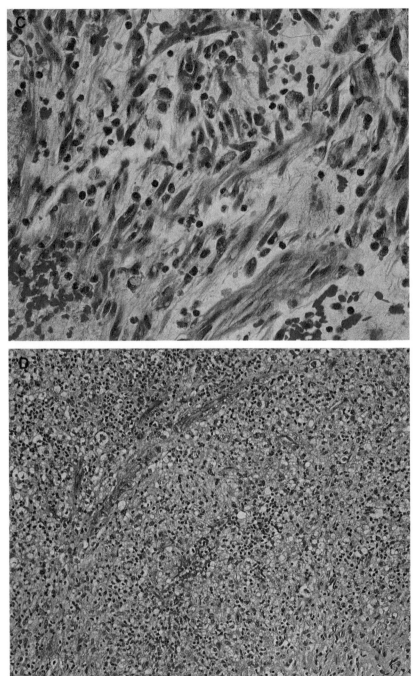

Fig. 21. (continued).

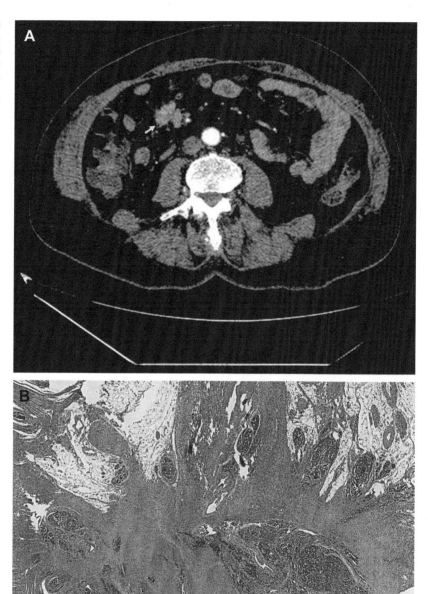

Fig. 22. Mesenteric mass in midgut NET. (*A*) An irregular mesenteric mass (indicated by a yellow arrow) at CT scan. (*B*) A section from the peripheral mass showing irregular contour and fibrosis.

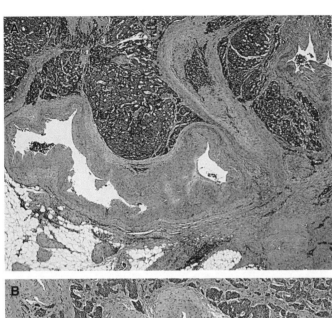

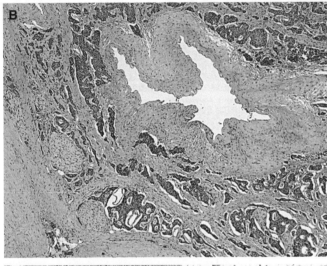

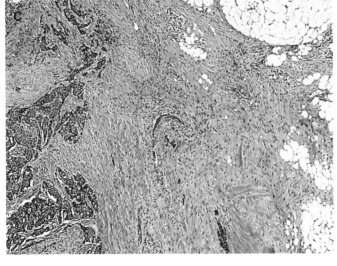

Fig. 23. Microscopic features of midgut NET. (*A*) A mesenteric vein containing tumor cells (*upper right*) (hematoxylin-eosin, original magnification ×20). (*B*) Entrapped artery and nerves (hematoxylin-eosin, original magnification ×40). (*C*) Fibrosis and chronic inflammation at periphery (hematoxylin-eosin, original magnification ×40).

REFERENCES

1. Hmoud B, Singal AK, Kamath PS. Mesenteric venous thrombosis. J Clin Exp Hepatol 2014;4(3):257–63.

2. Kolkman JJ, Geelkerken RH. Diagnosis and treatment of chronic mesenteric ischemia: an update. Best Pract Res Clin Gastroenterol 2017;31(1):49–57.

3. Barret M, Martineau C, Rahmi G, et al. Chronic mesenteric ischemia: a rare cause of chronic abdominal pain. Am J Med 2015;128(12):1363.e1-8.

4. Chin AB, Kumar AS. Behcet colitis. Clin Colon Rectal Surg 2015;28(02):99–102.

5. Hatemi I, Hatemi G, Celik AF. Gastrointestinal Involvement in Behçet Disease. Rheum Dis Clin North Am 2018;44(1):45–64.

6. Ebert EC. Gastrointestinal manifestations of Behçet's disease. Dig Dis Sci 2009;54(2):201.

7. Ngo N, Chang F. Enterocolic lymphocytic phlebitis: clinicopathologic features and review of the literature. Arch Pathol Lab Med 2007;131(7):1130–4.

8. Yantiss RK, Cui I, Panarelli NC, et al. Idiopathic Myointimal Hyperplasia of Mesenteric Veins. Am J Surg Pathol 2017;41(12):1657–65.

9. Sharma P, Yadav S, Needham CM, et al. Sclerosing mesenteritis: a systematic review of 192 cases. Clin J Gastroenterol 2017;10(2):103–11.

10. Kumar P, Malla S, Singh A, et al. Demystifying the mesenteric root lesions. Abdom Radiol (NY) 2019; 44(8):2708–20.

11. Fletcher CDM, Bridge JA, Hogendoorn P, et al, editors. WHO classification of tumours of soft tissue and bone. 4th edition. Lyon (France): IARC WHO; 2013. p. 33–43.

12. Pilotti S, Della Torre G, Lavarino C, et al. Molecular abnormalities in liposarcoma: role of MDM2 and CDK4-containing amplicons at 12q13–22. J Pathol 1998;185(2):188–90.

13. Pedeutour F, Suijkerbuijk RF, Forus A, et al. Complex composition and co-amplification of SAS and MDM2 in ring and giant rod marker chromosomes in well-differentiated liposarcoma. Genes Chromosomes Cancer 1994;10(2):85–94.

14. Meis-Kindblom J, Sjögren H, Kindblom LG, et al. Cytogenetic and molecular genetic analyses of liposarcoma and its soft tissue simulators: recognition of new variants and differential diagnosis. Virchows Arch 2001;439(2):141–51.

15. Weaver J, Downs-Kelly E, Goldblum JR, et al. Fluorescence in situ hybridization for MDM2 gene amplification as a diagnostic tool in lipomatous neoplasms. Mod Pathol 2008;21(8):943.

16. Weaver J, Rao P, Goldblum JR, et al. Can MDM2 analytical tests performed on core needle biopsy be relied upon to diagnose well-differentiated liposarcoma? Mod Pathol 2010;23(10):1301.

17. Henricks WH, Chu YC, Goldblum JR, et al. Dedifferentiated liposarcoma: a clinicopathological analysis of 155 cases with a proposal for an expanded definition of dedifferentiation. Am J Surg Pathol 1997; 21(3):271–81.

18. Elgar F, Goldblum JR. Well-differentiated liposarcoma of the retroperitoneum: a clinicopathologic analysis of 20 cases, with particular attention to the extent of low-grade dedifferentiation. Mod Pathol 1997;10(2):113–20.

19. Hasegawa T, Seki K, Hasegawa F, et al. Dedifferentiated liposarcoma ofretroperitoneum and mesentery: Varied growth patterns and histological grades—A clinicopathologic study of 32 cases. Hum Pathol 2000;31(6):717–27.

20. Mariño-Enríquez A, Fletcher CD, Dal Cin P, et al. Dedifferentiated liposarcoma with "homologous" lipoblastic (pleomorphic liposarcoma-like) differentiation: clinicopathologic and molecular analysis of a series suggesting revised diagnostic criteria. Am J Surg Pathol 2010;34(8):1122–31.

21. Patil DT, Rubin BP. Gastrointestinal stromal tumor: advances in diagnosis and management. Arch Pathol Lab Med 2011;135(10):1298–310.

22. Miettinen M, Lasota J. Gastrointestinal stromal tumors: pathology and prognosis at different sites. Semin Diagn Pathol 2006;23(2):70–83. Elsevier.

23. Reith JD, Goldblum JR, Lyles RH, et al. Extragastrointestinal (soft tissue) stromal tumors: an analysis of 48 cases with emphasis on histologic predictors of outcome. Mod Pathol 2000;13(5):577.

24. Lam MM, Corless CL, Goldblum JR, et al. Extragastrointestinal stromal tumors presenting as vulvovaginal/rectovaginal septal masses: a diagnostic pitfall. Int J Gynecol Pathol 2006;25(3):288–92.

25. Demetri GD. Targeting the molecular pathophysiology of gastrointestinal stromal tumors with imatinib. Mechanisms, successes, and challenges to rational drug development. Hematol Oncol Clin North Am 2002;16(5):1115–24.

26. Powell SM, Petersen GM, Krush AJ, et al. Molecular diagnosis of familial adenomatous polyposis. N Engl J Med 1993;329(27):1982–7.

27. Miyoshi Y, Ando H, Nagase H, et al. Germ-line mutations of the APC gene in 53 familial adenomatous polyposis patients. Proc Natl Acad Sci U S A 1992; 89(10):4452–6.

28. Caspari R, Olschwang S, Friedl W, et al. Familial adenomatous polyposis: desmoid tumours and lack of ophthalmic lesions (CHRPE) associated with APC mutations beyond codon 1444. Hum Mol Genet 1995;4(3):337–40.

29. Lazar AJ, Tuvin D, Hajibashi S, et al. Specific mutations in the β-catenin gene (CTNNB1) correlate with local recurrence in sporadic desmoid tumors. Am J Pathol 2008;173(5):1518–27.

30. Gerald WL, Ladanyi M, de Alava E, et al. Clinical, pathologic, and molecular spectrum of tumors associated with t (11; 22)(p13; q12): desmoplastic small

round-cell tumor and its variants. J Clin Oncol 1998; 16(9):3028–36.

31. Finke NM, Lae ME, Lloyd RV, et al. Sinonasal desmoplastic small round cell tumor: a case report. Am J Surg Pathol 2002;26(6):799–803.

32. Bismar TA, Basturk O, Gerald WL, et al. Desmoplastic small cell tumor in the pancreas. Am J Surg Pathol 2004;28(6):808–12.

33. Tison V, Cerasoli S, Morigi F, et al. Intracranial desmoplastic small-cell tumor: report of a case. Am J Surg Pathol 1996;20(1):112–7.

34. Ladanyi M, Gerald W. Fusion of the EWS and WT1 genes in the desmoplastic small round cell tumor. Cancer Res 1994;54(11):2837–40.

35. Coffin CM, Dehner LP, Meis-Kindblom JM. Inflammatory myofibroblastic tumor, inflammatory fibrosarcoma, and related lesions: an historical review with differential diagnostic considerations. Semin Diagn Pathol 1998;15(2):102–10.

36. Coffin CM, Hornick JL, Fletcher CD. Inflammatory myofibroblastic tumor: comparison of clinicopathologic, histologic, and immunohistochemical features including ALK expression in atypical and aggressive cases. Am J Surg Pathol 2007;31(4):509–20.

37. Griffin CA, Hawkins AL, Dvorak C, et al. Recurrent involvement of 2p23 in inflammatory myofibroblastic tumors. Cancer Res 1999;59(12):2776–80.

38. Cook JR, Dehner LP, Collins MH, et al. Anaplastic lymphoma kinase (ALK) expression in the inflammatory myofibroblastic tumor: a comparative immunohistochemical study. Am J Surg Pathol 2001; 25(11):1364–71.

39. Cessna MH, Zhou H, Sanger WG, et al. Expression of ALK1 and p80 in inflammatory myofibroblastic tumor and its mesenchymal mimics: a study of 135 cases. Mod Pathol 2002;15(9):931.

40. Bridge JA, Kanamori M, Ma Z, et al. Fusion of the ALK gene to the clathrin heavy chain gene, CLTC, in inflammatory myofibroblastic tumor. Am J Pathol 2001;159(2):411–5.

41. Yamamoto H, Yoshida A, Taguchi K, et al. ALK, ROS 1 and NTRK 3 gene rearrangements in inflammatory myofibroblastic tumours. Histopathology 2016; 69(1):72–83.

42. Antonescu CR, Suurmeijer AJ, Zhang L, et al. Molecular characterization of inflammatory myofibroblastic tumors with frequent ALK and ROS1 fusions and rare novel RET gene rearrangement. Am J Surg Pathol 2015;39(7):957.

43. Mariño-Enríquez A, Wang WL, Roy A, et al. Epithelioid inflammatory myofibroblastic sarcoma: an aggressive intra-abdominal variant of inflammatory myofibroblastic tumor with nuclear membrane or perinuclear ALK. Am J Surg Pathol 2011;35(1): 135–44.

44. Fata CR, Gonzalez RS, Liu E, et al. Mesenteric tumor deposits in midgut small intestinal neuroendocrine tumors are a stronger indicator than lymph node metastasis for liver metastasis and poor prognosis. Am J Surg Pathol 2017;41(1):128.

45. Roberts J, Gonzalez RS, Revetta F, et al. Mesenteric tumour deposits arising from small-intestine neuroendocrine tumours are frequently associated with fibrosis and IgG4-expressing plasma cells. Histopathology 2018;73(5):795–800.

46. Winant AJ, Vora A, Ginter PS, et al. More than just metastases: a practical approach to solid mesenteric masses. Abdom Radiol (NY) 2014;39(3):605–21.

Advances and Annoyances in Anus Pathology

Angela R. Shih, MD, Lawrence Zukerberg, MD*

KEYWORDS

• Anus • Anal cancer • Anal neoplasia • Anal infection

Key points

- The anus is composed of numerous types of epithelium and cell types, resulting in a very broad spectrum of disorders.
- Histologic changes associated with prolapse or hemorrhoids can mimic or disguise more sinister disorders.
- Recognition of unusual neoplastic and infectious lesions often requires additional clinical or histologic work-up.

ABSTRACT

Anal lesions are commonly mistaken clinically for prolapse or hemorrhoids but span a wide spectrum of disorders. Anal lesions include squamous, glandular, melanocytic, infectious, and lymphoid tumors. This article provides a broad overview of anal disorders and highlights specific issues that may hinder diagnosis.

OVERVIEW

The anus is defined by the internal sphincter muscle and extends from the lower valve of Houston to the anal verge. The dentate line is a wavy fold that is visible on gross examination and marks the lower two-thirds of the anal canal; it represents the embryologic junction between the hindgut and proctodeum. The anus contains multiple types of epithelium, including colonic epithelium, non-keratinizing squamous epithelium, transitional or cloacogenic epithelium, and true skin, giving rise to many types of lesions.

Because the most common clinical and pathologic findings in the anus are hemorrhoids and prolapse changes, these findings can occasionally mimic or disguise more sinister processes. For example, hemorrhoids may contain squamous dysplasia and koilocytosis. In contrast, infections (including condyloma acuminata and condyloma lata of syphilis) and Crohn disease may present with lesions clinically suspected to be hemorrhoids. Prolapse changes that are characterized by smooth muscle splaying, inflammatory stroma, and surface erosions and ulceration can at times entrap glandular epithelium, causing confusion regarding the presence of mucinous adenocarcinoma.

This article reviews the breadth of annoyances that can be seen at the anus and summarizes some of the advances in these areas.

ANAL SQUAMOUS LESIONS

ANAL INTRAEPITHELIAL NEOPLASIA

Over the past few decades, the terminology for anal intraepithelial neoplasia had been inconsistently used and often has not reflected the current understanding of human papillomavirus (HPV)–related pathogenesis. The Lower Anogenital Squamous Terminology (LAST) Project, sponsored by the College of American Pathologists and the American Society for Colposcopy and Cervical Pathology, provided recommendations to standardize the terminology across all

Department of Pathology and Laboratory Medicine, Massachusetts General Hospital, 55 Fruit Street, Boston, MA 02144, USA
* Corresponding author.
E-mail address: lzukerberg@mgh.harvard.edu

Surgical Pathology 13 (2020) 557–566
https://doi.org/10.1016/j.path.2020.06.002
1875-9181/20/© 2020 Elsevier Inc. All rights reserved.

surgpath.theclinics.com

anogenital tract sites as well as recommendations regarding appropriate usage of markers to drive therapy.[1]

At present, the terminology for anal dysplasia mirrors that of cervical dysplasia, which is where most of the published literature is focused. Although historically these intraepithelial lesions were divided into 3 grades, more current assessment of HPV-related biology supports a 2-tiered system. Analogous to cervical intraepithelial neoplasia, anal intraepithelial neoplasia (AIN) is now divided into low-grade squamous intraepithelial lesions (LSIL; composed of previously categorized AIN1) and high-grade squamous intraepithelial lesions (HSIL; composed of previously categorized AIN2 and AIN3). Low-grade lesions are generally self-limited HPV infections, and high-grade lesions have a risk of progression to carcinoma. The 2-tiered system improved interobserver variation, leading to more reproducible diagnoses.

The criteria for differentiating reactive atypia from LSIL and HSIL have been well established and rely on the identification of abnormal nuclear features, including increased nuclear size, irregular nuclear membranes, and increased nuclear-to-cytoplasmic ratios, often accompanied by mitotic figures. In general, LSIL is defined to have changes restricted to the lower third of the epithelium, whereas HSIL has dysplastic changes in the middle or superficial third of the epithelium. Koilocytic atypia, even in condyloma acuminatum, is classified as LSIL.

It is sometimes difficult to distinguish severe reactive changes from high-grade dysplastic changes, and this can be particularly true when hemorrhoids are present. There are specific circumstances in which immunohistochemistry for p16 is recommended to help further classify these lesions.[1] If the differential diagnosis is between reactive changes and HSIL, p16 is recommended to stratify these lesions into reactive changes and HSIL. In lesions that already have morphologic features of high-grade neoplasia (AIN2), immunohistochemistry for p16 is recommended to stratify these lesions into LSIL and HSIL. In both situations, reactive changes and LSIL show negative or weak/patchy staining, and HSIL shows strong diffuse block-positive staining. Importantly, staining is not recommended when the diagnosis is unequivocal, and is not useful in distinguishing between reactive changes and LSIL.

Equally important is to be cautious that other causes can mimic or coincide with squamous dysplasia, particularly highly reactive or infectious causes, which show highly abnormal nuclear features, including increased nuclear size and irregular nuclear contours. For example, a case of herpes simplex viral infection, shows nuclear features that mimic high-grade dysplasia with background koilocytosis; however, closer inspection shows characteristic viral inclusions, and the infection can be confirmed by immunohistochemistry (Fig. 1). Care must be taken to assess for other causes that might either mimic or coincide with squamous intraepithelial neoplasia.

MICROINVASIVE SQUAMOUS CELL CARCINOMA

In addition, the appropriate classification of superficially invasive squamous cell carcinoma can be difficult in certain contexts, particularly because the significance and definition in the anal canal have not been well defined. The LAST Project suggested the definition of superficially invasive squamous cell carcinoma in the anal canal that has been completely excised, as an invasive depth less than or equal to 3 mm from the basement membrane of the point of origin and a horizontal spread of less than or equal to 7 mm in length.[1] Microinvasion is most commonly identified as small invasive nests in the superficial mucosa, with surrounding desmoplasia or stromal reaction. Importantly, this should be differentiated from involvement of anal glands by dysplastic epithelium, which does not show the typical stromal changes of true invasion.

Identification of microinvasion can be particularly difficult in small and poorly oriented biopsies. In some situations, immunohistochemistry can occasionally be helpful. Cytokeratin 17 (CK17) has been evaluated in the spectrum of anal lesions and shows diffuse (or, less frequently, peripheral) staining in the invasive components, which has a sensitivity and specificity in invasive squamous cell carcinoma and invasive basaloid squamous cell carcinoma of 100% and 91%, respectively[2] (Fig. 2A, B). However, caution is necessary when pure basaloid variants of anal carcinoma are considered, because these carcinomas are negative for CK17. Historically, small cancers excised with clean margins have excellent outcomes, and the identification of this category of microinvasive carcinoma is important to promote conservative management in these patients.

ANAL CARCINOMA

Anal carcinoma is the most common carcinoma encountered in the anus. Endoscopically it may present as a polyp or hemorrhoid or as an ulcerated mass at the dentate line. Historically it was

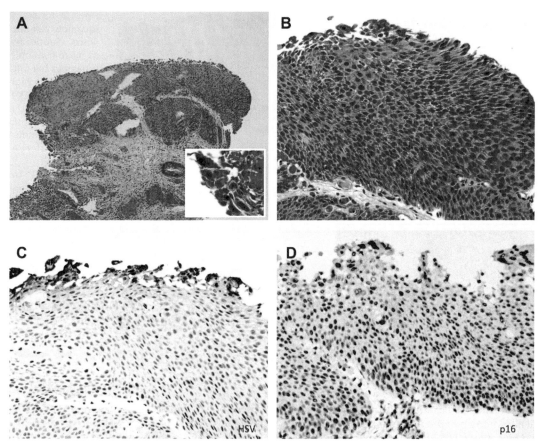

Fig. 1. Squamous atypia in herpes simplex virus infection. An anal biopsy shows atypical squamous epithelium with viral cytopathic changes of herpes simplex virus infection (hematoxylin-eosin, original magnification 40x [inset 400x]) (*A*). Another portion of the biopsy shows acanthotic squamous epithelium with loss of surface maturation and hyperchromatic nuclei (hematoxylin-eosin, original magnification 200x) (*B*). A herpes simplex virus stain is positive (HSV immunostain 200x) (*C*) and a p16 stain is negative (p16 immunostain 200x) (*D*).

called by a variety of names, such as keratinizing and nonkeratinizing squamous cell carcinoma, transitional cell carcinoma, cloacogenic carcinoma, adenosquamous carcinoma, and basaloid carcinoma, but now all are considered variants of squamous cell. It has been shown that prognosis and treatment depend on the stage and, to a lesser extent, the grade of the carcinoma. In addition, many tumors have mixed histology.

Most cases of anal squamous cell carcinoma are not diagnostically challenging, especially when the biopsy shows keratinizing or differentiated squamous cell carcinoma. One factor that makes biopsies challenging is small biopsy fragments and crush artifact. In such cases, evaluation of invasion can be difficult, and CK17 positivity can help.[2] For practical purposes, a request for additional material is critical if the patient is to be treated with chemoradiation therapy, as is now the standard of care.

Some histologic variants, such as basaloid squamous cell carcinoma, present diagnostic problems. Tumors diagnosed as basaloid squamous cell carcinoma are often misdiagnosed (**Fig. 2**C) In 1 study, review of 37 cases diagnosed as basaloid squamous cell carcinoma found that 27% were reclassified as basal cell carcinoma, melanoma, or neuroendocrine carcinoma.[3] The remaining basaloid squamous cell carcinomas were all positive for CK5/6 (27 of 27 cases) and p16 (27 of 27 cases), and all but 1 was positive for p40 (26 of 27 cases). In contrast, neuroendocrine carcinomas were all positive for synaptophysin and negative for CK5/6, p40, and p16. Similarly, melanomas were all positive for some melanoma markers, and negative for CK5/6, p40, and p16. Basal cell carcinomas of the perianal skin were separated out by retraction, but this feature is not reliable; the World Health Organization (WHO) classification scheme mentions that basaloid squamous cell carcinomas may show retraction artifact.[4] Staining for p16 and in situ hybridization for high-risk HPV can aid in separation of perianal skin basal cell carcinoma and anal basaloid squamous cell carcinoma. Given the

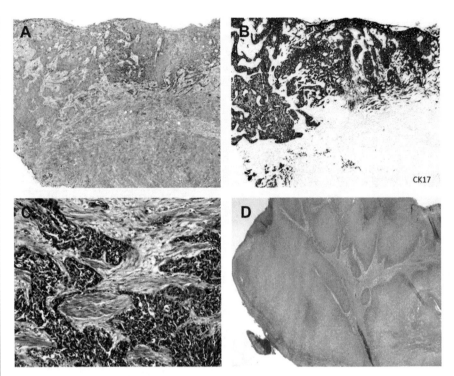

CK17

Fig. 2. Issues in squamous cell carcinoma. Subtle foci of microinvasion in squamous cell carcinoma can be highlighted by CK17 immunostain (*A*, *B*) (hematoxylin-eosin, original magnification 100x [for A]; cytokeratin 17 100x [for B]). Unusual histologic variants should be recognized, including basaloid squamous cell carcinoma (hematoxylin-eosin, original magnification 400x) (*C*) and verrucous carcinoma (hematoxylin-eosin, original magnification 20x) (*D*).

high incidence of misdiagnosis, undifferentiated or basaloid tumors of the anus should be characterized by immunohistochemistry. In addition, cases of basaloid squamous cell carcinoma have been misdiagnosed as recurrent colorectal carcinoma in some patients with a history of colorectal carcinoma, so CDX2 is also a useful marker.

A difficult issue in anal squamous cell cancers are tumors that have an exophytic growth pattern and are not clearly invasive (ie, do not show destructive stromal invasion). Biopsies of papillary squamous cell carcinoma create uncertainty if a definite invasive component is not seen. A diagnosis of papillary squamous cell carcinoma is appropriate, with a note saying stromal invasion cannot be evaluated.

Rarely, cases of squamous cell carcinoma have been described to arise from giant condylomas.[5,6] Verrucous carcinoma (formerly called giant condyloma of Buschke and Löwenstein) can be a large fungating lesion that clinically is invasive cancer[7,8] (**Fig. 2**D). However, histologically, it is a large, undulating, bland-appearing lesion without classic features of koilocytosis despite being secondary to HPV infection, often low-risk subtypes. The exophytic component shows acanthosis and papillomatosis and the endophytic component shows a broad pushing stromal-epithelial interface (see **Fig. 2**D). The low-power appearance is most important in making the diagnosis. The lesion

stains for p16 and CK17, supporting HPV infection and invasion. Complete excision is necessary for both these types of lesions.

ANORECTAL GLANDULAR LESIONS

HIDRADENOMA PAPILLIFERUM

Very rarely, a proliferation of the perianal glands can cause a benign cystic nodular lesion in the perianal region, called hidradenoma papilliferum. These lesions are most commonly found in middle-aged women in the vulvar region, but rare cases have been described in the anal region as well. The exact cell of origin is debated between apocrine sweat glands and anogenital mammary-like glands, but the morphology of the well-circumscribed nodule is distinctive with anastomosing tubules and papillary proliferation of columnar cells with abundant eosinophilic cytoplasm and prominent myoepithelial cells.[9–12] Because of their apocrine origin, the exact morphology of the cells can change with the menstrual cycle. It is common to see areas of secretory change. Immunohistochemistry reveals that the lesional cells are positive for both estrogen receptor (ER) and progesterone receptor (PR), which can be helpful if the diagnosis is in doubt. Because these lesions are benign, they can be managed with local excision with a good prognosis and a very low risk of local recurrence.

ANAL GLAND ADENOCARCINOMA

The anal glands are present in the submucosa, opening into the anal transitional zone, and, together with the anal ducts, have rarely been described to transform to adenocarcinoma. The largest series to date of anal canal adenocarcinoma identified 7 cases that have been defined as anal gland–type carcinoma, which histologically shows small haphazard glands with scant mucin production involving the anal wall without an intraluminal proliferation[13](Fig. 3A, B). These lesions seem to be universally positive for CK7, with loss of p63 and expression of CK5/6.[14] Occasionally, tumors involving the anal canal have significant morphologic overlap with more conventional colorectal-type adenocarcinoma, but these should be distinguished from true anal gland adenocarcinoma by both histology and immunohistochemistry.[13]

Complicating these findings is the fact that adenocarcinoma arising within an anorectal fistula has been well described, often in association with inflammation bowel disease. These tumors typically have the morphology of a well-differentiated colorectal-type adenocarcinoma.[15] Because it is difficult in these cases to distinguish an anal gland adenocarcinoma from other types, the diagnosis of anal gland adenocarcinoma should be restricted to tumors that are centered in the anal wall without any association with an anorectal fistula.

PAGET DISEASE

Extramammary Paget disease is a rare intraepithelial adenocarcinoma that often clinically presents in elderly patients as a skin lesion, and, like other extramammary sites, its classification in the anus has been divided into primary disease and secondary disease.

Primary Paget disease is composed of cases that seem to originate from the squamous epithelium and may not necessarily result in invasive disease (Fig. 3C). Although the cell origin is still unknown, several cell types have been proposed to be the initiating cell, including epidermal stem cells, adnexal stem cells, intraepidermal Toker cells, and apocrine glands.[16–19]

In contrast, secondary Paget disease consists of the intraepithelial growth of an adenocarcinoma whose primary site is known (most commonly colorectal in origin, followed by tubo-ovarian primaries).[20,21] The primary malignancy may not be clinically apparent at the time of presentation of Paget disease. Although exact numbers for primary and secondary Paget disease are not known, studies have indicated that perhaps more than 50% of patients with perianal Paget disease may have another primary.[22]

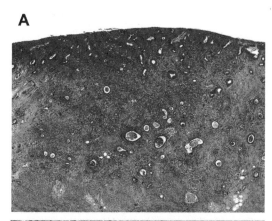

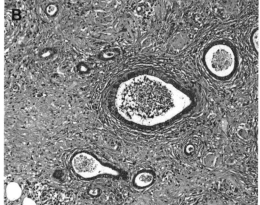

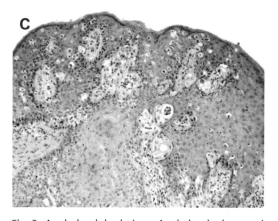

Fig. 3. Anal glandular lesions. Anal gland adenocarcinoma is rare but typically presents with small haphazard glands with scant mucin production involving the anal wall without an intraluminal proliferation (hematoxylin-eosin, original magnification 40x [for A]; hematoxylin-eosin, original magnification 200x [for B]) (*A*, *B*). Paget disease shows intraepithelial growth of an adenocarcinoma, which may be primary or secondary and may show focal invasion (hematoxylin-eosin, original magnification 100x) (*C*).

Consequently, patients with perianal Paget disease should be carefully screened for a visceral malignancy that could serve as a primary site, and, on occasion, immunohistochemistry may be informative in pointing to a possible primary site. Although CK7 seems to be universally positive in cases of anal Paget disease, CK20 staining seems to be variably positive.[23,24] Commonly, CK20 is positive when associated with more conventional colonic adenocarcinoma, although occasional cases of CK20-positive staining have been seen in primary Paget disease as well. In addition, most cases of primary Paget disease have been positive for gross cystic disease fluid protein. However, these immunohistochemical findings are only suggestive, and adequate clinical screening should be implemented to exclude the possibility of secondary Paget disease.

Recently, literature on the long-term outcomes in patients with perianal Paget disease has shown that there is an increased risk for developing invasive adenocarcinoma in patients with perianal Paget disease.[25] Although there were limited numbers, there is a suggestion that survival is similar whether the Paget disease was primary or secondary, possibly because there is a risk of invasive disease in primary Paget disease. In addition, overall survival was similar between patients treated with wide local excision and local excision, regardless of the status of the surgical margin. Consequently, the presence of perianal Paget disease, regardless of type or treatment modality, likely warrants close follow-up.

ANORECTAL MELANOCYTIC LESIONS

ANORECTAL MELANOMA

Anorectal malignant melanoma is a rare but highly malignant tumor that is misdiagnosed in a significant number of patients as hemorrhoids or polyps.[26] Mucosal melanomas often show a high degree of histologic variability, ranging from an epithelioid to spindled morphology, and can be amelanotic.[27,28] Because of the challenge in accurate recognition and diagnosis, most of these lesions are diagnosed at a late stage and have poor outcomes[28] (**Fig. 4**).

Immunohistochemistry is critical for diagnostic confirmation, and any combination of S100, HMB45, Melan A, and Mart1 can be used. In addition, although there is some genetic overlap in cutaneous and mucosal melanomas, anorectal melanoma seems to have a lower frequency of *BRAF* mutations.[29,30] Surgical resection (either wide local excision or abdominoperineal resection, if the anal sphincter cannot be spared) and

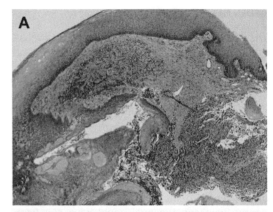

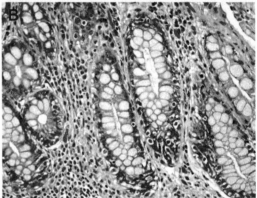

Fig. 4. Anal melanoma. This anal biopsy shows a subepithelial proliferation of neoplastic cells, which are confirmed on immunohistochemistry to be melanoma (hematoxylin-eosin, original magnification 40x) (*A*). On occasion, melanoma can also show colonization of glandular crypts (hematoxylin-eosin, original magnification 400x) (*B*).

radiotherapy remain mainstays of treatment, but adjuvant therapeutic options have been increasingly used in recent years in the metastatic setting.[31,32] Advanced mucosal melanoma treated with immunologic checkpoint inhibitors have been shown to have a small increase in survival[33]

Because surgical resection with clear margins remains an important mainstay treatment modality and an independent factor for overall survival, the appropriate evaluation of margins becomes important. Margin evaluation in this setting can be challenging because of potential morphologic overlap between residual melanoma in situ (MIS) and benign melanocyte hyperplasia. Adding to the difficulty is that the density of normal melanocytes in the anorectal mucosa has only recently been established as a mean of 1.4 melanocytes per 100 epithelial cells in the glandular mucosa and 3.6 melanocytes per high-power field (HPF) in the squamous mucosa by Microphthalmia-associated transcription factor (MITF) immunostain.[34] Notably, there was no difference based on race, and the nuclear morphology of these melanocytes in normal mucosa was banal, even when focally extending up to the midlevel epithelium.

The most reliable features in distinguishing residual MIS from hyperplasia include melanocyte nuclear atypia and near-confluent growth. MIS is composed of a confluent and nested proliferation of cytologically atypical melanocytes with some pagetoid spread. These features can be highlighted by immunohistochemistry (in particular, MITF), which can be helpful in distinguishing MIS from hyperplasia in peritumoral mucosa. Benign melanocytic hyperplasia adjacent to the tumor was found to have increased melanocytes, with a mean density of 10 melanocytes per 100 epithelial cells in the glandular mucosa and 1.8 melanocytes per HPF in the squamous mucosa.[34] Given the increase from the background mucosa, increase in melanocytic density should be interpreted with caution and only in conjunction with cytologic and architectural features (nuclear atypia and confluent growth) to differentiate hyperplasia from residual MIS.

INFLAMMATORY AND LYMPHOID LESIONS

INFLAMMATORY LESIONS

The anal biopsies often contain inflammation and lymphoid aggregates. Most lymphoid aggregates are benign. Often, large organized lymphoid aggregates with germinal centers are seen; these have been referred to as the anal-rectal tonsil, after an organizing lymphoid structure in rats termed the rectal tonsil.[35] The rectal tonsil may be secondary to infection (such as chlamydia) or immune disorders (such as Crohn disease). Reactive germinal centers are present underneath anal mucosa. It is important on biopsies to appreciate the reactive germinal centers. Biopsies from the anus may be crushed and contain large lymphoid cells, suggesting large cell lymphoma. B-cell marker staining and a high KI67 may serve to reinforce an erroneous diagnosis. The biopsy may be sampling a reactive germinal center. A follicular dendritic cell (FDC) marker, such as cluster of differentiation (CD) 21, should be performed. If there are FDC fibers present among the large lymphoid cells in a biopsy, clinicians should be cautious of making a diagnosis of lymphoma; instead, additional biopsies should be requested, because the biopsy may simply represent a sampled reactive germinal center.

Nonspecific chronic inflammation in anal biopsies may be caused by irritation, prolapse, and stercoral injury. However, if the overlying mucosa is intact and there is a moderately dense lymphoid infiltrate (occasionally with admixed neutrophils), a diagnosis of Crohn disease should be considered. Although Crohn disease may present with anal

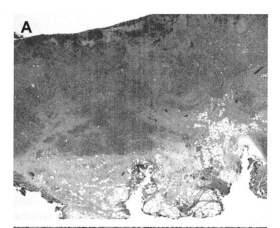
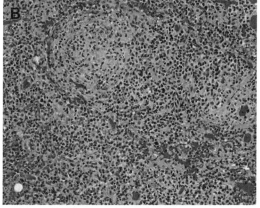
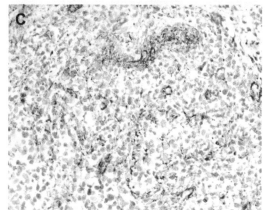

Fig. 5. Anal syphilis. Anal syphilis often shows a dense mononuclear inflammatory infiltrate with surface erosion and numerous plasma cells (hematoxylin-eosin, original magnification 40x [for A]; hematoxylin-eosin, original magnification 200x [for B]) (*A, B*). A spirochete immunohistochemical stain is necessary to highlight organisms (Spirochete immunostain 200x) (*C*).

skin tags, anal fissures, and nonspecific anal symptoms, primary anal presentation of Crohn disease is common.[36] Finding granulomas in the anus should strongly suggest Crohn disease, unless an infectious cause is readily apparent. Biopsies with a moderately dense chronic inflammation or germinal centers in the absence of HPV infection or recent instrumentation/trauma may also represent Crohn disease. Finding even rare giant cells admixed with the inflammation strengthens that association.

INFECTIOUS LESIONS

According to a new report from the Centers for Disease Control and Prevention, the rates of the sexually transmitted diseases gonorrhea, chlamydia, and syphilis have increased greatly in the United States. Dense plasma cell proliferations often suggest lymphoma and are characteristic of marginal zone lymphoma, but should raise the possibility of anal syphilis (either primary or secondary syphilis). Histologic features that support anal syphilis include a dense plasma cell infiltrate, plasma cells in and around nerves or vascular structures, and a vascular proliferation with prominent endothelial cells and endothelial swelling.[37,38] Immunostaining for kappa and lambda should show polytypic plasma cells. Spirochete immunostain should always be performed on plasma cell infiltrates in the anus. Importantly, a Steiner stain for spirochetes is not sensitive; even biopsies teeming with spirochetes on a spirochete immunostain may be negative on Steiner stain (Fig. 5).

Chlamydia also is common in the anus. Clinically, it can present as ulcerative proctitis or as anorectal ulceration. On histology, it can have a variety of appearances, ranging from nonspecific neutrophilic inflammation to reactive germinal centers without neutrophils or ulceration. Characteristically, there are hyperplastic germinal centers with focal overlying erosion or ulceration. No stain is available to aid in diagnosis, so a high index of

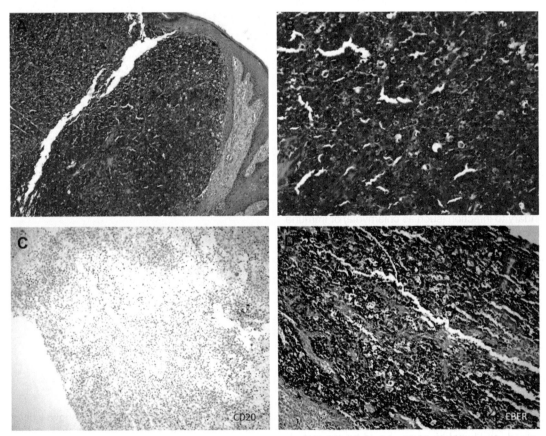

Fig. 6. Anal plasmablastic lymphoma. This biopsy shows a densely cellular proliferation of highly atypical malignant cells beneath the squamous epithelium (hematoxylin-eosin, original magnification 40x [for A]; hematoxylin-eosin, original magnification 400x [for B]) (*A, B*). Although the cells are negative for CD20, in situ hybridization for EBER is positive (CD20 immunostain 200x [for C]; EBER in situ hybridization 200x [for D]) (*C, D*). This biopsy also showed marked kappa light chain predominance over lambda light chain.

suspicion should be communicated to the gastroenterologist, who can perform a nucleic-acid amplification test swab.

LYMPHOMA

Lymphomas in the anus are usually diffuse large B-cell lymphomas.[39] As mentioned earlier, do not make a diagnosis on crushed small biopsies. Even gene rearrangement studies may show clonality if a germinal center was biopsied. Plasmablastic lymphoma often occurs in the anus, especially in immunocompromised individuals. The appearance is that of a high-grade neoplasm such as large cell lymphoma or plasmacytoma. They are usually CD20 negative and express CD138. Lack of CD20 may be confusing and suggest carcinoma or another neoplasm. These lymphomas are always Epstein-Barr virus (EBV) positive, and EBV-encoded small RNA (EBER) positivity should suggest this diagnosis (**Fig. 6**). Therefore, EBER is critical in the diagnostic work-up and should be performed on all lymphomas or plasma cell neoplasms occurring in the anus. Plasmacytomas are always EBER negative.

Occasionally, cases of small B-cell lymphoma occur in the anus. Marginal zone lymphoma can occur and is difficult to diagnose, because benign lymphoid aggregates are often present in reactive anal biopsies. Finding monotypic plasma cells is the most helpful feature in making this diagnosis. Rarely, follicular lymphoma or mantle cell lymphoma may occur in the anus, typically as part of generalized gastrointestinal tract involvement by lymphoma.

SUMMARY

Although often overlooked, the anus is a gastrointestinal site that has a broad range of disorders. The presence of squamous epithelium, glandular epithelium, and lymphoid tissue at this site lends itself to lesions that overlap extensively with genital cutaneous disorders, glandular disorders, infectious disorders, and lymphoid neoplasia.

The most common findings in the anus are hemorrhoids and prolapse changes, but these findings can mimic and mask a large variety of other lesions. An understanding of the breadth of annoyances that can be seen at the anus is important for general pathology.

DISCLOSURE

None.

REFERENCES

1. Darrragh T, Colgan TJ, Cox TJ, et al. The lower anogenital squamous terminology standardization project for HPV-associated lesions. Int J Gynecol Pathol 2013;32(1):76–115.
2. Nazarian RM, Primiani A, Doyle LA, et al. Cytokeratin 17: an adjunctive marker of invasion in squamous neoplastic lesions of the anus. Am J Surg Pathol 2014;38(1):78–85.
3. Graham RP, Arnold CA, Naini BV, et al. Basaloid squamous cell carcinoma of the anus revisited. Am J Surg Pathol 2016;40(3):354–60.
4. WHO Classification of Tumours Editorial Board, editor. WHO classification of tumours: digestive system tumours. 5th edition. Lyon (France): International Agency for Research on Cancer; 2019.
5. Wells M, Robertson S, Lewis F, et al. Squamous carcinoma arising in a giant peri-anal condyloma associated with human papillomavirus types 6 and 11. Histopathology 1988;12(3):319–23.
6. Sturm JT, Christenson CE, Uecker JH, et al. Squamous-cell carcinoma of the anus arising in a giant condyloma acuminatum. Dis Colon Rectum 1975; 18(2):147–51.
7. Chu QD, Vezeridis MP, Libbey PN, et al. Giant condyloma acuminatum (Buschke-Lowenstein tumor) of the anorectal and perianal regions. Dis Colon Rectum 1994;37(9):950–7.
8. Boshart M, zur Hausen H. Human papillomaviruses in Buschke-Löwenstein tumors: physical state of the DNA and identification of a tandem duplication in the noncoding region of a human papillomavirus 6 subtype. J Virol 1986;58(3):963–6.
9. Cheong J, Lee C, Young C. Hidradenoma papilliferum: an unusual benign perianal tumour. BMJ Case Rep 2018;2018, bcr-2017-220354.
10. Cooper WL. Hidradenoma of the anal canal. Arch Surg-chicago 1965;90(5):716–9.
11. Daniel F, Mahmoudi A, de Parades V, et al. An uncommon perianal nodule: Hidradenoma papilliferum. Gastroenterol Clin Biol 2007;31(2):166–8.
12. Filho E, Formiga F, Miotto S, et al. Perianal hidradenoma papilliferum. J Coloproctology 2018;38(1):70–2.
13. Hobbs C, Lowry M, Owen D, et al. Anal gland carcinoma. Cancer 2001;92(8):2045–9.
14. Lisovsky M, Patel K, Cymes K, et al. Immunophenotypic characterization of anal gland carcinoma: loss of p63 and cytokeratin 5/6. Arch Pathol Lab Med 2007;131(8):1304–11.
15. Wong N, Shirazi T, Hamer-Hodges D, et al. Adenocarcinoma arising within a Crohn's-related anorectal fistula: a form of anal gland carcinoma? Histopathology 2002;40(3):302–4.
16. Jones RE, Austin C, Ackerman BA. Extramammary Paget's disease. Am J Dermatopathol 1979;1(2):101–32.

17. Regauer S. Extramammary Paget's disease-a proliferation of adnexal origin? Histopathology 2006; 48(6):723–9.

18. Marucci G, Betts CM, Golouh R, et al. Toker cells are probably precursors of Paget cell carcinoma: a morphological and ultrastructural description. Virchows Arch 2002;441(2):117–23.

19. Mazoujian G, Pinkus G, Haagensen D. Extramammary Paget's disease–evidence for an apocrine origin. An immunoperoxidase study of gross cystic disease fluid protein-15, carcinoembryonic antigen, and keratin proteins. Am J Surg Pathol 1984;8(1):43–50.

20. Chanda JJ. Extramammary Paget's disease: Prognosis and relationship to internal malignancy. J Am Acad Dermatol 1985;13(6):1009–14.

21. Marchesa P, Fazio VW, Oliart S, et al. Long-term outcome of patients with perianal Paget's disease. Ann Surg Oncol 1997;4(6):475–80.

22. Billingsley KG, Stern LE, Lowy AM, et al. Uncommon anal neoplasms. Surg Oncol Clin N Am 2004;13(2): 375–88.

23. Smith K, Tuur S, Corvette D, et al. Cytokeratin 7 staining in mammary and extramammary Paget's disease. Mod Pathol 1997;10(11):1069–74.

24. Goldblum JR, Hart WR. Perianal Paget's disease. Am J Surg Pathol 1998;22(2):170–9.

25. Isik O, Aytac E, Brainard J, et al. Perianal Paget's disease: three decades experience of a single institution. Int J Colorectal Dis 2016;31(1):29–34.

26. Weyandt G, Eggert A, Houf M, et al. Anorectal melanoma: surgical management guidelines according to tumour thickness. Br J Cancer 2003;89(11):2019–22.

27. Belli F, Gallino GF, Vullo LS, et al. Melanoma of the anorectal region The experience of the National Cancer Institute of Milano. Eur J Surg Oncol 2009; 35(7):757–62.

28. Iddings DM, Fleisig AJ, Chen SL, et al. Practice patterns and outcomes for anorectal melanoma in the USA, reviewing three decades of treatment: is more extensive surgical resection beneficial in all patients? Ann Surg Oncol 2010;17(1):40–4.

29. Maldonado JL, Fridlyand J, Patel H, et al. Determinants of BRAF mutations in primary melanomas. J Natl Cancer Inst 2003;95(24):1878–90.

30. Cohen Y, Rosenbaum E, Begum S, et al. Exon 15 BRAF Mutations Are Uncommon in Melanomas Arising in Nonsun-Exposed Sites. Clin Cancer Res 2004;10(10):3444–7.

31. Nilsson P, Ragnarsson-Olding B. Importance of clear resection margins in anorectal malignant melanoma. Br J Surg 2010;97(1):98–103.

32. Droesch JT, Flum DR, Mann GN. Wide local excision or abdominoperineal resection as the initial treatment for anorectal melanoma? Am J Surg 2005; 189(4):446–9.

33. Vecchio M, Guardo L, Ascierto PA, et al. Efficacy and safety of ipilimumab 3mg/kg in patients with pretreated, metastatic, mucosal melanoma. Eur J Cancer 2014;50(1):121–7.

34. Tse JY, Chan MP, Zukerberg LR, et al. Assessment of melanocyte density in anorectal mucosa for the evaluation of surgical margins in primary anorectal melanoma. Am J Clin Pathol 2016;145(5):626–34.

35. Farris AB, Lauwers GY, Ferry JA, et al. The rectal tonsil: a reactive lymphoid proliferation that may mimic lymphoma. Am J Surg Pathol 2008;32(7): 1075–9.

36. Gray B, Lockhartmummery H, Morson B. Crohn's disease of the anal region. Gut 1965;6(6):515–24.

37. Tse JY, Chan MP, Ferry JA, et al. Syphilis of the aerodigestive tract. Am J Surg Pathol 2018;42(4): 472–8.

38. Arnold CA, Roth R, Arsenescu R, et al. Sexually transmitted infectious colitis vs inflammatory bowel disease: distinguishing features from a case-controlled study. Am J Clin Pathol 2015;144(5): 771–81.

39. Swerdlow SW, Campo E, Harris NL, et al, editors. WHO classification of tumours of haematopoietic and lymphoid tissues. 4th edition. Lyon (France): International Agency for Research on Cancer; 2017.

Moving?

Make sure your subscription moves with you!

To notify us of your new address, find your **Clinics Account Number** (located on your mailing label above your name), and contact customer service at:

Email: journalscustomerservice-usa@elsevier.com

800-654-2452 (subscribers in the U.S. & Canada)
314-447-8871 (subscribers outside of the U.S. & Canada)

Fax number: 314-447-8029

Elsevier Health Sciences Division
Subscription Customer Service
3251 Riverport Lane
Maryland Heights, MO 63043

*To ensure uninterrupted delivery of your subscription, please notify us at least 4 weeks in advance of move.